IMMUNOLOGY

Basic Concepts, Diseases, and Laboratory Methods

IMMUNOLOGY

Basic Concepts, Diseases, and Laboratory Methods

J. Helen Cronenberger, PhD, MT(ASCP)
Associate Professor
Department of Medical Allied Health Professions
Department of Pathology
School of Medicine
University of North Carolina at Chapel Hill
Chapel Hill, North Carolina

J. Charles Jennette, MD
Associate Professor
Director of Immunopathology
Department of Pathology
School of Medicine
University of North Carolina at Chapel Hill
Chapel Hill, North Carolina

APPLETON & LANGE
Norwalk, Connecticut/San Mateo, California

0-8385-8880-8

Prentice-Hall of Australia, Pty. Ltd., Sydney
Prentice-Hall Canada, Inc.
Prentice-Hall Hispanoamericana, S.A., Mexico
Prentice-Hall of India Private Limited, New Delhi
Prentice-Hall International (UK) Limited, London
Prentice-Hall of Japan, Inc., Tokyo
Prentice-Hall of Southeast Asia (Pte.) Ltd., Singapore
Whitehall Books Ltd., Wellington, New Zealand
Editora Prentice-Hall do Brasil Ltda., Rio de Janeiro

Library of Congress Cataloging-in-Publication Data

Cronenberger, J. Helen.
   Immunology: basic concepts, diseases, and laboratory methods.

   Bibliography: p.
   1. Immunodiagnosis. 2. Immunology. 3. Immunologic diseases. I. Jennette, J. Charles. II. Title. [DNLM: 1. Immunologic Diseases—diagnosis. 2. Immunologic Technics. WD 300 C947i]
RB46.5.C76 1987   616.07'9   87–33269
ISBN 0–8385–8880–8

Designer: Steven M. Byrum
Production Editor: John Robert Hirschfeld

Contents

Preface

Immunology is one of the most rapidly growing areas in clinical laboratory science. Every section of the clinical laboratory is involved with some aspects of immunology, especially the application of immunologic and serologic methods. Examples of immunologic methods that are commonly used in clinical laboratories are serologic tests for exposure to pathogens performed in the serology laboratory, rapid identification of bacteria and viruses in cultures by immunofluorescence microscopy performed in the microbiology laboratory, latex particle agglutination assays for rheumatoid factor performed in the immunology laboratory, blood typing and crossmatching performed in the blood bank, quantitation of blood hormone levels by radioimmunoassay (RIA) and enzyme immunoassays performed in the chemistry laboratory, assays for coagulation factor inhibitors performed in the coagulation laboratory, identification of antibody-coated bacteria in the urine performed in the urinalysis laboratory, classification of leukemias by immunofluorescence microscopy and flow cytometry performed in the hematology laboratory, and identification of tumor markers by immunoenzyme microscopy performed in the anatomic pathology laboratory. Therefore, an understanding of immunology is required for anyone who is generating or making use of clinical laboratory data.

The immune system is intimately involved in both disease prevention and disease induction. For example, deficient immune function predisposes to life-threatening infections. Conversely, too much immune reactivity leads to the development of allergies. A knowledge of normal and abnormal immune system functioning is required to understand these and many other important diseases.

This book covers all aspects of clinical immunology, with special emphasis on immunologic methods used in clinical laboratory medicine and on immune-mediated diseases that are frequently diagnosed and evaluated by immunologic methods. Many books cover various components of this body of information, for example books on basic immunology, serology, and immunopathology. But to our knowledge this is the only book that addresses all these aspects.

We begin by presenting an overview of the immune system (Chap. 1) to provide a basis for beginning discussion of the interconnected and circuitous events that comprise the immune response. Next, nonimmune body defenses (Chap. 2) are covered to put them into perspective with immune defenses. As a prelude to the discussions of immunologic techniques throughout the rest of the book, Chapters 3 and 4 present the physiologic, biochemical, and methodologic principles that underlie immunologic assay procedures and the laboratory evaluation of the immune system. The next seven chapters discuss lymphocytes and lymphoid tissues (Chap. 5), immune deficiency diseases (Chap. 6), lymphocytic leukemias and lymphomas (Chap. 7), T lymphocyte immune responses and T cell-mediated inflammation (Chap. 8), B lymphocyte activation and antibody synthesis (Chap. 9), complement and other humoral mediators of inflammation (Chap. 10), and antibody-mediated injury and autoimmunity (Chap. 11). The final two chapters (Chaps. 12 and 13) present the immune defense against and immunologic evaluation of some bacterial, fungal, viral, parasitic, rickettsial, and chlamydial infections.

The organization and content of this book were chosen on the basis of years of teaching immunology in clinical laboratory science courses. It provides a theoretical and practical basis for understanding the normal immune system, the role of the immune system in disease production, and the application of immunologic methods in clinical laboratory medicine.

J. Helen Cronenberger, PhD, MT(ASCP)

J. Charles Jennette, MD

Section I

The Body's Defense Systems

Chapter
1 An Overview
of the Immune System

OBJECTIVES

1. To describe the characteristics of the immune system that distinguish it from other defense mechanisms.
2. To briefly describe morphology, tissue distribution, embryonic development, and activation of lymphocytes.
3. To discuss the role of the immune system in immunodeficiency, inflammatory, allergic, autoimmune, and lymphoproliferative diseases.
4. To comment on some of the laboratory procedures used to evaluate the immune system.

Illustrative Case

An 18-year-old woman developed a sore throat, fever, and swollen glands in her neck. When she viewed her oropharynx with a mirror, she saw that her mucosa was reddened, and her tonsils were enlarged with a few white splotches on their surfaces. She did not go to a physician. The sore throat and fever disappeared after about a week.

After an additional week she noted that her urine had become tea-colored. She went to her physician, who elicited the history of the lymphadenopathy and pharyngitis beginning approximately 2 weeks earlier but who observed no residual abnormalities in the pharynx at the time of examination. The physician did find an elevated blood pressure (BP).

Microscopic examination of the urine revealed hematuria. Chemical analysis of the urine demonstrated substantial proteinuria. Chemical analysis of the blood serum showed azotemia and hypocomplementemia. Evaluation of serum demonstrated high titers of antibodies to streptococcal antigens, specifically antistreptolysin O and anti-DNAse B. Culture of the pharyngeal swab grew out a group A β-hemolytic streptococcus.

DISTINGUISHING CHARACTERISTICS OF THE IMMUNE SYSTEM

The *immune system* is one of the defense mechanisms that the body uses to fend off potentially injurious agents. There are other, nonimmune defense mechanisms, such as the physical barrier provided by the skin and mucous membranes and the inflammatory response, that also play an essential role in the body's ability to deter foreign agents. These nonimmune defenses will be discussed in Chapter 2. Immune defense has three major characteristics that distinguish it from nonimmune defense: (1) preferential attack on nonself rather than self, (2) specificity, and (3) memory.

Under most circumstances the immune system attacks foreign, or *nonself*, substances but not one's own tissues, or *self*. This discrimination between self and nonself is obviously an advantageous characteristic that serves to eliminate foreign invaders present within our bodies and thus intimately admixed with our own tissues. It was once thought that the normal immune system was totally incapable of attacking self. However, current evidence indicates that the immune system does have the ability to attack one's own tissues, but normally this potential is held in check by a complex control mechanism.

The *specificity* of the immune system results from its ability to recognize particular molecular configurations on what is to be attacked. The receptors that carry out this recognition can be present in molecules called *antibodies (immunoglobulins)* in the body fluids or on the surface membrane of *lymphocytes*. The substance that is recognized as foreign (nonself) is called an *antigen*. The portion of the antigen that specifically interacts with the immune system receptors is called an *epitope* or antigen determinant. An immune response occurs only when lymphocyte receptors recognize an antigen by interacting with specific epitopes. Thus to be able to respond to the myriad antigens in the environment, the immune system must generate a vast array of receptors, each having a different specificity.

The immune system is said to have *memory* because once it has come in contact with a given antigen, it will respond quicker and to a greater degree on subsequent exposures to that same antigen (Fig. 1–1). This more rapid and enhanced response on re-exposure to an antigen is called an anamnestic or *secondary response*. The initial reaction to first contacting an antigen is called a *primary response*. This greater efficiency of the immune system in responding to previously contacted antigens is the basis for *immunization* and *vaccination*. For example, an individual is inoculated with antigens from an infectious microorganism (e.g., measles virus vaccine), or inactive forms of toxins (e.g., diphtheria toxoid), so that an effective anamnestic response will occur if immune resistance to this potentially disease-producing agent is ever required. There-

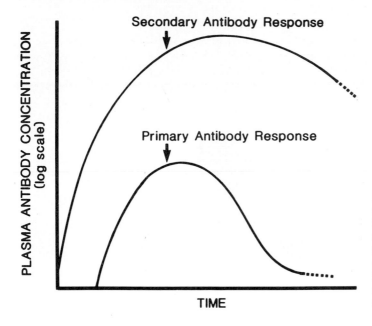

Figure 1-1. Primary Versus Secondary Antibody Response. Plasma antibody concentration as a function of time after initial antigen exposure (primary antibody response) compared to subsequent antigen exposure (secondary antibody response).

after re-exposure to the immunizing antigen will result in a rapid secondary response that will protect against disease.

THE TISSUES OF THE IMMUNE SYSTEM: LYMPHOCYTES

Lymphocytes are the cells responsible for carrying out immune responses. They are small, round cells with scanty cytoplasm and dense nuclei (Fig. 1-2). They are present in blood and lymphatic vessels, lymphoid tissues, and the interstices of many tissues. Of the leukocytes in the blood of healthy individuals, approximately 35% are lymphocytes, 60% are granulocytes, and 5% are monocytes. Lymphocytes circulate throughout the body within blood and lymphatic vessels. They can pass from the microvasculature into the interstitial fluid of most tissues. Lymphocytes can exit the interstitium by entering *lymphatic vessels* that carry lymphocyte-rich fluid, *lymph*, back to the venous circulation. Therefore lymphocytes are continually moving through the body in search of foreign invaders.

At strategic locations, there are larger accumulations of lymphocytes, referred to as lymphoid tissues. The *spleen* is a lymphocyte-rich organ straddling the blood stream, while the *lymph nodes* are in an analogous position along the lymphatic vessels. Both of these tissues are also rich in cells that ingest (phagocytose) material. Most of these *phagocytes* are derived from the differentiation of blood monocytes into *macrophages,* also called *mononuclear phagocytes.* These mononuclear phagocytes can ingest debris without the assistance of the immune system, but their phagocytic activity is greatly

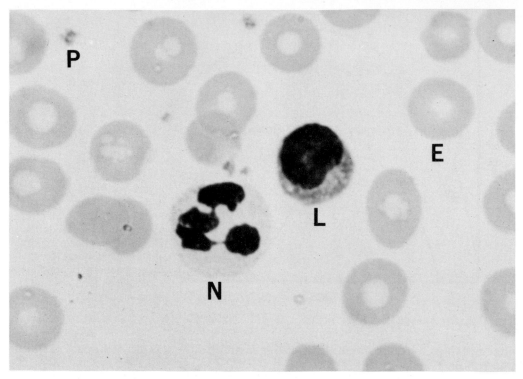

Figure 1-2. Blood Cells. Wright's-stained blood smear showing a lymphocyte (L), neutrophil (N), erythrocytes (E), and platelets (P) (original magnification ×2000).

enhanced and made specific through the assistance of lymphocytes and their products. Macrophages also function as one type of *accessory cell (antigen-presenting cell)*. Such cells assist lymphocytes in responding to antigens, probably by phagocytosing antigens and then presenting antigen epitopes on their surfaces for recognition by lymphocyte receptors.

In the spleen blood circulates through many small channels called sinusoids. Here blood cells and plasma come into contact with mononuclear phagocytes and lymphocytes, thus providing maximum opportunity for immune responses. The lymphocytes are organized into cuffs around the small splenic arteries.

Lymphocyte-rich lymph enters lymph nodes through afferent lymphatic vessels and exits through an efferent lymphatic vessel (Fig. 1-3). Inside lymph nodes lymphocytes percolate through masses of lymphocytes and accessory cells organized into particular zones based upon function and state of activation. The outer portion of a lymph node has the densest population of lymphocytes and is called the *cortex*. The inner portion, called the *medulla*, contains many sinuses lined by mononuclear phagocytes. These sinuses coalesce to form the efferent lymphatic vessels.

Foci of lymphoid tissue are located immediately beneath the mucosa of the respiratory and gastrointestinal (GI) tracts to provide immune defense against foreign sub-

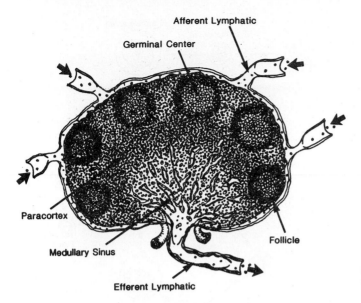

Afferent Lymphatic

Germinal Center

Paracortex

Medullary Sinus

Efferent Lymphatic

Follicle

Figure 1-3. Diagram of Lymph Node.

stances that breach the mucosal barriers. The largest foci are found in the oropharynx and include the palatine tonsils and pharyngeal tonsils or adenoids.

When there is an immune response to an antigen, lymphoid tissues in the region of the body where antigen recognition occurs become swollen as a result of lymphocyte accumulation and proliferation. For example, during viral or bacterial pharyngitis, the tonsils and lymph nodes under the jaw and in the neck are often enlarged. These are indications that the immune system is responding to an antigenic challenge.

Lymphocyte Development

As with all mature tissues of the body, the lymphocytes arise from primitive, undifferentiated precursors, *stem cells,* during embryogenesis. Lymphocyte stem cells differentiate from stem cells that give rise to all blood cells. Lymphocyte stem cells differentiate into two major lineages of lymphocytes, *T lymphocytes* and *B lymphocytes* (Fig. 1-4). Each lineage carries out a different kind of immune response.

T lymphocytes are so named because their differentiation occurs in a lymphoid organ called the *thymus,* which is found in the neck and upper chest. The thymus is a pyramid-shaped organ that is largest in proportion to body weight at birth and undergoes extensive atrophy after puberty. It is densely populated by developing T lymphocytes, *thymocytes,* that are released into the circulation once they mature.

The location or source of the inductive influence that directs B lymphocyte differentiation is not known in mammals, although it is known in birds to be a gut-associated lymphoid organ called the *bursa of Fabricius.* In mammals B lymphocyte differentiation probably occurs in the fetal liver and bone marrow.

During differentiation T and B lymphocytes must develop specific receptors for antigen recognition. These receptors are glycoproteins that are manufactured in the cytoplasm and are inserted into the cell membranes so that their antigen-binding sites

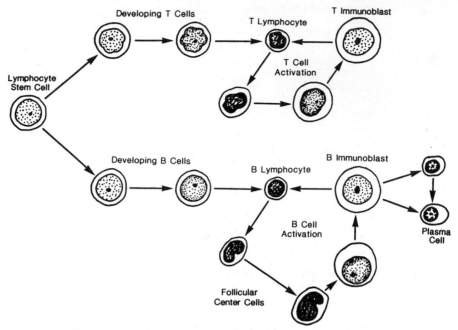

Figure 1-4. Diagram of Lymphocyte Ontogeny and Activation.

are available to bind noncovalently to the specific antigen epitope for which they have specificity. Any one lymphocyte expresses only one type of antigen-binding site, thus there must be a population of lymphocytes produced to express each of the multitude of receptor specificities required to respond to the myriad varieties of antigens.

Lymphocyte Activation

Once mature T and B lymphocytes are released into the circulation and begin moving through the body, they are ready to respond to the specific antigens to which their receptors can bind. The interaction of antigens with lymphocyte receptors is often facilitated by initial processing of the antigen by accessory cells, such as mononuclear phagocytes. Subsets of T lymphocytes are important regulators of immune responses to most antigens. *Helper T lymphocytes* augment immune responses, while *suppressor T lymphocytes* inhibit immune responses.

When antigen epitopes bind to lymphocyte receptors, a signal is generated that leads to morphological and functional transformation of the lymphocyte (Figs. 1–5 and 1–6). To proliferate and express additional genetic information, the densely packed nuclear chromatin of the lymphocyte opens up, resulting in a large, low-density nucleus in a cell much larger than the unstimulated lymphocyte. This process of lymphocyte activation is called *blast transformation,* and the resultant cell is called an *immunoblast.*

T immunoblasts give rise to a clone of T lymphocytes having binding sites specific for the antigen that induced the blast transformation (Fig. 1–5). Thus the number of

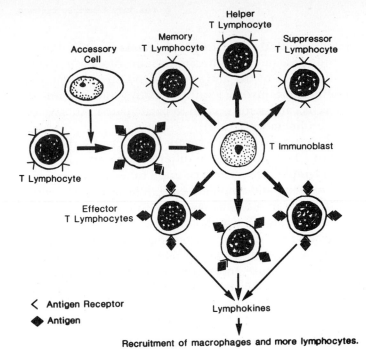

Figure 1-5. T Lymphocyte Function. T lymphocyte antigen recognition, blast transformation, clonal expansion, and production of functionally heterogeneous T lymphocyte subsets.

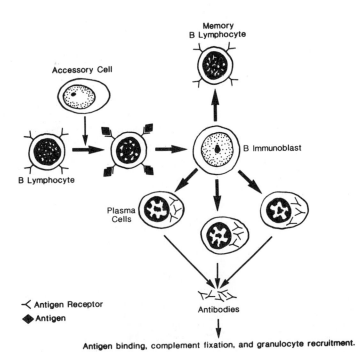

Figure 1-6. B Lymphocyte Function. B lymphocyte antigen recognition, blast transformation, and production of memory B cells and antibody-secreting plasma cells.

T lymphocytes capable of interacting with that particular antigen is amplified by the process of blast transformation and subsequent proliferation. Some of the resultant T lymphocytes become involved with attack of the antigens that initiated the immune response (effector T cells), some become involved with regulating the immune response (helper and suppressor T cells), and some remain to participate in subsequent anamnestic responses to the antigen (memory T cells).

B immunoblasts give rise to B lymphocytes with receptor specificity for the stimulating antigen (Fig. 1–6). In addition, their progeny can differentiate into cells with a morphology differing from that of lymphocytes. These cells are called *plasma cells* and are oval, with an eccentric, round nucleus, and abundant basophilic cytoplasm, with a prominent Golgi region. This difference in morphology between B lymphocytes and plasma cells is due to differing functions. Most B lymphocytes are functioning as recognition units of the immune system and are therefore expressing membrane receptors. Plasma cells are produced to carry out the effects of an immune response, i.e., are effector cells. Their function is to manufacture and secrete antibodies with the same antigen-binding site as that of the B lymphocyte membrane receptor that initially bound antigen and initiated the immune response. Because of this extensive protein synthesis, their cytoplasm is rich in RNA and therefore basophilic, and because of their secretory activity, the Golgi apparatus is large.

Antibody (immunoglobulin) molecules are composed of four polypeptide chains joined by disulfide bonds (Fig. 1–7). Each molecule contains two identical larger chains, *heavy chains,* and two identical smaller chains, *light chains.* There are two types of light chains, κ and λ, and five types of heavy chains, γ, α, μ, δ, and ε. Each antibody molecule has one type of light chain and one type of heavy chain. Based on the type of heavy chain present, antibodies are divided into five *classes (allotypes),* IgG, IgA, IgM, IgD, and IgE.

Immunoglobulin chains are divided into *constant* and *variable* regions. The constant regions of all heavy chains of one type (e.g., gamma) have similar amino acid sequences, and the constant regions of all light chains of one type (e.g., kappa), have

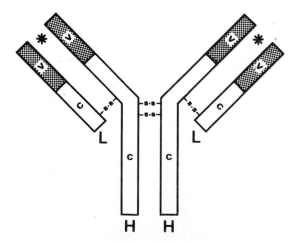

Figure 1–7. Antibody Molecule. Diagram of an antibody molecule showing two heavy chains (H) and two light chains (L), variable (V) and constant (C) regions, and two antigen-binding sites (∗).

similar amino acid sequences. The amino acid sequences of the variable regions of heavy and light chains, however, vary extensively among antibody molecules. The antigen-binding sites of an antibody molecule are located between the variable regions of the heavy and light chains (Fig. 1–7). The constant regions of the heavy chains are responsible for mediating most of the biological events that are set into motion when antibodies bind to antigens.

In lymph nodes (Fig. 1–3) a majority of the B lymphocytes are located within the cortex in nodular aggregates called *follicles.* These follicles usually have a central area, called a *germinal center,* where the B lymphocytes, called *follicular center cells,* are undergoing blast transformation. Plasma cells typically accumulate in the medulla, adjacent to the sinuses, where they are strategically located to release antibodies into the efferent lymph. T lymphocytes predominate in the interfollicular and deep cortical, *paracortical,* areas. A majority of the lymphocytes moving through the lymph nodes and circulating in the lymph and blood are T lymphocytes.

When T lymphocytes respond to antigens, the effector elements that result from blast transformation and subsequently interact with the antigens are cells, i.e., more T lymphocytes (Fig. 1–5). Therefore T lymphocyte-mediated responses to antigen are called *cell-mediated* or *cellular immune responses.* When B lymphocytes respond to antigens, the effector elements that result from blast transformation and subsequently interact with the antigens are molecules, i.e., antibodies (Fig. 1–6). Therefore B lymphocyte-mediated responses to antigens are called *humoral* or *antibody-mediated immune responses.*

Once T and B lymphocytes have contacted an antigen and have undergone blast formation and proliferation, there is an increased number of lymphocytes with receptors for that antigen. Even after the antigen is eliminated during a primary response, a greater number of lymphocytes specific for that antigen are present compared to the number present prior to initial antigen exposure. These residual specific lymphocytes are called *memory cells* and are the source of secondary or anamnestic immune responses.

DISEASE INDUCTION BY THE IMMUNE SYSTEM

Activation of the immune system is a calculated risk. Obviously in most instances the benefits outweigh the risks, or this system would not have evolved. The importance of immune responses is underscored by the substantial amount of genetic code utilized to produce the vast array of antigen recognition sites available for initiating immune responses.

Abnormal functioning of the immune system will produce disease, but even normal functioning contributes to the tissue injury in many diseases. Disease induction by the immune system can be categorized on the basis of (1) too little immune response (immune deficiency diseases), (2) appropriate immune response (some inflammatory diseases), (3) too much immune response (allergic diseases), (4) misdirected immune response (autoimmune diseases), and (5) cancers of the immune system (lymphocytic leukemias and lymphomas) (Table 1–1).

TABLE 1-1. THE ROLE OF THE IMMUNE SYSTEM IN DISEASE INDUCTION

Type of Immune Response	Type of Associated Disease	Example
Appropriate	Inflammatory	Tuberculosis
Too little	Immune deficiency	DiGeorge's syndrome
Too much	Allergic	Hay fever
Misdirected	Autoimmune	Lupus erythematosus
Neoplastic	Lymphoma and leukemia	Burkitt's lymphoma

IMMUNE DEFICIENCY DISEASES

Without an adequate immune system the body does not fare well against infectious microorganisms or abnormal cells. Antibodies, and therefore B lymphocytes, are most important in defending against bacteria while T lymphocytes are most important in defending against viruses, fungi, rickettsiae, and intracellular bacteria such as mycobacteria. Thus if the immune system is deficient, an individual is predisposed to infectious diseases.

Immune deficiency can either be *congenital,* i.e., present at birth, or *acquired.* Congenital immune deficiency can either be familial, i.e., due to an inherited genetic defect or nonfamilial, i.e., due to a disturbance of lymphocyte differentiation occurring in utero but not dictated by inherited genetic information. The nature and severity of a congenital immune deficiency is determined by the site and degree of disruption of lymphocyte differentiation during ontogeny.

If the precursor stem cell for both T and B lymphocytes does not generate either lineage of lymphocytes, the result is *severe combined immune deficiency* (SCID). Infants with this disease will die of infection unless they are totally isolated from microorganisms or an immune system is provided by transplantation of bone marrow hematopoietic cells. This latter option is complicated by the fact that the transplanted lymphoid cells may recognize the recipient as nonself, leading to graft versus host disease.

If only T lymphocyte development is deficient, a *cell-mediated immune deficiency* results. One example is *DiGeorge's syndrome,* in which there is abnormal embryogenesis of tissues arising from the third and fourth pharyngeal pouches. Since the lip, ears, aortic arch, parathyroid glands, and thymus all arise from these structures abnormal development can lead to aberrant facial structure, congenital heart disease, hypoparathyroidism, and deficiency of thymus-induced T lymphocyte development. The thymus is absent (thymic aplasia), or very small (thymic hypoplasia), in such individuals.

Complete congenital absence of B lymphocytes results in no antibody production. Once the temporary protection afforded by maternal antibodies that have crossed the placenta is lost, an infant is susceptible to fatal infections. Because most of the plasma gamma globulins are immunoglobulins (antibodies), this immune deficiency state is called *agammaglobulinemia,* meaning no gamma globulins in the blood. Partial or selective congenital defects in antibody production can result in *hypogammaglobulinemia* (reduced antibodies) or *dysgammaglobulinemia* (abnormal antibody production).

Disturbance of control mechanisms that modulate immune responses can also produce immune deficiencies. For example, too few helper T lymphocytes or too many suppressor T lymphocytes can result in reduced functioning of B lymphocytes leading to hypogammaglobulinemia.

Acquired immune deficiencies are much more common than congenital immune deficiencies and often do not result in as severe a defect in immune defense. Acquired immune deficiencies can be produced by infections or cancers that suppress lymphocyte production or function, by depletion of lymphocytes or antibodies through abnormal lymphatic drainage, by increased protein and antibody loss into the gut or urine, and by drugs that destroy lymphocytes. Some drugs inadvertently suppress the immune system as an unwanted side effect of treatment. Physicians sometimes administer drugs to reduce unwanted immune responses that are producing inflammatory or autoimmune diseases.

INFLAMMATORY DISEASES

Inflammation occurs in a tissue when, in response to injury, leukocytes are attracted and accumulate, release molecular mediators, and activate other molecular mediators in the plasma and interstitial fluid. These molecular mediators can produce increased blood flow, causing erythema; increased vascular permeability, causing increased fluid in the tissue (edema); and accumulation of more leukocytes, causing pus formation or induration. An immune response to an antigen may induce inflammation. There are also nonimmune mechanisms capable of inducing inflammation. For example, a bacterial infection in the skin can produce immune-mediated inflammation, but burning the skin will produce non-immune-mediated inflammation.

Inflammation can be induced by either antibody-mediated or cell-mediated immune responses. In the former, granulocytes are the major inflammatory cells called in; while in the latter, macrophages and lymphocytes are the major inflammatory cells attracted.

The most important mediator molecules participating in most forms of antibody-induced inflammation are the *complement* proteins. These are a group of plasma proteins that are activated by both immune and nonimmune mechanisms. Certain resultant complement fragments are chemotactic for granulocytes (polymorphonuclear leukocytes), i.e., they attract granulocytes to the site of complement activation. This attraction is predominantly for neutrophils rather than eosinophils and basophils. When antibodies bind to antigens in tissues, complement is activated and neutrophils accumulate. Granulocytes are phagocytic and contain lytic enzymes in cytoplasmic organelles called lysosomes. They have membrane receptors for certain complement components and for a nonantigen-binding region of antibody molecules. Neutrophils can thus bind to antigen–antibody or antigen–antibody–complement complexes and then ingest and degrade them. If the antigen is part of an infecting microorganism, the pathogen can be destroyed by this mechanism. Granulocytes can be sloppy eaters and can die. In both instances lytic enzymes are released at the site of the immune-mediated inflammation and produce tissue injury.

Even when due to an appropriate humoral immune response, immune-mediated inflammation can contribute to the injury produced during a disease. For example, an antibody-mediated immune response to *Streptococcus pneumoniae* infecting a lung will lead to production of antistreptococcal antibodies. These antibodies will bind to streptococcal antigens and activate complement, leading to influx of granulocytes and inflammation of the lung (i.e., bacterial pneumonia; Fig. 1–8). Without an adequate immune response, however, the bacterial infection would overwhelm the host. Thus immune-mediated inflammation directed against a bacterial lung infection is usually beneficial in the long run to the individual, but it may kill the individual if too much lung injury occurs during the inflammatory process.

Antibodies binding to antigens in the circulation can also produce disease if these *immune complexes* deposit in tissues, e.g., blood vessel walls, and incite inflammation. Alternatively, antigens and antibodies can deposit in tissue uncomplexed and then form immune complexes in situ leading to tissue inflammation.

Lymphokines are the most important molecular mediators participating in inflammation initiated by cell-mediated immune responses. Lymphokines are released by antigen-stimulated effector T lymphocytes (Fig. 1–5). Unlike the antibody molecules

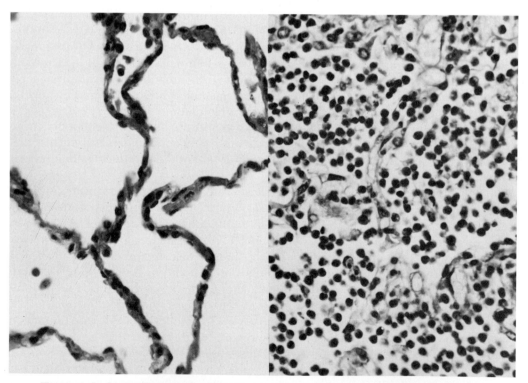

Figure 1–8. Acute Pneumonia. Micrographs of normal lung (alveolar walls and air spaces, *left panel*) and lung with acute bacterial pneumonia showing polymorphonuclear leukocytes filling the air spaces (*right panel*) (H&E, original magnification ×500).

released by effector B lymphocytes and plasma cells, lymphokines do not bind specifically to antigens. They function as mediators of inflammation and, therefore, in this respect, are somewhat analogous to complement. However, unlike activated complement, which attracts predominantly granulocytes to the site of an antibody-mediated immune response, lymphokines attract predominantly macrophages and lymphocytes to the site of a cell-mediated immune response. Lymphokines can attract macrophages to the site of T lymphocyte interaction with antigen, inhibit macrophage migration away from the site once they are there, stimulate proliferation of macrophages, and activate macrophages so that they aggressively phagocytose and degrade materials at the site of inflammation. Macrophages, with their lytic enzymes and phagocytic capacity, play an analogous role in cell-mediated immune injury to that played by granulocytes in antibody-mediated immune injury. Some T lymphocytes can kill cells directly, but most cell death resulting from T lymphocyte activation is produced by macrophages.

Viral hepatitis is an example of a disease resulting from an appropriate cell-mediated immune response to a viral infection of the liver. Liver cells infected with virus display viral antigens on their membranes. The foreign antigens are recognized by T lymphocytes, which undergo blast transformation and produce more T lymphocytes expressing the same antigen-binding sites. The T lymphocytes can then release lymphokines when viral antigens bind to their receptors. These lymphokines mediate the accumulation of lymphocytes and macrophages in the liver, resulting in liver inflammation (hepatitis) that destroys the virally infected cells as well as some innocent bystander cells (Fig. 1-9). If the virus can be eradicated without too much liver damage, the individual will survive.

ALLERGIC DISEASES

Allergic diseases (allergies) result from a greater degree of immune response than would be appropriate for a given antigen challenge. This is also called *hypersensitivity,* although this term is sometimes used to designate anamnestic immune responses in general.

For a person not allergic to poison ivy, rubbing the skin against this plant causes no injury. However, when the skin of an individual who is allergic to poison ivy comes in contact with this plant, inflammation of the skin, called contact dermatitis, occurs. This is a cell-mediated immune response resulting from antigen recognition by T lymphocytes. The antigen that stimulates the immune response in this example is actually a combination of a small molecular moiety from the poison ivy, called a *hapten,* and a protein in the skin, called a *carrier.* Haptens alone are not able to stimulate immune responses, but they are when conjugated to carrier molecules.

Some of the most common allergic diseases are the result of antibody-mediated rather than cell-mediated immune responses. Different classes of antibodies are primarily involved in the induction of different types of inflammation. *IgG* and *IgM* are classes of antibodies that are able to activate complement and therefore induce immune-mediated inflammation by classical complement activation. Many forms of

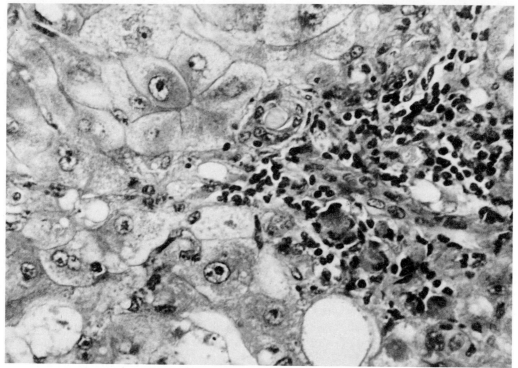

Figure 1-9. Hepatitis. Micrograph of liver infected with hepatitis-B virus showing an area of inflammation produced by the cell-mediated immune response to the viral infection (H&E, original magnification ×600).

antibody-mediated allergy are induced by *IgE*. IgE does not activate complement but induces inflammation by a different mechanism. Examples of IgE-mediated allergy include hay fever, hives, some forms of asthma, and anaphylactic shock. Individuals who are prone to this form of allergy are said to have *atopy*.

In atopic individuals certain antigens, called *allergens*, stimulate B lymphocytes to proliferate and transform into plasma cells that secrete IgE antibodies (Fig. 1-10). The constant regions of IgE antibodies are able to attach to receptors on the surface of tissue *mast cells*. Mast cells with membrane-bound IgE use the antigen-binding sites of the antibodies to specifically bind the allergen that initially induced the IgE production. Mast cells have numerous cytoplasmic granules that contain molecular mediators, such as histamine, that have effects on blood vessels, smooth muscle, and secretory glands. Mast cells release the contents of their granules when membrane-bound IgE binds allergens, and they also secrete additional mediators not packaged in the granules. When released these mediators can cause increased vascular permeability, vascular dilation, contraction of nonvascular smooth muscle, increased gland secretion, and influx of eosinophilic granulocytes.

For example, a person who develops hay fever due to exposure to a certain kind

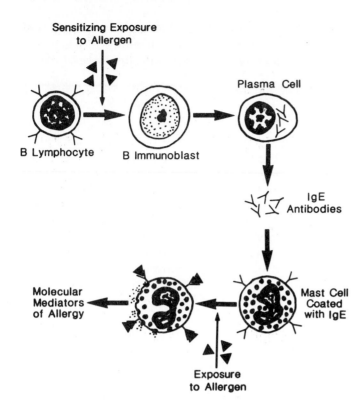

Figure 1-10. IgE-Mediated Allergy. Mechanism of allergen-induced, IgE-mediated, mast cell release of molecular mediators of allergy.

of pollen will have IgE-coated mast cells with specificity for that allergen in the ocular and nasopharyngeal mucosa. When the IgE on these mast cells binds the pollen allergen, mediator molecules are released from the granules into the mucosa of the eyes and nasopharynx. The resultant vascular dilation leads to increased blood flow and redness. Increased secretion induced in mucosal glands leads to a runny nose and watery eyes. Thus the symptoms and signs of hay fever are produced.

Antibody-mediated allergy is also called *immediate hypersensitivity*, and cell-mediated allergy is referred to as *delayed hypersensitivity*. This nomenclature is based on the time required to develop the inflammatory effects after antigen exposure in an allergic individual. Because mast cells coated with IgE are already present at the site of the allergic response, and because they release their mediator molecules immediately upon allergen binding, the resultant inflammatory changes occur within seconds or minutes of allergen exposure. In contrast, the inflammation induced by a cell-mediated response to an allergen is delayed by the time required for T lymphocyte binding of the allergen, lymphokine release, macrophage and additional lymphocyte migration into the site of inflammation, and macrophage activation. These events usually reach a maximum only after several days.

This immediate versus delayed response to antigens is the basis for skin testing to determine the presence and nature of immune reactivity toward a given antigen. The appropriate allergen injected into the skin of an individual with an IgE-mediated allergy will immediately produce a red, swollen lesion. Mycobacterial antigen injected into the skin of an individual who has had a mycobacterial infection will produce a raised, hard lesion due to a cell-mediated immune response only after several days.

AUTOIMMUNE DISEASES

Normally immune responses against one's own tissues are substantially suppressed by the control mechanisms of the immune system. In some individuals, however, this control is inadequate. Such individuals are said to have *autoimmunity* and may develop *autoimmune disease.* Autoimmune disease can be produced by cell-mediated or antibody-mediated autoimmune responses, although the latter are more commonly recognized.

The mechanisms of tissue injury by the immune system are the same for induction of appropriate immune injury, allergic immune injury, or autoimmune injury. For example, appropriate antibody attack on mismatched transfused red blood cells (RBCs) leads to a transfusion reaction that utilizes the same mechanisms as the autoimmune attack on one's own RBCs in autoimmune hemolytic anemia. In both instances antibodies bind to antigens on the surface of the RBCs and subsequently activate complement. Activated complement then lyses the cells. Also receptors for immunoglobulin and complement on phagocytes lead to phagocytosis of the RBCs that are coated with antibodies and complement.

Autoimmunity can lead to a wide variety of diseases by attack on tissues, cells, or molecules. For example, autoantibodies to skin antigens can produce dermatitis, autoantibodies to RBCs can produce hemolytic anemia, and autoantibodies to insulin can produce a rare form of diabetes mellitus.

LYMPHOCYTIC LEUKEMIAS AND LYMPHOMAS

As in all other tissues of the body, cancers can arise in the tissue of the immune system, i.e., the lymphocytes. Neoplasms are uncontrolled growths of cells, and cancers are malignant neoplasms that are able to spread throughout the body and can ultimately lead to death. In *lymphocytic leukemias* the neoplastic lymphocytes proliferate extensively in the bone marrow and typically enter the blood in large numbers, thus the term leukemia. In addition to lymphocytic leukemias there can be leukemias derived from other blood cell lineages, e.g., granulocytic leukemia. In *lymphomas* the earliest and most extensive proliferation of neoplastic lymphocytes occurs outside the bone marrow, most often within lymph nodes. However, in advanced cases both lymphocytic leukemias and lymphomas can become widely distributed throughout the body.

Many different types of lymphocytic leukemias and lymphomas are recognized based on the morphological and functional characteristics of the neoplastic lymphocytes. In general there are categories of lymphocytic neoplasms that correspond in morphology and physiology to each of the stages of T and B lymphocyte maturation and blast transformation depicted in Figure 1–4. Thus some lymphoid neoplasms resemble primitive lymphoid stem cells (e.g., acute lymphoblastic leukemia), some resem ble lymphocytes undergoing blast transformation (e.g., follicular center cell lymphoma), and some resemble mature effector cells (e.g., multiple myeloma, a neoplasm composed of plasma cells; Fig. 1–11).

LABORATORY EVALUATION OF THE IMMUNE SYSTEM

Because the immune system plays such an important role in defense and the induction of many different types of diseases, laboratory methods for evaluating its status are important for proper patient management. Many medical laboratories perform tests that analyze certain aspects of the immune system. In addition, many laboratory procedures not directed at evaluating the immune system utilize the great specificity of antibodies as a means of identifying and quantitating unknown substances in patient samples. For example, radioimmunoassays (RIAs), enzyme-linked immunoassays, immunodiffusion, immunoelectrophoresis, and immunohistochemistry are frequently used laboratory procedures that make use of reagent antibodies.

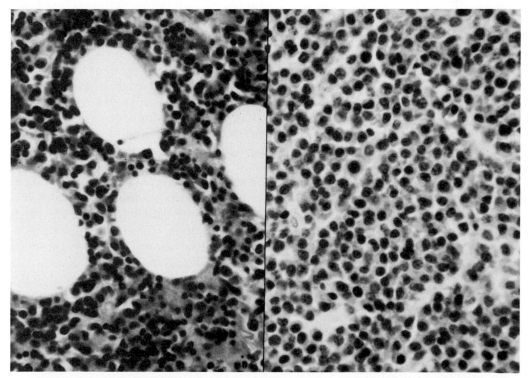

Figure 1–11. Multiple Myeloma. Micrographs of normal bone marrow with heterogeneous hematopoietic cells and several large fat cells (*left panel*) and marrow completely replaced by a mass of neoplastic plasma cells in a patient with multiple myeloma (*right panel*) (H&E, original magnification ×500).

Laboratory analysis of lymphocytes is a means of assessing the immune system. Lymphocytes in the blood can be quantified and qualitatively analyzed. Quantification can be performed by a variety of automated instruments or by visual counting. The microscopic morphology of lymphocytes in blood smears is most often evaluated after Giemsa or Wright's staining (Fig. 1–1). Special staining can be used to identify particular lymphocyte subsets. The most extensive lymphocyte subcategorization can be accomplished with staining using reagent antibodies specific for lymphocyte subsets. The binding of these antibodies to lymphocytes is visualized by linking the antibodies to substances that can be seen on microscopic examination or by an automated cell counter. In this case antibodies are being used as laboratory probes to identify specific cell types. This technique takes advantage of the fact that lymphocytes express different antigenic membrane proteins dependent upon their stage of maturation and differentiation. These proteins can be identified by staining lymphocytes with labeled antibodies specific for the various lymphocyte membrane proteins. This technique can be used on lymphocytes in tissue biopsy specimens (Fig. 1–12) or lymphocytes from the blood.

There are also in vitro functional assays that can evaluate the physiologic activity of lymphocytes. For example, helper T lymphocytes can be shown to promote B lymphocyte function, while suppressor T lymphocytes will inhibit B lymphocyte function.

Quantification, identification of membrane marker proteins, functional analysis, and morphological examination of lymphocytes in blood, other body fluids, and tissue can yield information that is important for diagnosis and management of many diseases in which the immune system plays a role. Congenital and acquired immune deficiency diseases will have characteristic quantitative or qualitative defects in certain lymphocyte subsets. Many infectious diseases, especially viral infections, will manifest typical quantitative or morphological alterations in blood lymphocytes. Characterization of the neoplastic lymphocytes is an integral part of diagnosing and directing therapy for lymphocytic leukemias and lymphomas.

Antibody analysis, usually performed on serum, is an important means of assessing the activity of the B lymphocyte limb of the immune response. Abnormally low levels of antibodies are found in some forms of immune deficiency, while very high levels of antibodies can be present in patients with certain types of B lymphoid neoplasms, especially multiple myeloma. The branch of laboratory medicine known as *serology* seeks to identify the presence of increased levels of antibodies to a particular microorganism as evidence for infection by that microorganism. By examining the changes over time in the amount and class of antibody in the serum, a conclusion can often be reached as to whether the infection occurred in the past or is ongoing. Identification of autoantibodies in the serum is a method for diagnosing antibody-mediated autoimmune diseases. Blood bank technologists evaluate serum antibodies to confirm patient blood types and also to determine the presence of antibodies that could attack transfused blood.

Since complement is activated and consumed during some antibody-mediated inflammatory reactions, quantitative and functional analysis of complement proteins is used to diagnose and assess the activity of some immune-mediated diseases.

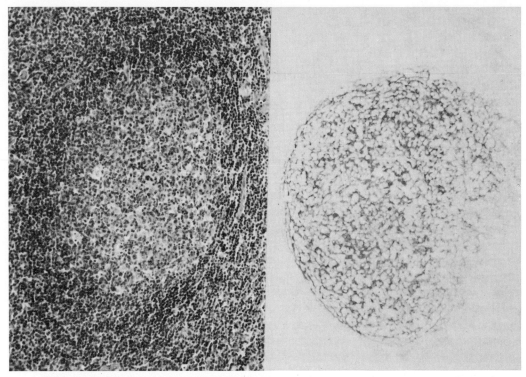

Figure 1-12. Specific Immunostaining. Micrographs of lymph node cortex comparing the appearance of a follicle and the surrounding cells after routine staining (H&E, *left panel*) with specific staining for cells in germinal centers (*right panel*) (original magnification ×170).

T lymphocyte reactivity can be tested by evaluating responses to antigens and *mitogens* (substances that stimulate proliferation). This can be done in vivo by injecting antigens into the skin and evaluating the degree of resultant inflammation. Alternatively, this can be done in vitro by first isolating viable lymphocytes, then incubating them with antigens or mitogens and assessing the degree of blast transformation, lymphokine production, or proliferation.

Discussion of the Illustrative Case

The case described at the beginning of this chapter illustrates the two-edged sword of the immune system. The immune system plays a beneficial role in defending against foreign invaders, but it can also participate in disease production.

The patient described successfully overcame a streptococcal infection of the pharynx by mounting an antibody-mediated immune attack that destroyed the invading microbial pathogens. The serologic identification of antistreptolysin O and antiDNAse B, both antibodies against streptococcal antigens, documented the streptococcal infection. Some residual bacteria were identified by culture, but the resolution of the pharyngeal inflammation indicated that the infection had been overcome. The symptoms and signs of the pharyngitis were the side effects of both the injurious products of the bacteria and the immune attack on the streptococci. In the pharyngeal mucosa the union of antibodies with streptococcal antigens led to inflammation induced by complement activation and recruitment of granulocytes. The granulocytes phagocytosed and destroyed the antibody-coated and antibody-complement–coated bacteria but coincidentally caused local tissue injury. The white splotches on the mucosa were accumulations of granulocytes and debris (pus). The enlarged tonsils and cervical lymph nodes resulted from extensive, follicular, B lymphocyte blast transformation and proliferation as well as phagocytosis by medullary macrophages of debris draining through afferent lymphatics from the site of inflammation.

Why is there blood and protein in the urine? This resulted from the deposition from the circulation of immune complexes containing antistreptococcal antibodies and streptococcal antigens into the renal glomeruli. When the immune complexes localized in the glomerular capillaries, they activated complement and attracted granulocytes. This glomerular inflammation (glomerulonephritis) led to injury of the capillaries, allowing passage of proteins and RBCs into the urine. The reduction of filtration of wastes from the plasma resulted in the build up of nitrogenous wastes, azotemia. The consumption of complement by binding to the immune complexes lowered plasma levels and led to hypocomplementemia.

Once the source of additional antigen was eliminated by the immune-mediated inflammatory process in the pharynx and the immune complexes were eliminated by the inflammatory process in the glomeruli, the glomerulonephritis resolved. Within two months the patient had no signs or symptoms of kidney disease.

QUESTIONS

1. What three major characteristics of the immune system distinguish it from other nonimmune defense systems?

2. Why do not all lymphocytes have the same morphology?

3. In a lymph node near the site of a bacterial infection, which region would be most expanded, cortical follicles or paracortex; and why?

4. In a child with congenital absence of the thymus, what kind of immune response would be most severely deficient?

5. After touching a poison ivy plant, why does it take several days for an allergic individual to develop the maximum symptoms?

Chapter 2 Nonimmune Defense Systems

OBJECTIVES

1. To outline nonimmune external defenses.
2. To outline nonimmune internal defenses.
3. To discuss polymorphonuclear leukocytes and their role in nonimmune defense.
4. To describe and discuss macrophages and their role in nonimmune defense.
5. To describe natural killer cell activity.
6. To describe the nonimmunologic activation of complement and its role in defense.
7. To discuss the nonimmune initiation of the inflammatory response.
8. To discuss amplification of the inflammatory response.

Illustrative Case

A 4-year-old male child was playing in the kitchen when he spilled a large pot of boiling water over his head, shoulders, and the front of his body. On evaluation at the hospital he was found to have third-degree and deep second-degree burns over 30% of the body surface. He was admitted to the burn-care ward where routine wound care, thermal regulation, and fluid and electrolyte management were instituted. He was given immunization against tetanus but was not placed on prophylactic antibiotics other than Sulfamylon cream.

The patient did well until two weeks after admission, when he had the abrupt onset of increased fever, chills, and mental disorientation. Wound cultures obtained just prior to and at the time of onset of symptoms grew numerous colonies of *Pseudomonas aeruginosa*. The patient was begun on therapy with appropriate antibiotics, and blood was sent to the microbiology laboratory for culture. Over the following day the patient developed progressive hypotension, oliguria, tachycardia, tachypnea, and mental obtundation. Blood culture grew *P aeruginosa*. The *P aeruginosa* previously isolated from the wound was found to be sensitive to the antibiotics being administered.

Over the next week the patient's symptoms and signs of sepsis resolved. Blood cultures became negative, and wound cultures showed a progressive decline in Pseudomonas colonies.

INTRODUCTION

Nonimmune defense systems are those protective systems of the body that are not dependent upon lymphocyte activation. They do not require previous exposure to a pathogen to be effective and are innately present in all normal newborns. Nonimmune defense systems are sometimes referred to as nonspecific defense systems because they are effective against most agents potentially harmful to the body.

Immune defense systems, in contrast, are those protective systems of the body that are developed only after an exposure to a specific agent that initiates lymphocyte stimulation. After exposure, time is required for the immune response to become effective. These systems are *specific* because they are directed primarily against that one agent that induced their development.

Nonimmune body defense systems may be divided into *external nonimmune defense systems* and *internal nonimmune defense systems.* External nonimmune defense systems are those that are effective on body surfaces exposed to the external environment. These surfaces include the skin, eye, mucous membrane-lined respiratory tract, alimentary tract, intestinal tract, and genitourinary tract. Internal defenses are those that are effective within the sterile environment of the body, i.e., the tissues and blood. The external defenses protect the internal body against direct exposure to the surrounding environment. Entry into the sterile internal body is gained only by penetration of the external defenses.

NONIMMUNE EXTERNAL DEFENSES

The *skin* is the most important nonimmune external defense and covers the entire body. This physical barrier of epithelial cells extends and covers all invaginations of exterior body surfaces, e.g., the alimentary canal, the respiratory tract, the genitourinary tract. Particular anatomical areas of the skin contain other cells that provide specialized nonimmune external defenses.

Cornified and stratified epithelial cells of the skin form a physical barrier to prevent potential pathogens from entering and colonizing the fertile environment of the internal body. The dead outer layer of the skin is constantly being shed and replaced with cells grown in the lower levels of the skin. Constant shedding of the epithelium eliminates surface bacteria that may have accomplished the initial step of infection, i.e., attachment to living cells. Dryness of the skin prevents growth of moisture-requiring fungus. A common example of fungal growth where skin dryness is not maintained is athlete's foot, which occurs in the moist areas between the toes. In addition to the above defenses afforded by the skin, *secretions* of the sebaceous glands contain bactericidal and fungicidal substances. Together these defenses of the skin provide a very effective protection to the body from infection.

An outer physical barrier of cells also protects normal eyes from infection. In addition, eyes have *tearing,* a flushing action that rids the eye of surface contaminations. Besides the physical flushing action, tearing provides *lysozyme,* which is bactericidal against most gram-positive bacteria. When tearing is deficient, as in Sjögren's syndrome, there is a predisposition to ocular infections.

The body's outer epithelial layer covers and protects the oral cavity. Cells in this area secrete *saliva,* which contains several nonimmune defense agents. One is bactericidal lysozyme discussed above. Another is glycolipids that competitively inhibit attachment of bacteria to the oral epithelium and thus prevent infection.

In the upper respiratory tract, *nasal hairs* act as filters to prevent larger particles from being inhaled. *Nasal secretions* contain lysozyme and other antimicrobial substances. The *mucous membranes* that line the entire respiratory tract are layers of epithelial cells plus cells producing a viscous secretion termed *mucus.* Mucus is an adhesive substance that sticks to the surface of the epithelium. Most bacteria and viruses must attach to living cells to secure nutrition to support their growth. Mucus physically prevents microbes from approaching live, underlying epithelial cells and from setting up residence. Also, mucus contains glycoproteins and lipoproteins that are capable of binding to viral surfaces and neutralizing the virus. *Ciliated epithelial cells* along the respiratory tract have cilia constantly waving upward toward the pharynx. Particles that pass the nasal hair filtration stick to the viscous mucus. Waving cilia move the mucus and trapped particles upward. As they move upward to the pharynx, mucus and particles clump together and are eventually either swallowed, coughed out, or spit out. In the lower respiratory tract phagocytic cells called *alveolar macrophages* move along the air spaces (alveoli) and scavenge. These cells phagocytize microbes or particles that have evaded the defenses of the upper respiratory tract and entered the alveoli. After engulfment normal macrophages will kill most of the internalized organisms and degrade these and other phagocytized debris.

Epithelial cell lining, mucus, and secretions are also characteristics of the alimentary tract. Passing down the alimentary tract, other nonimmune defenses are effective. In the stomach, a *low pH* deters survival of most microbes. In the small intestines *digestive secretions* prevent bacterial growth. As the colon is approached, the amount of microbial growth increases, and innocuous, indigenous flora of the lower intestinal tract and colon are a major deterrent to the establishment of new pathogenic microorganisms. *Indigenous microbial flora* inhabiting the surface of epithelial body linings occupy physical space and use available nutrients to leave little opportunity for new potential pathogens to thrive. Inappropriate or extended use of antibiotics can increase the risk to certain types of infection by reducing this indigenous flora. Throughout the intestinal tract the action of *peristalsis* propels food and associated bacteria out of the body.

The genitourinary tract is lined with mucous membranes. In addition, the washing motion of the *urine flow* is an important nonimmune defense that flushes away microorganisms. Urine itself has a low pH that inhibits the growth of most microorganisms. It also contains bactericidal lysozyme. The external opening of the urinary tract is in contact with the microorganisms of the external environment. If urine flow is reduced, these microbes may gain entrance to the urinary tract and cause infection.

All of the above nonimmune external defense systems (Table 2–1) are functional in normal individuals and usually prevent microbes from entering the fertile, sterile environment of the internal body. Any malfunction of these defenses is an opportunity for pathogens to infect the body. For example, cuts or breaks in the skin allow bacteria to freely penetrate the broken barrier. A few microorganisms have unique properties that enable them to penetrate the intact external defense systems. If microorganisms do penetrate the external defenses, the body has immune and nonimmune internal defenses to seek out and destroy the invaders.

NONIMMUNE INTERNAL DEFENSES

Beneath the protective layer of epithelial cells lining the body's surface is the internal, sterile body. This nutritive environment is optimal for the growth and replication of many organisms. Most microorganisms that gain entry into this internal, sterile body would grow and multiply if not controlled. Because it is not uncommon for an individual to experience breaks or cuts in the skin, the body's internal defenses are important for survival. In this section the discussion of internal defenses will be limited to the nonimmune ones; however, the immune defenses, which will be presented in subsequent chapters, should not be forgotten.

Neutrophilic Polymorphonuclear Leukocytes (Neutrophils)
Neutrophils are the most abundant type of circulating white blood cell (WBC) and are one of the most important nonimmune internal defenses. Deficiencies in function of

TABLE 2–1. SUMMARY OF THE EXTERNAL AND INTERNAL NONIMMUNE DEFENSES

External nonimmune defenses	Internal nonimmune defenses
Outer body surfaces	Neutrophil
Epithelial barrier	Macrophage
Dryness	NK cell
Sloughing, dead cells	Complement
Secretions	Inflammation
Tearing	C-reactive protein
Invaginated body surfaces	
Mucous membrane	
Macrophages	
Cilia motion	
pH	
Peristalsis	
Normal flora	
Urination	

this cell predispose to many diseases. Neutrophils originate in the bone marrow and once released into the blood survive for only about 6 days. There is a constant turnover in the circulating neutrophil population. Normally the number of circulating neutrophils is about 7000 to 10,000 per cubic millimeter. Additional neutrophils are found in the tissues and adhering to blood vessel walls. The total number of circulating neutrophils is increased in most bacterial infections as part of the body's effort to protect itself. An increase in circulating neutrophils is termed *neutrophilia* and is useful to the clinician as an indicator of bacterial infection. During infection or other acute inflammatory process, neutrophils leave the blood vessels (Fig. 2–1) by first marginating at the endothelial surfaces of vessels and then working their way between the endothelial cells lining the vessel wall. This migration of neutrophils through the vessel walls is termed *diapedesis.* Once outside the vessels, neutrophils migrate through the

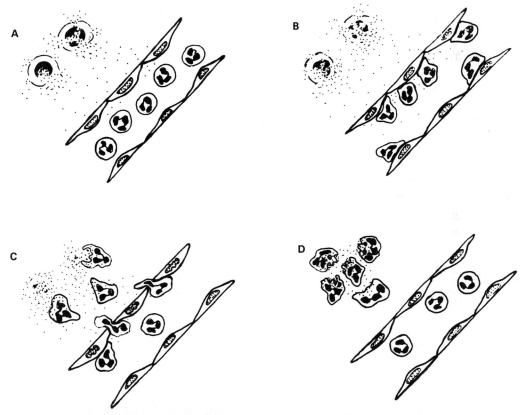

Figure 2–1. Diapedesis During Nonimmune Inflammatory Response. A. Injury to tissue cells and vessel with circulating neutrophils in same area. **B.** Margination of neutrophils in response to a chemotactic gradient formed from released intracellular contents and their action to initiate the complement system. **C.** Diapedesis of neutrophils in response to chemotaxins and anaphylotoxins. **D.** Cleaned-up tissue area after neutrophils have migrated to the area, phagocytized, and degraded the debris.

tissues, attracted by chemotactic substances produced in the area of infection. Upon reaching the infected site the neutrophils engulf (phagocytose) organisms and debris. Internalized microorganisms are normally killed and degraded.

Because there are some diseases in which neutrophils are adequate in number but inadequate in function, laboratory science has developed procedures to evaluate their functional activity. Clinical laboratory assays of neutrophil phagocytic function divide phagocytic activities into (1) chemotaxis, (2) phagocytosis, and (3) killing.

Chemotaxis is the directed motion of a leukocyte toward an increasing chemical gradient. This movement requires energy that is supplied through normal anaerobic glycolysis of adenosine triphosphates (ATPs) generated via the Krebs' cycle. Actin within the leukocyte is polymerized to rearrange the cytoskeleton. ATPs are consumed in supplying energy for contraction of myosin around these microfilaments in the cytoskeleton to result in movement. Locomotion allows the neutrophil to approach foreign particles in preparation for phagocytosis. Chemotaxins are substances that induce chemotaxis. Fragments of molecules released during activation of certain plasma proteins, especially those in the complement, fibrinolysis, and kinin systems, are potent neutrophil chemotaxins. Neutrophils themselves are stimulated by phagocytosis to produce arachidonic-acid–derived leukotrienes some of which are chemotaxins that attract more neutrophils. Figure 2–2 is an outline of the possible arachidonic metabolites resulting from activation of cell-membrane–associated phospholipase. Pertubation of the neutrophil membrane activates membrane phospholipases to release free arachidonic acid from membrane phospholipids. Arachidonic acid may then be metabolized via the lipoxygenase or the cyclo-oxygenase pathways. The former route produces a series of molecules called *leukotrienes,* some of which are chemotaxins, especially leukotriene B4, and others of which are anaphylatoxins. The latter route of arachidonic acid metabolism produces a series of molecules called *prostaglandins,* some of which are anaphylatoxins and *thromboxanes,* which have a role in initiating coagulation.

Immunologists have identified specific substances and conditions that suppress chemotaxis. Certain viruses (e.g., Herpes simplex and influenza) cause temporary defects in neutrophil locomotion. *Lazy leukocyte syndrome* is a disease in which neutrophils demonstrate deficient chemotaxis leading to inability of the phagocyte to reach the site of infection and therefore an inability to perform phagocytosis and killing. Individuals with this syndrome succumb to repeated bacterial infections. *Chemotactic factor inhibitor* (CFI) is a normal serum α or β globulin present in miniscule amounts in healthy individuals. Such conditions as Hodgkin's disease, sarcoidosis, systemic lupus erythematosus, and lepromatous leprosy cause increased concentrations of CFI and resultant suppression of neutrophil chemotaxis.

Phagocytosis may be divided into an *attachment* and an *internalization* phase. *Attachment* is the physical association of a neutrophil with the particle to be phagocytosed. The neutrophil has several specific receptors integrated into its surface membrane. Particles having molecules that react with the specific receptors become physically held in juxtaposition to the neutrophil by these molecules, which act as a bridge between the particles and the neutrophils. This association promotes phagocytosis by holding the particle in place until internalization can occur. An example of a nonimmune

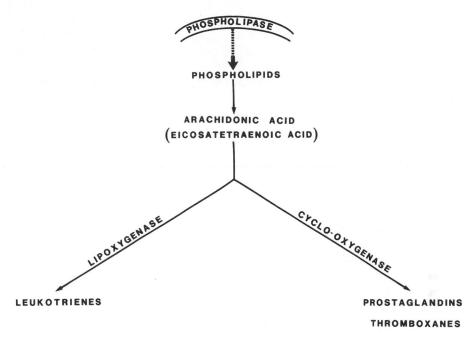

PHOSPHOLIPASE

PHOSPHOLIPIDS

ARACHIDONIC ACID
(EICOSATETRAENOIC ACID)

LIPOXYGENASE

CYCLO-OXYGENASE

LEUKOTRIENES

PROSTAGLANDINS

THROMBOXANES

Figure 2-2. Arachidonic Acid Metabolites and Their Actions. Pertubation of membranes of phagocytes activates membrane-associated phospholipase. This enzyme acts upon cellular phospholipids to release the free fatty acid arachidonic acid (eicosatetraenoic acid). Arachidonic acid may be metabolized via the lipoxygenase route to form leukotrienes or via the cyclo-oxygenase route to form prostaglandins and thromboxanes. The particular type and quantity of arachidonic acid product depends upon the cell type involved and the environmental influences upon that cell. The biological role of arachidonic acid metabolism is still the subject of intensive research; however, the following sentences seem to summarize emerging knowledge in this area. Leukotrienes are a group of biologically active proteins so named because they were originally found in leukocytes. Various leukotrienes mediate smooth muscle contraction, vasodilation, and chemotaxis. Prostaglandins are a group of naturally occurring fatty acids. Individual prostaglandins mediate aggregation of platelets, vasoconstriction, vasodilation, bronchoconstriction, and disaggregation or inhibition of aggregation of platelets. Thromboxanes are produced mostly in platelets. They mediate aggregation of platelets and vasoconstriction.

molecule that coats particles and combines with specific receptors on the neutrophil is a product of complement activation, e.g., C3b. Molecules that enhance phagocytosis by coating particles to be phagocytosed and combining with specific receptors on the membrane of the phagocyte are *opsonins*. The coating of a particle with opsonins is *opsonization*.

Internalization of particles into the phagocyte is depicted in Figure 2–3. Pseudopodia are extended around the particle and eventually completely encircle it. The membrane projections fuse to leave an internalized particle completely surrounded by cell membrane. This internalized particle within a vesicle is termed a *phagosome*.

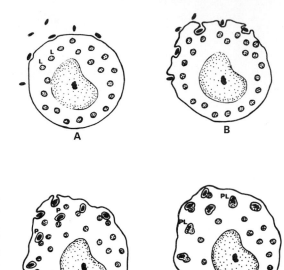

Figure 2-3. Phagocytosis. This figure depicts the steps in phagocytosis. **A.** Chemotaxis or approaching particle to be ingested. **B.** Attachment of particle and extension of pseudopodia. **C.** Ingestion of particle as a membrane-bound phagolysosome. **D.** Fusion of phagosome and lysosome into a phagolysosome and subsequent exposure of particle to lysosomal contents, which degrade and/or kill particle.

Scattered throughout the cytoplasm of the neutrophil are *lysosomes*, which are membrane-bound organelles filled with enzymes. A phagosome and lysosome fuse together to form one larger membrane-bound *phagolysosome*. At this point the internalized particle is exposed to all the proteases, lipases, glycoases, and other enzymes found inside the lysosome. This process of internalization requires energy that is supplied via the normal anaerobic glycolytic pathway and the Krebs' cycle, as shown in Figure 2–4.

Concomitant with internalization, normal neutrophils alter their metabolism and shift to the *hexose-monophosphate pathway* (HMP) of glycogen catabolism. There is an accompanying tremendous consumption of oxygen. Both of these alterations in metabolism lead to the conversion of O_2 to highly reactive *microbicidal products*, as shown in Figure 2–4. *Glucose-6-phosphate dehydrogenase* allows branching of glycolysis to the HMP, which produces NADPH as a by-product. In order for the HMP to continue, NADP must continually be made available by the oxidation of NADPH to NADP. Oxygen is converted via interaction with NADPH and the enzyme *NADPH oxidase* to the very active superoxide radical and hydrogen peroxide. Both of these products are bactericidal agents. H_2O_2 then reacts with a superoxide to form the oxidizing hydroxyl ion and singlet oxygen. Both of these products are bactericidal. Hydrogen peroxide and halide ions (C1, I) are used as substrates by myeloperoxidase to form hypohalite, which is an important bactericidal agent. These bactericidal products, produced by increased oxygen consumption, are in descending order of microbicidal potency:

1. Hypohalite ion
2. Hydroxyl radical
3. Hydrogen peroxide

4. Superoxide radical
5. Singlet oxygen

Almost any pertubation of the normal neutrophil membrane may initiate conversion to the HMP with a burst of oxygen consumption. Adherence of particles to the neutrophil in the absence of phagocytosis is one example.

Neutrophils contain two kinds of granules. In a Wright's-stained smear these appear blue (azurophilic granules) or clear (neutrophilic granules). The former are called primary granules because they appear first during neutrophil maturation; the latter are called secondary granules. *Primary granules* are lysosomes and contain hydrolytic enzymes, myeloperoxidase, lysozyme, and cationic proteins. They are the source of the myeloperoxidase for the microbicidal hypohalite formation. Hydrolytic enzymes of these granules degrade phagocytosed particles upon phagolysosome formation. The lysozyme degrades cell walls of gram-positive bacteria. Cationic proteins bind to cellular proteins to alter the microbe's metabolism and promote cell death. *Secondary gran-*

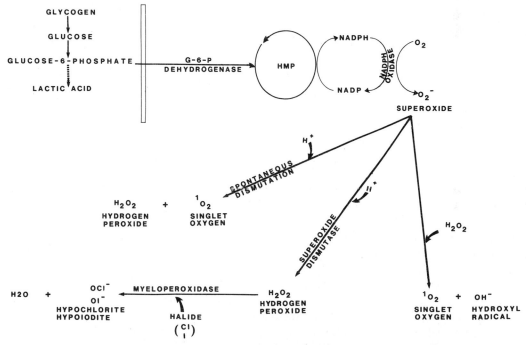

Figure 2–4. Glycogenolysis in the Neutrophil During Normal and Active Phagocytic States. Normally phagocytes catabolize glycogen to lactic acid. Phagocytosis stimulates normal phagocytes to shift to catabolizing glycogen via the HMP. The HMP generates NADPH and needs NADP to continue. NADPH is oxidized to NADP with the concomitant generation of the highly reactive and microbicidal superoxide anion. Additional microbicidal products generated are H_2O_2 in the presence of halide to the strong microbicidal hypohalide. Various diseases associated with defects in phagocytosis can be related to defects in glycogenolysis involving the HMP route and the associated generation of microbicidal products.

ules are smaller in size and contain lactoferrin but no myeloperoxidase. There is controversy over what lytic enzymes are in secondary granules. Lactoferrin binds iron, which is essential for most bacterial growth. Lactoferrin-bound iron is unavailable for bacteria, and thus the bactericidal effect of lactoferrin is mediated by depriving the organisms of vital iron. Cathepsin G cleaves a complement protein into a piece that stimulates release of lysosomal enzymes and a piece that acts as an opsonin to enhance phagocytosis.

Defects in the normal activity of neutrophils cause several diseases. *Chronic granulomatous disease* (CGD) is an X-linked recessive disease in which the individual's phagocytes exhibit normal chemotaxis and phagocytosis but do not accomplish postphagocytic killing. Individuals with this disease have repeated episodes of severe bacterial infections, often by normally nonpathogenic or mildly pathogenic organisms. One morphological characteristic of this disease is the accumulation of macrophages around infections, thus forming granulomas. The defect in killing is due to a lack of ability to switch to the HMP and to generate the bactericidal products generated by oxygen consumption. Experimental data suggest that the defect is in NADPH oxidase. Patients with this disease usually fare relatively well during infections with catalase-negative bacteria; however, they suffer repeated infections with catalase-positive bacteria. The reason is that most bacteria generate H_2O_2, which may then be converted to bactericidal hypohalite forms by the neutrophil's myeloperoxidase. Catalase-positive bacteria degrade the H_2O_2 that they generate, but catalase-negative bacteria do not. Therefore, even though the neutrophil cannot provide H_2O_2 for hypochlorite formation, some bacteria assist with their destruction by synthesizing and providing H_2O_2 to the neutrophil's myeloperoxidase. Streptococci are catalase negative and are readily killed by CGD patients. Staphylococci are catalase positive and survive postphagocytosis to infect CGD patients.

A similar disease is *G-6-P dehydrogenase deficiency*. The absence of this enzyme prevents the postphagocytic switch to the HMP. This disease is not X-linked. Patients with G-6-P dehydrogenase deficiency also have hemolytic anemia. *Job's syndrome* is another similar disease in which neutrophils cannot execute a HMP shift and therefore cannot mediate postphagocytic killing. This disease has not been biochemically defined, and perhaps it is a variant of CGD.

Chédiak–Higashi syndrome is characterized by the presence of large cytoplasmic granules in neutrophils and platelets. Patients have albinism and photophobia. Recurrent bacterial infections are common due to ineffective postphagocytic killing. HMP is intact, and oxygen burst metabolism occurs, but the large abnormal primary granules cannot release their myeloperoxidase. Death due to overwhelming infection occurs in most patients during childhood. These patients also have demonstrated reduced activity in another cell type involved in nonimmune defense, the natural killer (NK) cell.

Myeloperoxidase deficiency is a complete lack of this enzyme in the neutrophil. Patients with this disease have decreased postphagocytic killing; however, there is killing via other mechanisms not requiring myeloperoxidase. This disease is associated with a much better prognosis than is CGD.

Another disease associated with neutrophil dysfunction is *lazy leukocyte syndrome.*

TABLE 2-2. DISEASES ASSOCIATED WITH DEFECTS IN PHAGOCYTOSIS AND CORRELATION TO GLYCOGENOLYSIS INVOLVING THE HMP

Disease	HMP/O_2 Consumption Burst	Myeloperoxidase	Other
Chronic granulomatous disease	−	+	Probably absent or deficient NADPH oxidase
Job's syndrome	−	+	Not sure
G-6-P dehydrogenase deficiency	−	+	No G-6-P dehydrogenase
Chédiak–Higashi syndrome	+	+	Myeloperoxidase not released from granules
Lazy leukocyte	+	+	Deficient chemotaxis
Myeloperoxidase deficiency	+	−	No myeloperoxidase

This condition results from deficient chemotaxis of the neutrophil. Patients suffer repeated bacterial infections and usually have neutropenia.

Table 2–2 summarizes these diseases of neutrophil dysfunctions and notes the biochemical deficiencies associated with them. Neutrophil function may also be adversely affected by other conditions. For instance, chronic infections, Hodgkin's disease, diabetes mellitus, and alcoholic cirrhosis tend to decrease chemotaxis. Burns and sickle cell disease are known to depress phagocytosis. Drugs can affect neutrophil function. Corticosteroids, for example, inhibit release of lysosomal contents and slow phagocytosis. Anesthetics are well-known depressors of phagocytosis.

Macrophages (Mononuclear Phagocytes)

Monocytes are mononuclear leukocytes that originate in the bone marrow and are later released into the circulation. Their half-life in circulation is about the same as that of the neutrophil. Monocytes in the blood are actually immature cells that are in transit to the tissues or to fixed sites along specialized vessels. Once they reach these locations monocytes mature into macrophages. They are so named because they are large and actively phagocytic. Macrophages located in tissue are often called *histiocytes*. Those that localize along blood and lymphatic vessels are sometimes called *reticuloendothelial cells*. These are most numerous in the liver, where they are called *Kupffer's cells*. Those that localize in the lung tissue are called alveolar macrophages.

Macrophages are found in either a *resting stage* or an *active stage*. Active macrophages accomplish phagocytosis more rapidly, have more cytoplasmic lysosomes, and kill phagocytosed microbes or cells more rapidly than resting macrophages. One important asset of the activated macrophage, or "angry macrophage," is that it will attack all foreign cells. This activated macrophage is, therefore, nonspecific in its action, as are all of the nonimmune defenses. Substances that are known to activate macrophages from the resting stage include double-stranded nucleic acids, bacterial endo-toxins, interferon, and products of neutrophils.

Like the neutrophil, the macrophage also performs the steps of phagocytosis with a shift to HMP and a burst of oxygen consumption. Lysosomal contents are released both into phagosomes and outside the cell, just as with the neutrophil. Leukotrienes, prostaglandins, and thromboxanes are synthesized during pertubation of macrophage membrane, just as with pertubation of the neutrophil membrane.

The activated macrophage synthesizes and secretes molecules termed *monokines* that include most components of the complement and the coagulation systems. By-products from the activated complement system are chemotaxins for macrophages as well as for neutrophils. Endogenous pyrogen (EP; interleukin 1) is a monokine that affects the hypothalmus and the thermoregulatory system to induce the fever that is associated with most infections and inflammatory responses. Many bacterial and viral species grow poorly at these higher temperatures. In addition to its thermoregulatory effect, EP stimulates HMP metabolism with production of microbicidal products. Another monokine is interferon, which is inhibitory to viral replication and growth of cancer cells. Some monokines, including interleukin 1, are essential for lymphocyte immune responses, and will be discussed in Chapters 8 and 9.

Natural Killer Cells

Another cell provides the body with an immediate nonimmune defense that is espe-cially effective against foreign cells such as virus-infected cells or cancer cells. No prior exposure to foreign cells is required for this cell to be active. This cell is the *NK cell* and is believed to be an important body defense against cancer. Exact origin and devel-opment of the NK cell has not yet been established. The NK cell has been classified as a lymphocyte that is neither a T nor a B type. NK cells are also referred to as *large granular lymphocytes* (LGL) because they are larger and have more cytoplasmic azurophi-lic granules than most B and T lymphocytes.

Various agents and conditions influence NK cell activity. X-irradiation, cyclophos-phamide, and hydrocortisone reduce activity, while aspirin and interferon enhance activity. Decreased NK activity has been observed in patients who develop spontaneous tumors and in patients suffering from systemic lupus erythematosus and multiple scle-rosis. Recipient NK cell activity correlates with survival of bone marrow transplants.

Complement System, C-Reactive Protein

The complement system consists of more than a dozen blood proteins that, once acti-vated, sequentially interact with one another to produce by-products that mediate a number of biological functions. Nonimmune activation of complement via the classi-cal pathway may be accomplished with DNA, C-reactive protein (CRP), and trypsin-like enzymes released from phagocytes or from damaged tissue cells. CRP is synthesized in the liver. Inflammation can stimulate up to a 1000-fold increase in synthesis. Labora-tory measurement of CRP is therefore a means of monitoring inflammation. CRP can bind to microorganisms, activate complement, and mediate phagocytosis and degrada-tion. Nonimmune activation of complement via the alternate pathway may be accomplished with lipopolysaccharides (LPS), cobra venom, microbial cell walls, and plasmin from the fibrinolytic system that dissolves clots.

Defenses mediated via by-products resulting from complement activation are

1. *Opsonization:* Coating of particles to enhance their subsequent phagocytosis
2. *Chemoattraction:* Chemical attraction of neutrophils and macrophages
3. *Anaphylotoxic effects:* Vessel dilation, smooth muscle contraction (including bronchoconstriction), and degranulation of mast cells and basophils
4. *Virus neutralization:* Binding to virus and covering sites on the virus that are requisite for attachment to cell and pathogenesis
5. *Cell lysis:* Disruption of cell membrane leading to cell death and release of intracellular contents

Activation of the complement system ultimately results in cell lysis. Normal cells as well as foreign cells are lysed. The complement system and direction of its lytic action toward selected cells via antibodies is discussed in Chapter 10.

Inflammatory Response

Any injury to tissue, whether by microbial invasion, by physical damage, or by physiologic damage, induces a response by the body to destroy the cause of the damage and to repair the injury. This reaction is termed the *inflammatory response.* Typical characteristics of inflammation are local heat, redness, swelling, pain, and loss of function.

The series of events constituting the inflammatory response involves the defense systems previously discussed in this chapter (Table 2–3). Initial tissue injury by cutting, trauma, burning, or microbial invasions results in cell rupture and release of intracellular contents, which include chemotactic agents and complement-activating agents. Neutrophils respond to chemotaxins by margination or adherance to the endothelial lining of blood vessels. Complement by-product anaphylotoxic agents promote vasodilation. Fluid escapes into the inflammatory site to cause *edema.* As a chemotactic gradient is created, neutrophils diapedese into the injured tissue and proceed to actively phagocytose and degrade foreign materials. Lysosomal contents are released extracellularly and act upon the involved area. All the events previously discussed as being

---

TABLE 2–3. EVENTS IN NONIMMUNE INFLAMMATORY RESPONSE[a]

1. Cell disruption by trauma to tissue and outpouring of cell contents
2. Activation of complement
3. Chemoattraction of neutrophils
   Margination, diapedesis, and migration of neutrophils to site
   Phagocytosis, degradation, and release of lysosomal contents
4. Amplification via coagulation system, fibrinolytic system, kinin system, and complement system

---

[a]*The major difference between this nonimmune inflammatory response and the immune inflammatory response discussed in Chapter 1 is the means and the substances involved in the original activation of complement and the generation of chemotaxins.*

initiated by phagocytosis also occur. Thereafter, actively phagocytosing neutrophils will rid the area of foreign or injured material, will produce chemotaxins to attract more phagocytes, will produce anaphylotoxins to amplify the inflammatory response, and will activate complement to produce complement-associated amplification of the inflammation. The coagulation system is activated to form a fibrin thrombi in vessels and masses of fibrin to fill in tissue defects. Later in inflammation macrophages migrate into the site and eventually replace the neutrophils if the injurious event has not been terminated. Because they are most numerous in the earlier phases of inflammation, neutrophils are called acute inflammatory cells. Because they are most numerous during the late phases of inflammation and during persistent inflammation, macrophages are called chronic inflammatory cells.

At sites of inflammation several biological systems—the kinin, coagulation, fibrinolytic, and complement systems—are activated and provide amplification for each other as well as for inflammation. These inflammatory mediator systems are further discussed in Chapter 10. Figure 2–5 emphasizes the interaction of these systems and their enhancement of the inflammatory response. The *kinin system* consists of several normal blood proteins and a series of reactions resulting in the end product *bradykinin,* which is a mediator of chemotaxis, vessel dilation, smooth muscle contraction, and pain. This system may be activated by lysosomal enzymes and by the complement, the coagulation, and the fibrinolytic systems.

COMPLEMENT SYSTEM	CLOTTING SYSTEM	KININ SYSTEM	FIBRINOLYSIS SYSTEM

Figure 2–5. Amplification of Inflammatory Response. Once intracellular constituents and/or phagocytic lysosomal contents are released for extended periods, inflammatory response occurs. The complement system, the clotting system, the kinin system, and the fibrinolytic system are all activated and activate one another. Mediators synthesized as by products of the complement and kinin systems produce the clinical signs of the inflammatory response: swelling, redness, heat, and pain. Thus these four systems continually stimulate each other and amplify the inflammatory response.

Complement system	A group of normal serum proteins that, when activated, lead to lysis of cells and production of products that mediate opsonization, anaphylaxis, chemotaxis, increased vascular permeability, smooth muscle contraction, and viral neutralization.
Coagulation system	A group of blood and platelet factors and proteins that interact to produce an insoluble clot.
Kinin system	A group of normal blood proteins, the activation of which leads to the formation of bradykinin, which mediates contraction of smooth muscles, increased vascular permeability, increased mucous gland secretions, and pain.
Fibrinolytic system	Dissolves clots via the enzymatic action of plasmin produced by activation of the normal blood protein plasminogen.

The kinin and coagulation systems amplify each other. The *coagulation system* consists of blood proteins that interact to produce *thrombin,* which can, in turn, activate the complement system. Activated coagulation factors activate the *fibrinolytic system,* which is a series of blood proteins that can be activated to dissolve thrombi. The fibrinolytic system can then activate the complement system. In summary, once any of these systems is activated via the inflammatory response, they are all activated, and the inflammatory response is enhanced many fold.

Although the inflammatory response has been discussed in terms of a defense system, continued and uncontrolled inflammation can be damaging to the body. Corticosteroids are used therapeutically to decrease the inflammatory response. These drugs decrease margination of neutrophils to the vessel walls and therefore migration out into the inflamed areas. They inhibit chemotaxis, phagocytosis, postphagocytic killing, and suppress immune responses. Aspirin is another drug that decreases the inflammatory response, in part, by decreasing synthesis of prostaglandins that potentiate the inflammatory response.

Discussion of the Illustrative Case

A major problem in the management of extensive, deep burns is infection. Other problems include loss of fluid and electrolytes through the burn wound and loss of cutaneous thermal control. Infections are caused primarily by the loss of the skin barrier, which functions as an important nonimmune defense mechanism. There is a contribution from a comparatively mild acquired immunodeficiency that includes reduced plasma immunoglobulin levels and depressed cell-mediated immune reactivity.

The patient developed gram-negative sepsis caused by *P aeruginosa.* The Pseudomonas colonized the surface of the wound, grew into the underlying debris and tissue, and entered the circulation. Toxins released by this pathogen then produced the signs and symptoms of sepsis. Thus in an individual with a relatively intact immune defense, the extensive loss of one form of nonimmune defense can lead to life-threatening infections.

QUESTIONS

1. List and discuss the importance of the body's external nonimmune defense systems.
2. In the case of the burned patient, what should that patient's internal nonimmune defenses be accomplishing?
3. Outline the metabolism associated with phagocytosis, and associate specific metabolic problems with diseases involving the phagocyte.
4. What role, if any, do macrophages and NK cells play in nonimmune defense against invasion by foreign cells?
5. A patient experiences a severe and traumatic leg injury during a motorcycle accident. Relate the subsequent series of events of inflammatory response and CRP production.

Section II

Introduction to Laboratory Immunologic Methods

3 Isolation of Blood Cellular Elements and Evaluation of Phagocytes

OBJECTIVES

1. To discuss general considerations for isolating different cells from whole blood.
2. To outline the steps in isolation of erythrocytes, neutrophils, lymphocytes, and monocytes.
3. To discuss the principles of two screening assays for overall function of phagocytes.
4. To discuss the principles of assays for specific phagocytic functions: chemotaxis, ingestion, and killing.

Illustrative Case

A 5-year-old boy was admitted to the hospital with fever; enlarged, tender, cervical nodes; and multiple skin abscesses and granulomas. He had a history of repeated severe episodes of respiratory infections and otitis media beginning during his first year of life. His laboratory data included:

WBC	$15,000/mm^3$
Differential count	72% Polymorphonuclear leukocytes
	20% Lymphocytes
	5% Monocytes
	2% Eosinophils
	1% Basophils

Urinalysis	Normal
Total immunoglobulins	Elevated
CH_{50}	Normal
Serum Protein electrophoresis	Normal
Skin test against Candida antigens	Positive
T lymphocyte enumeration	Normal
ConA stimulation	Normal
Abscess culture	*Staphylococcus epidermidis*
Nitroblue tetrazolium test	Negative, no reduction
Leukotaxis test	Normal

GENERAL CONSIDERATIONS

To evaluate the status of the immune and nonimmune defense systems by laboratory methods, it is sometimes necessary to isolate a particular population of cells from the blood. For example, mononuclear cells are separated from erythrocytes and granulocytes for quantification of lymphocyte subtypes. Granulocytes are isolated for functional assays. Erythrocytes are isolated from animal blood for use as reagents in rosetting to identify T lymphocytes. There are some general considerations to keep in mind during the isolation and assay of whole blood cellular elements.

Handling of living cells should be done using sterile technique to prevent bacterial contamination that could interfere with cell assays or cause cell death. Containers and liquids, such as syringes, test tubes, tissue culture dishes, pipettes, saline, and tissue culture medium to which the cells are exposed, should be sterile. Drawing of whole blood into and subsequent transfer from a syringe should be done slowly and through a large bore needle (i.e., 18-gauge). Thereafter transfer of cellular elements should be either by pouring or with pipettes having a large orifice. When using pipettes take up and deliver the cell suspension slowly and with little pressure to prevent physical stress and damage to the cells.

Whole blood, if allowed to stand, will coagulate and form a clot of fibrin entrapping the cellular elements (red cells, white cells, and platelets). A clear supernatant serum separates above the clot of fibrin and cells (Fig. 3–1). *Serum* is blood minus the cellular elements and the coagulation factors that have become part of the clot. When isolating cellular elements of blood, an anticoagulant must be added immediately upon drawing to prevent these cellular elements from becoming entrapped in the clot. Heparin is the anticoagulant of choice for most viable cell studies. After the anticoagulant and whole blood are mixed and allowed to sit, the erythrocytes settle to the bottom with a thin layer of leukocytes settling on top of them (Fig. 3–1). Atop both these layers will be clear plasma. *Plasma* is whole blood minus the cellular elements, or serum plus the coagulation factors.

Anticoagulants should be free of preservatives because preservatives interfere with and inhibit normal cell function. Some commercial heparin contains added pre-

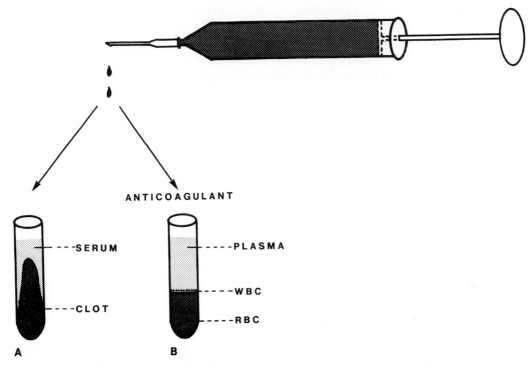

Figure 3-1. Serum Versus Plasma. A. Freshly drawn blood allowed to sit at room temperature will form a clot and supernatant serum. The clot formation removes the clotting factors and the cellular elements from the serum. Blood cells are trapped within the fibrin net and are not retrievable for laboratory studies. **B.** Anticoagulant prevents clot formation. Freshly drawn blood mixed with an anticoagulant and allowed to set at room temperature yields plasma, a sedimented layer of erythrocytes, and a layer of leukocytes. Clotting factors remain in the plasma. Blood cells are easily retrieved for laboratory studies.

servatives. It is therefore a good idea to check with the supplier before purchasing to be sure that the anticoagulant is free of preservatives. Other substances that will interfere with live cell assays are traces of detergents or other cleaning compounds. Chromate ions are notorious for their adverse effect upon viable cell studies. It is best to use disposable glassware, plasticware, and pipettes to ensure the absence of traces of detergent or other cleaning compounds.

Only physiologic solutions (solutions that are isotonic or which have the same pH and total ionic concentration as body fluids) should be used to wash and suspend living cells. Commonly used buffered physiologic saline solutions are Hanks' balanced saline solution (HBSS) and phosphate-buffered saline (PBS). If cells are exposed to either hypertonic or hypotonic solutions for any length of time, their membranes lose integrity and the cells lyse. Erythrocytes will interfere with some leukocyte assays and therefore must be removed. A short exposure of the cellular isolate to hypertonic am-

monium chloride solution is performed to lyse and remove erythrocytes. In our laboratories, however, we have found this treatment to be of limited value.

When sedimentation of cells by centrifugation is required, it should be at slow
speed. Centrifuges can roughly be divided into three major categories according to
the speed at which they rotate: (1) slow speed, (2) high speed, and (3) ultra speed. The
IEC PR6000 is an example of a slow-speed centrifuge and has a maximum rotation of
6000 rpm. High-speed centrifuges such as the Spinco JA21 rotate at speeds up to
21,000 rpm. Ultra-speed centrifuges (ultracentrifuges) rotate up to 70,000 rpm. Choice
of centrifuge is dependent upon the relative centrifugal force (RCF) units (g) needed.
A nomogram may be used to calculate gravitational units (g). This is a graphic correlation of rotating radius (r), relative centrifugal force (g), and revolutions per
minute(rpm). If any two of the three values are known, the third can be calculated.
The general formula for RCF is:

$$g = \frac{4\ r^2/3600}{981}\ r\ (rpm^2) = 1.1 \times 10^{-5}r\ (rpm^2)$$

Note RCF varies directly as the r and as the square of rpm. During centrifugation
particles in a fluid are sedimented toward the bottom of the spinning container in
relation to the factors of RCF, specific gravity and viscosity of fluid, buoyant density,
and size and shape of the particles. Essentially the more dense the particle the faster
it settles. The larger the surface area of the particle, the greater its buoyant density,
and the greater its resistance to settling down through the fluid. Varying the g and/or
the fluid in which cells are suspended allows different cells to remain suspended while
others are pelleted down. Another important consideration in centrifuging is the selection of the containers into which the cells are placed. Normal glass will not withstand
a g > 2000. A higher g will crush the glass. Therefore heavy wall or reinforced glass
or plastic containers are used when using higher g forces.

Washing is a part of most laboratory procedures involving cells. This term means
to centrifuge the suspended cells, decant the resultant supernatant, and resuspend the
pelleted cells. Pelleted cells are resuspended by adding fresh physiologic liquid to the
pellet, dislodging the pellet, and mixing gently and thoroughly, e.g., slowly drawing
the mixture into and out of a large orifice pipette. Erythrocytes are usually pelleted
by centrifugation at 4°C and 500 × g for 20 minutes. Leukocytes are usually pelleted
at 250 × g. Washing is used to resuspend cells in a different solution than they are
in, to remove undesired substances from the suspension liquid, or to remove unwanted
substances that are noncovalently absorbed to the cell surface.

Because isolation of cells is a long process involving several steps, it is a good
practice to evaluate the *viability* of the final cell isolate before proceeding with the
actual assay. Trypan blue is a vital stain (the dye is excluded from living cells but is
taken up by dead cells) that may be used. One may visually count the percentage of
total cells without dye. Trypan blue should be suspended in a physiologic solution.
Addition of a nonphysiologic trypan blue solution to a cell isolate could result in a
final nonphysiologic solution causing cell death and falsely low estimates of viability.

Another consideration that must be borne in mind when isolating phagocytes is that these cells readily adhere to glass and plastic surfaces. In fact, this characteristic is utilized to separate and isolate macrophages from other cellular elements. To prevent inadvertent adherence and thus loss of phagocytic cells during isolation, all containers, pipettes, etc. should be silicone coated. Commercial products are available for this purpose. Well-dried and clean glassware is submerged or filled with a silicone solution and allowed to sit. The glassware is then drained and air dried.

Depending upon the length of time the assay requires, various media may be used to sustain viable cells. Tissue culture medium is a physiologic medium that contains nutrients to support cell metabolism. Buffered physiologic saline will preserve the integrity of the cells; however, it does not provide nutrients for metabolic activity. Cells must have available nutrients if they are to be metabolically active, e.g., carry out phagocytosis, or if they are to synthesize and secrete molecular products, e.g., monokines and lymphokines. One commonly used tissue culture medium is RPMI 1640. As yet undefined ingredients essential for cell activities are found in fetal calf serum (FCS), which is added to the RPMI for many laboratory procedures involving cells.

ISOLATION OF WHOLE BLOOD CELLULAR ELEMENTS

Erythrocytes

For isolation of erythrocytes (Fig. 3–2 A), sodium citrate is usually the anticoagulant of choice. A mixture that is used for erythrocyte isolation and that contains sodium citrate is *Alsever's solution*. Whole blood is drawn into the Alsever's solution and is mixed well. The blood–Alsever's is then centrifuged. Supernatant plasma and the thin layer of leukocytes are drawn off with a pipette and discarded. Red cells are washed with physiologic saline solution until the supernatant is colorless.

The isolated red cells may then be processed in different ways and used for various assays such as hemagglutination. Some procedures treat the erythrocytes with *tannic acid* to cause their membranes to absorb antibodies or antigens to which they are subsequently exposed. The resultant red cell, then, is a large carrier with exposed antigen or antibody on its surface. These coated red cells may be mixed with preservatives such as isotonic formalin to extend their shelf life far beyond that which they would have without the preservative. Tanned red cells without preservatives may be used for about 3 to 7 days. When the cells are no longer good, excessive hemolysis and clumping of cells is evident. It is a good practice to wash any red cell preparation immediately prior to using to rid the preparation of old, hemolyzed cells or aggregated cells that could interfere with the testing. Untreated erythrocytes are also used as reagents in several assays. Rabbit erythrocytes, for instance, are used as the indicator system in complement fixation assays, and sheep erythrocytes are used to identify T lymphocytes.

Neutrophils

For neutrophil isolation (Fig. 3–2 B), whole blood is drawn into a syringe having a large bore needle (18-gauge) and containing a solution of citrate, dextrose, and heparin. The syringe is stood on end and allowed to sit for 1 hour. Erythrocytes settle to the bottom.

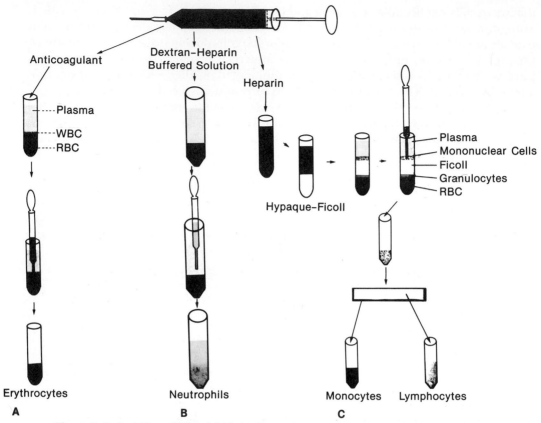

Figure 3-2. Isolation of Blood Cellular Elements. A. Erythrocytes. Blood is drawn into anticoagulant, is mixed well, and is allowed to sit so that the supernatant plasma may be decanted. The erythrocytes may then be washed and diluted to a given concentration. **B. Neutrophils.** Fresh blood is drawn into a dextran, anticoagulant-buffered solution and allowed to sit at 37°C. The supernatant is recovered and centrifuged to yield a pellet of WBC. The pellet is washed and diluted to desired concentration. **C. Monocytes-Lympho-cytes.** Fresh blood is diluted and layered onto Hypaque-Ficoll. Cells are aspirated into a centrifuge tube and washed to eliminate Hypaque-Ficoll and platelets. Washed cells are poured onto a plastic tissue culture dish and incubated. Lymphocytes are in the supernatant and may be collected by pouring off. Monocytes adhere to the tissue culture dish and are recovered by scraping off. Cells may be centrifuged, washed, and diluted to desired concentrations.

Due to the density of the dextrose solution, the neutrophils remain suspended in the plasma instead of settling out in a thin layer on top of the erythrocytes as they do in freshly drawn blood mixed with only an anticoagulant. The plasma, containing sus-pended neutrophils, is then slowly expelled through the large bore needle and col-lected in a centrifuge tube. The dextrose-plasma is centrifuged to sediment the neutro-phils. Cold isotonic solution is used to wash the neutrophils and rid them of platelets. The neutrophils are counted and diluted to appropriate concentrations for upcoming assays.

Lymphocytes and Monocytes (Mononuclear Cells)

Isolating lymphocytes involves the differential sedimentation of blood cell components through a hypaque-ficoll density gradient during centrifugation. Ficoll-Paque (Pharmacia, Piscataway, N.J.) is an example of a commercial mixture for isolating lymphocytes. It is an aqueous solution of Ficoll 400 (highly branched synthetic polymer of sucrose and epichlorohydrin, MW 400,000) and diatrizoate sodium (MW 636). When mixed together these ingredients form a solution of low viscosity and high density. Both the density and viscosity of the gradient affect the centrifugal separation of cells centrifuged through it. Diatrizoate is a sodium salt of 3,5-diacetamido-2,4,6-trilodobenzoic acid and is light sensitive; therefore the Ficoll-Paque should be stored in the dark.

Diluted whole blood mixed with heparin is carefully layered onto Ficoll-Paque in a centrifuge tube. Alternatively, the Ficoll-Paque can be introduced beneath the diluted blood using a long needle. The tube is then centrifuged at a speed, time, and temperature recommended by the manufacturer of the separating medium, with resulting fractions as noted in Figure 3–2 C. The lymphocyte layer is collected by aspiration and is centrifuged and washed to rid the cells of contaminating platelets, Ficoll-Paque, and plasma. It is important to correctly dilute the blood sample, to carefully layer the blood sample onto the Hypaque-Ficoll without disturbing the gradient surface, and to centrifuge at the exact g force, time, and temperature recommended. Any deviation will reduce the recovery of cells. Good separation conditions should yield a 50% recovery of cells with 95% viability.

From the mononuclear cell pellet obtained by the above method, one may isolate either lymphocytes or monocytes. There are commercially available density gradient media that are advertised to centrifugally separate lymphocytes and monocytes in a manner analogous to that just described. Most commonly, the monocyte's property of adhering to glass and plastic surfaces can be used to either rid a monocyte–lymphocyte suspension of monocytes or to collect the monocytes. If *lymphocytes* are desired, a monocyte–lymphocyte suspension is plated onto a plastic tissue culture dish and incubated for several hours. Afterwards the supernatant lymphocytes are poured off into a centrifuge tube and are centrifuged and washed to give a lymphocyte pellet. The monocytes are left behind, adhering to the plastic plate. If *monocytes* are desired, the supernatant from the above incubated tissue culture plate is discarded, and the monocytes are scraped from the plastic surface with a rubber-coated rod (rubber policeman) into a centrifuge tube. The cells are centrifuged and washed to give a pellet of monocytes.

With the development of very specific monoclonal antibodies, a variety of other techniques are now available for isolating lymphocytes or monocytes. For instance, columns made of inert beads coated with antibodies for a certain type of lymphocyte can be prepared. A mixture of leukocytes is then passed through the column to which only that type of lymphocyte is bound. All other cell types pass out through the column with the effluent. Then the column is washed with a buffer of either lower pH or higher ionic concentration to detach the bound lymphocytes that are collected in that effluent. A similar column may be made with antibodies specific for monocytes. Alternatively, after isolating the mononuclear cells (lymphocytes and monocytes) from the hypaque-ficoll, antimonocyte antibody plus complement could be added to destroy all monocytes, or complement plus antilymphocyte antibody could be added to destroy lymphocytes.

LABORATORY ASSAYS FOR PHAGOCYTIC FUNCTION

Malfunction of phagocytes is one important cause of recurrent pyogenic infections. In patients with phagocytic defects, it is necessary to evaluate the phagocytic function of leukocytes to identify the cause of the dysfunction. As discussed in Chapter 2, the process of phagocytosis may be divided into several discrete steps. Laboratory assays of a patient's phagocytes are designed to evaluate the cells' general metabolic integrity, to evaluate their ability for chemotaxis, to evaluate their ability to ingest particles, and to evaluate their ability to accomplish postphagocytic killing. Neutrophils are most often evaluated; however, monocytes and macrophages may also be analyzed. As described previously, neutrophils and monocytes are isolated from whole blood. After leaving the blood and entering body tissues, monocytes mature into macrophages, which are difficult to isolate for functional studies. Macrophages for analysis can be collected from bronchopulmonary lavage, but this is done very rarely. Assay techniques for evaluation of neutrophils and monocytes are the same, except that incubation times for the monocyte are extended about three times longer.

Screening Assays

Phagocytic uptake and postphagocytic killing ability (as reflected by hexose monophosphate [HMP] products) may be simultaneously evaluated by a *two-color flow cytometric assay*. Ingestion of fluorescent beads of propidium iodide (PI) and oxidization of 1′, 7′-dichlorofluorescein diacetate (DCFH/DA) allow this simultaneous evaluation. Phagocytes are incubated with soluble DCFH/DA that readily diffuses into isolated neutrophils where it is hydrolyzed into an insoluble form and is trapped within the cells. The phagocytes are then stimulated with phorbol mytristate acetate (PMA). Normal cells will oxidize the colorless DCFH to a fluorescent green that may be analyzed in the flow cytometer. Simultaneously, PI beads that have been opsonized with C3b and Abs are incubated with the phagocytes. Once ingested the PI beads emit a red fluorescence that may also be evaluated on the flow cytometer. Neutrophils from patients with defective phagocytic function will have a lower percentage of cells demonstrating green and/or red fluorescence when compared with neutrophils from normal individuals.

Another clinical laboratory assay to evaluate killing ability of phagocytes is the *nitroblue tetrazolium test* (NBT test). This is a screening test for evaluating the overall function of a population of phagocytes and is used in smaller laboratories where flow cytometry analyzers are not available. It encompasses oxygen-dependent but not oxygen-independent postphagocytic microbicidal product formation. In the assay phagocytes from a patient are incubated in tissue culture medium containing latex particles and NBT. It is necessary to concomitantly perform the assay on control phagocytes from a normal individual. As the particles are engulfed by the cells, a metabolic shift to the HMP pathway occurs, and there is a respiratory burst of oxygen-dependent metabolism with production of microbicidal products. NBT is reduced to a blue color during the oxygen-dependent metabolism. Hydrochloric acid is added to stop the reaction, and the incubation mixture is centrifuged. After discarding the supernatant, pyridine is used to extract the dye from the phagocytes. Spectrophotometric quantitation of reduced dye is performed at 550 nm. If all phagocytic functions and oxidative metabolism are normal in the patient, the NBT will be quantitatively reduced to the same extent as it is in the control or normal cells. This screening procedure measures the metabolic integrity of phagocytes, including motility to the latex particles, ingestion of the particles, and HMP product formation. The NBT is a rapid assay compared to other phagocytic assays, and it requires no special equipment. A modification of the NBT is to visually count the cells to estimate that percentage containing blue dye. The NBT test value is abnormally low in patients with phagocytic abnormalities, such as chronic granulomatous disease, myeloperoxidase deficiency, and glucose-6-phosphatase deficiency. Other conditions that have been associated with abnormally low NBT test values are cancer and treatment with corticosteroids and other immunosuppressive agents. A few conditions, such as malaria, have been associated with abnormally elevated NBT assay levels.

Chemiluminescence is another method for general screening of phagocytic function. This procedure follows the same logic as that for the NBT test in that the phagocytes are incubated with latex or other particles to stimulate ingestion, which, in turn, initiates HMP metabolism. The HMP metabolism generates high-energy oxygen products that emit light that can be detected in a scintillation counter. Some laboratories perform chemiluminescence assays on whole blood and eliminate the isolation of phagocytes before the assay.

Chemotaxis Assays

Evaluation of the mobility of phagocytes in the presence of a chemoattractant can be useful in diagnosing some phagocytic defects. One screening assay is shown in Figure 3-3. A tissue culture dish containing a layer of agar is used. Wells are cut in a configuration as shown in the figure, and agar is removed from the circles. Phagocytes are placed in one well, a chemoattractant (e.g., complement factor C3a or synthetic N-formylmethionyl peptides) is placed in a second well, and a control of saline is placed in the third well. The dish is placed in a moisturized chamber and incubated from several hours to overnight. The diameter of cell migration is measured for each well. A similar dish assay is set up for patient and one for normal phagocytes. Measured diameters are compared.

Older methods which are now rarely used are the Rebuck skin window (in vivo)

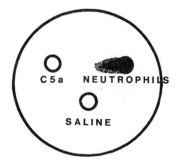

Figure 3-3. Chemotaxis Assay. Wells are cut in a layer of agar. One well is filled with the phagocytes; one well is filled with a chemotaxin, i.e., C5a; and a third well is filled with saline. After 24 hours the agar is examined for migration of phagocytes out of the well toward the chemotaxin, as compared to that toward the control, nonchemotactic substance, saline.

and the Boyden chamber (in vitro). For the *Rebuck skin window* test, a small area of skin is abraded and covered with a glass coverslip that is later removed and examined for adherent leukocytes. The *Boyden chamber* technique measures migration of leukocytes into a porous filter separating a suspension of leukocytes from a chemoattractant solution. We shall not discuss either of these methods in detail here, because they are usually not used in the clinical laboratory. In fact, it is a rare clinical laboratory that will do more than the general screening assays for phagocytic function.

Ingestion Assays

Uptake of particles by phagocytic ingestion may be evaluated by incubating particles and phagocytes and then either estimating disappearance of particles from incubation mixture or estimating accumulation of particles within phagocytes. The uptake varies with the ratio of phagocytes to particles and with the type and size of the particles. Phagocytosis can be enhanced by opsonizing particles with antibodies or complement. Therefore these parameters are determined for optimal activity and, thereafter, are held constant from assay to assay. During incubation it is important to constantly agitate the phagocytes and particles to ensure maximum contact.

Particles are prepared in different ways so that their uptake or disappearance can be evaluated by (1) visually counting cells containing ingested particles, (2) extracting and spectrophotometrically measuring the concentration of dye-marked particles, or (3) measuring the radioactivity of radioisotope-labeled particles. Any of these evaluation methods is performed after incubating particles and phagocytes in tissue culture medium under CO_2.

For visual counting, phagocytes may be incubated in a 1 : 10 (phagocyte : bacteria) ratio with a fresh overnight culture of *Staphylococcus aureus*. Samples of the incubation mixture are taken at 0 time and at 30-minute intervals for 2 hours. The samples are immediately centrifuged to sediment the cells and are washed once. Cells are smeared onto a coverslip, are allowed to dry, and are stained with Wright's stain. Percentage of cells containing ingested bacteria is determined microscopically.

For spectrophotometric measuring, lipopolysaccharide from *Escherichia coli* is coated with oil-red O by briefly sonicating the two together. These sonicated particles are then incubated with anti-*E coli* serum to coat them with antibody immediately before performing the ingestion assay. Particles are incubated with phagocytes, and aliquots are taken at 0 time and at 30-minute intervals for 2 hours. N-ethylmaleimide is immediately added to each aliquot to inhibit metabolism and thus stop phagocytosis. Aliquots are centrifuged. The cell pellet is washed once, extracted with dioxane, and analyzed for absorbance in a spectrophotometer.

For radioisotope labeling, albumin is reacted with iodine-125 (I-125) and then incubated with antialbumin antibodies. Radioactive, antibody-coated albumin and phagocytes are incubated together. Aliquots are taken at 0 time and at 30-minute intervals for 2 hours. Aliquots are centrifuged, washed once, and counted in a scintillation counter for quantifying uptake of particles by phagocytosis.

Killing Assays

Chapter 2 discussed those abnormal phagocytic conditions in which bacteria are ingested but are not killed postingestion because of deficiency in the oxygen-dependent metabolism and the synthesis of bactericidal products. It is helpful to the clinician to know whether the phagocytic cells of patients suffering from repeated infections are capable of killing ingested organisms. There are conditions in which the NBT test is normal; however, there is no production of bactericidal substances. There are also conditions in which effective killing of bacteria occurs in the absence of HMP metabolism. For instance, in chronic granulomatous disease (CGD) some ingested microorganisms may produce hydrogen peroxide, which is metabolized by the cell to form bactericidal products. In this sense these microorganisms are self-destructive by providing the phagocytes with the missing essential substance for microbicidal product formation.

   To measure the killing ability of phagocytes, fresh cultures of S aureus are incubated in tissue culture medium containing fresh serum and phagocytes. It is important to keep the ratio of phagocytes to bacteria at about 1 : 3 to 1 : 10. If the phagocytes are overloaded or ingest too many bacteria, they may become metabolically inert, and killing will not occur. As with particle uptake assays, incubation is carried out under CO_2 and with a constant mixing (preferably inversion) of the incubation mixture. Aliquots and cover slip smears are taken at 0 time and at 30-minute intervals for 2 hours. Pour plates and colony counts are performed on all aliquots after serially diluting the aliquots with water. The water causes hypotonic lysis of the leukocytes to free viable bacteria. Smears are stained with Wright's stain to determine that uptake of bacteria has occurred. Any phagocyte defect that depresses ingestion will directly affect the killing assay. Figure 3–4 shows a graph of colony counts from a killing assay.

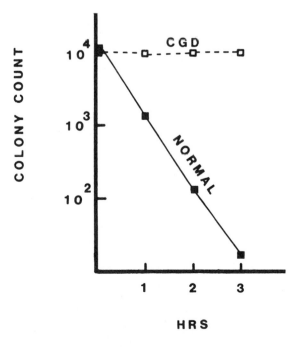

Figure 3-4. Postphagocytic Killing Assay. Blood is drawn from the suspected CGD patient and from a control, normal individual. Neutrophils and serum are isolated from fresh blood and incubated with an overnight culture of S aureus. At 0 hour, 1 hour, 2 hours, and 3 hours incubation, aliquots are taken from each of the patient and control mixtures. Colony counts are performed on serial dilutions in water. Results from a CGD patient and a normal control are shown.

Discussion of the Illustrative Case

The patient had normal values in most assays. There was an elevated white blood cell (WBC) count, elevated total gamma globulin, and abnormal chemotaxis. Physical examination revealed multiple skin lesions, which were cultured. *S epidermidis* was found to be the infecting organism. This young boy's history included repeated infections with usually nonpathogenic organisms, indicating some body defense system was not functioning properly. Assays for complement (CH$_{50}$ assay), B cell (immunoglobulin assay), and T cell (ConA stimulation, helper/suppressor T cell ratio, Candida skin test) were normal. An abnormal NBT test suggested chronic granulomatous disease, which is what this patient had. Defective neutrophil function of many types, including chronic granulomatous disease, is typically characterized by recurrent and prolonged infections that respond poorly to antibiotic therapy, often involve the skin and mucous membranes, and frequently are caused by staphylococci. Although some promising approaches to altering basic neutrophil defects are being developed, current management relies heavily upon aggressive treatment of the infections with antibiotics.

QUESTIONS

1. List and discuss general considerations that apply to isolation of all cell types.

2. Draw a flowchart, and explain each step for the isolation of lymphocytes from whole blood.

3. Describe how one would evaluate the viability and percent recovery for a lymphocyte isolate.

4. List and discuss the principles of assays to evaluate the various functions of phagocytes.

Chapter 4

General Concepts of Immunologic and Serologic Assays

OBJECTIVES

1. To relate the immune response to antibody production and to the logic for performing immunologic and serologic assays.
2. To discuss the physical chemical properties essential to antibody–antigen binding and to state the optimal conditions for in vitro binding.
3. To understand the principles of the major types of immunologic and serologic assays and to know the relative sensitivities of the assays.

Illustrative Case

An 18-year-old female was seen with complaints of fever, sore throat, lethargy, tender lymphadenopathy in the neck, and afternoon headaches. Relevent findings on initial examination and laboratory workup were lymph adenopathy and splenomegaly; lympocytosis with many atypical, large lymphocytes; normal urinalysis; and a negative monospot test for infectious mononucleosis heterophile antibodies. Further laboratory assays were ordered, and the results were:

Antigen	IgG Titer	IgM Titer
Cytomegalovirus	1 : 20	0
Epstein–Barr virus	0	1 : 80
Toxoplasma	0	0

One week later a repeat heterophile antibody test was positive.

THE IMPORTANCE OF IMMUNOLOGIC ASSAYS

Immunology is the study of all aspects of the immune system, including in vitro antigen–antibody interactions. *Immunologic tests* are those tests that utilize components of the immune system, e.g., antibodies and lymphocytes, as reagents. The most frequently used clinical laboratory immunologic tests involve the measurement of an antigen–antibody interaction (Table 4–1). *Serology* is the study of antibodies and antigens in serum by immunologic tests. Immunologic tests can be designed to measure either the antibody or the antigen. The major factor that makes antibodies so useful in laboratory assays is their great specificity for the antigen that stimulated their production. There are also immunologic assays that use antigen receptors on T lymphocytes to react with antigens. These tests will be discussed in later chapters dealing with T lymphocytes.

Immunologic assays that are based on antigen–antibody interactions are common in all areas of the clinical laboratory. By assessing the presence and nature of an immune response against an infecting microorganism, serologic assays play an essential role in the diagnosis and management of patients with infectious diseases. For example, enzyme immunoassay (EIA) for IgM anti-Toxoplasma antibodies is used in the laboratory diagnosis of toxoplasmosis. Immunologic assays are used in the microbiology laboratory to identify microorganisms in patient specimens and cultures at an earlier time than could be done by culture, colony isolation, and identification. Thus a more rapid diagnosis is provided, and earlier institution of appropriate therapy is possible. For example, immunofluorescence microscopy is used to confirm a diagnosis of Legionnaires' disease by identifying *Legionella pneumophila* bacteria in sputum. The

TABLE 4-1. MAJOR TYPES OF IMMUNOLOGIC ASSAYS AND RELATIVE SENSITIVITIES

Assay	Sensitivity (mg/ml)
Lattice	
Immunoelectrophoresis	500
Immunofixation electrophoresis	100
Ouchterlony	50
Radial immunodiffusion	50
Rocket electrophoresis	50
Flocculation	20
Agglutination	15
Complement fixation	10
Counter immunoelectrophoresis	3
Nonlattice	
Nephelometry	1
Fluorescence immunoassay	0.1
Enzyme immunoassay	0.001
Radioimmunoassay	0.001

great specificity and sensitivity of immunologic assays has led to widespread applications for quantitation of chemical constituents in patient samples, most often using automated nephelometry, EIA, or radioimmunoassay (RIA). For example, quantitation of the thyroid hormones T_3 and T_4 by RIA is used to evaluate thyroid gland function. Immunologic assays are such an integral part of blood banking that this discipline of laboratory medicine is called immunohematology. For the routine typing and cross-matching of donor and recipient blood and the identification of allospecific antibodies, blood bank technology relies heavily on immunologic assays. In the hematology laboratory reagent monoclonal antibodies are routinely used to identify different types of leukocytes. For example, in the classification of leukemia, fluorescence-activated cell sorting and immunofluorescence microscopy are used to identify the binding of antibodies to specific types of leukocytes. In the immunology laboratory immunologic assays are used to evaluate the immune system itself. Antibodies, lymphocytes, and accessory systems such as phagocytes and complement are analyzed, often by assays that rely on antigen–antibody interactions (i.e., immunologic assays).

The future promises continued extension of the use of immunologic assays in all areas of the clinical laboratory. Because the specificity of an antibody for the antigen that induced its formation is the key behind most immunologic assays, it is essential to understand the physiology and biochemistry of antigen–antibody interactions to optimally perform these assays.

INFECTION-INDUCED ANTIBODY PRODUCTION

Upon initial exposure to an antigen, there are no specific antiantigen antibodies in an individual's serum. Of particular value in the serologic diagnosis of infectious diseases are antibodies against those antigens that are either part of a pathogenic microorganism or are a secreted product of a pathogenic microorganism. Normally within about 2 to 5 days of initial exposure to microorganisms, antibodies (products of the humoral immune response) can be detected in the infected individual's serum. There are different types (classes) of antibodies that have different functions and appear at different times during the course of an infection. The biochemical properties and functions of these different immunoglobulin classes will be discussed in detail in Chapter 9. IgM (Fig. 4–1) is the first or earliest antibody class to appear in the serum after initial exposure to antigen. Later, IgG antibodies appear. If the antibodies are successful in enabling the infected person's body to overcome and recover from the infection, the IgM serum levels will become undetectable within 3 to 12 months. Detectable IgG levels, however, usually remain for an extended period of years.

Upon re-exposure to an antigen, memory cells respond immediately. These are precursors of antibody-producing cells that are primed to respond to antigen without a latent period. IgM reappears in the serum, and IgG concentration increases for several weeks after reinfection. After a few months IgM will again disappear from the serum, whereas IgG concentration will plateau and remain at a level higher than the plateau level after initial exposure to antigen. Each new infection or re-exposure is

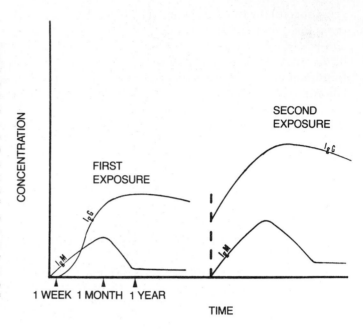

Figure 4–1. Antibody Appearance in Serum After a First and a Second Exposure to the Same Ag. IgM is the first type of Ab to be detected after a new antigen stimulates the immune system. Seven days later IgG is detectable in the serum. The level of IgM peaks at about 30 days and drops to low levels within 1 year. IgG peaks about 35 to 40 days and maintains its level for an extended period of time. Any subsequent exposure to the same Ag stimulates increased levels of IgM and IgG within a day. In the secondary exposure the peak levels of IgM and of IgG are higher, and the long-time, sustained level of IgG is higher.

marked by appearance of IgM and elevation of IgG. Antigen concentrations in serum and changes in class and concentration of specific antibodies are the bases of many clinical laboratory serologic assays for infection.

If the patient is suspected of suffering from an early infection to which the immune system has not had time to produce antibodies, an assay for some antigen associated with the pathogenic organisms may be performed. This principle is used for detecting infections that are potentially detrimental and even lethal before an immune response can occur. Examples of assays to detect antigens prior to the presence of identifiable antibodies are those for the causative agents of meningitis (*Streptococcus pneumoniae, Neisseria meningitidis,* group B streptococci, and *Hemophilus influenza*). These pathogens may cause death before the immune system is able to manifest an antibody response. Antibiotic therapy against these infections must be administered within 24 to 48 hours of onset of symptoms to prevent death. The immunologic diagnosis of these infections by antigen identification is therefore extremely important.

Because IgM is the earliest or first type of antibody to be produced after exposure to an antigen, detection of specific IgM antibodies indicates that a patient is experiencing a new infection or a reinfection. For example, patients with early symptoms of infectious mononucleosis will have IgM antibodies to Epstein–Barr virus (EBV); however, the IgG heterophile test will be negative. It is helpful to show the presence of IgM antibodies to differentiate the disease from more serious diseases with similar symptoms.

Not only is IgM the first type of antibody to appear upon exposure to an antigen, but it is also the first and essentially only type of antibody that a newborn can produce. Because newborns usually are not exposed to antigens in their protected environment, any substantial concentration of IgM in a newborn suggests it has experienced an intrauterine infection. The newborn immune system is not completely developed at birth and is incapable of synthesizing IgG and other types of antibodies. IgG is present in newborns, but it is maternal IgG that has crossed the placenta to the infant's blood. Because of its molecular properties, IgG is the only type of antibody that can cross the placental barrier.

Ongoing infection is detected by increasing titers of antibody to the infecting organisms. For example, in the Weil–Felix test for rickettsial disease, two serum samples are collected 7 to 10 days apart beginning immediately after onset of symptoms. An increased titer of antibodies in the second or later sample is diagnostic for the disease.

Some diseases resulting from infections can occur after the organism has been eliminated and the symptoms of the initial infection have disappeared. Because IgG levels remain for long periods, demonstration of IgG antibodies (Abs) to a specific pathogen substantiates past presence of the pathogen suspected of causing a postinfectious disease process. An example is the identification of anti-DNAse antibodies produced against DNAse that is secreted by infecting streptococci. These organisms play a role in causing scarlet fever. This disease often appears after symptoms of the pathogenic streptococcal infection have disappeared. The antecedent infection can be documented, however, by serologic detection of increased anti-DNAse antibodies.

FACTORS INFLUENCING ANTIGEN–ANTIBODY INTERACTIONS

Growing numbers of clinical immunochemical assays are not employed to evaluate a patient's immune response but rather to analyze a particular antigen. These assays take advantage of the specific binding of an antibody with its complementary antigen. In immunologic assays many factors can effect antigen–antibody binding.

Molecular Considerations

To maximize the opportunity for combination of antibody with antigen, reaction conditions must be carefully set and controlled. Antibodies are glycoproteins. Antigens are usually proteins but may have carbohydrate, nucleic acid, or lipid components. Binding of antigen with antibody is dependent upon the physical and chemical properties of these molecules. The noncovalent forces holding antigen and antibody together include hydrogen bonding, ionic or electrostatic bonding, hydrophobic bonding, and Van der Waals bonding.

Protein properties that are important in optimizing conditions for antigen and antibody combination are their ionizable side chains, their hydrophobic regions, and their solubility. Proteins are composed of amino acids that have amino, carboxyl, and other reactive side chains. The pH of the solvent in which the protein is suspended influences side-chain ionization. This plays a major role in the ionic binding between antigen and antibody. Beginning at a low pH, which has a high $[H^+]$ concentration, and adding $[OH^-]$, which produces a higher pH and lower $[H^+]$, the carboxyl and amino side chains lose their associated H^+. Figure 4–2 shows these conversions and

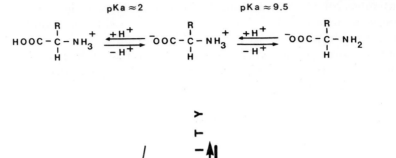

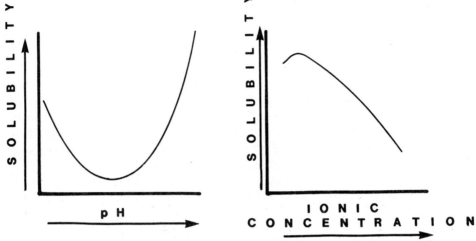

Figure 4–2. Effect of Solvent Upon Antibody Properties. The pH of the solvent in which Abs are suspended affects the charge of the amino acid side chains Ab. As the pH is increased (to about 2.0), the COOH side chains lose their H^+ to become negatively charged (COO^-). At about 7.5 the Ab has a net charge of 0 because it has NH_3+ and COO^- charges. This is the pI. Then as the pH is further increased, a H^+ is lost from the NH_3+ at about 9.5 to give a net negative charge. Solubility of Ab is minimal at its pI. An ionic strength of 0.154mol/L is that concentration that is optimal for solubility of Abs.

lists the average pKa of each. An amino acid at a pH below its pKa would have a H^+ associated with the side chain of that particular pKa. An amino acid at the pH of the pKa would have half of its side chains with an associated H^+ and half of them without. The pI is that pH at which the protein has a net neutral charge due to equal quantities of positive and negative changes. At physiologic or normal body pH (7.35 to 7.45), most amino side chains are ionized. Therefore at physiologic pH the protein side chains are maximally charged with COO^- and $NH3^+$.

Another important feature of proteins is their hydrophobic regions rich in amino acids with aromatic side chains, i.e., phenylalanine and tyrosine. Natural occurrence of aromatic amino acids is rare compared to that of the other amino acids. In the presence of both hydrophilic and hydrophobic groups, hydrophobic groups preferentially associate with each other in an attempt to exclude hydrophilic groups, water, and hydrophilic solvents. The hydrophobic nature of the protein affects its solubility in polar and apolar solvents. The greater the hydrophobicity of the protein, the greater its solubility in nonpolar solvents and the less its solubility in polar or hydrophilic solvents.

Carbohydrate moieties influence the net charge and solubility of antigens and antibodies. Carbohydrates are highly soluble in water and therefore enhance hydrophilicity and solubility of proteins in hydrous solvents. Some carbohydrates, such as sialic acid (N-acetyl-neuraminic acid), contain side chains that are ionized depending upon the pH in which they are dissolved. These carbohydrate moieties of glycoproteins are attached via a serine, asparagine, hydroxylysine, or threonine residue. All human antibodies contain a carbohydrate moiety. There are rare antigens that are largely or solely carbohydrate in nature.

Nucleic acids are composed of units of nucleotides that contain bases, ribose or deoxyribose, and phosphates. These components are ionizable and contribute toward the net charge of the proteins in which they are found. Nucleic acids are largely insoluble in water but soluble in salt solutions. Nucleic acids may be antigenic determinants themselves, as in patients with systemic lupus erythematosus who have autoantibodies against their own native DNA. Nucleic acids alone cannot stimulate an immune response—they must be associated with other molecules, i.e., proteins.

Lipids contain fatty acids and phosphate groups that are ionizable and thus affect the net charge of lipoproteins. Many bacterial antigens, for example cell walls, are highly lipid in nature and are largely insoluble in hydrophilic or polar solvents. Lipid components decrease solubility in water or water-based solvents and enhance solubility in nonpolar solvents. Lipids alone do not stimulate an immune response.

SOLVENT AND SAMPLE PROCESSING CONSIDERATIONS

The solvent in which the antigen–antibody reaction is performed determines solubility of antigen and antibody. This should be maximized to allow free association of the molecules. Solvents in which antibodies are dissolved may be changed by dialysis or by passage through molecular sieve columns. Among those factors affecting solubility is ionic strength. Antigens and antibodies, in general, are most soluble in physiologic salt solutions, 0.154 mol/L, and are insoluble at higher or lower ionic concentrations. Ionic strength may be calculated by the formula:

$$M = \frac{1}{2} \sum_i c_i Z_i^2$$

where M is the total molar concentration (mol/L) when c_i is the molar concentration of the ith ionic species and Z_i is the charge of the ith species. The pH of the solvent also affects solubility. Physiologic pH (7.35 to 7.45) is optimal for most antigen–antibody systems. Looking at the pKa values for chargeable side chains, one sees that physiologic pH is also that pH at which maximum charge exists. The greater the number of charges on the side chains, the greater the ionic bonding opportunity between antigen and antibody.

Some solvents may contain ingredients that are incompatible with procedures. Many buffers used in commercial reagents contain ethylenediaminetetraacetic acid (*EDTA*), a chelating agent that binds cations. If assays involving complement are to be performed, EDTA must be avoided, because the cations Ca^{++} and Mg^{++} are required for the complement cascade activation. Disodium and dipotassium salts of EDTA are also commonly used anticoagulants that act by binding calcium ions that are essential for blood coagulation. Another solvent ingredient to be avoided is sulfhydryl reagent, which is required to preserve enzyme activities in some commercial preparations. Sulfhydryl agents may denature antibodies and are therefore to be avoided if possible.

Sample Processing

Serum or plasma should be frozen and thawed only once. Multiple freezing and thawing of samples denatures proteins. It is best to perform an assay as soon as possible after collecting a sample and to avoid freezing and thawing.

Many serologic assays require patient sample to be heated at 56°C for 30 minutes to inactivate complement and other serum proteins that interfere with some procedures. The heating should be performed immediately before the assay is begun. If the serum is stored after heating and the assay is done at a later date, the serum should be reheated. Heating at 56°C denatures one of the types of antibodies, immunoglobulin E (IgE). IgG, IgM, IgD, and IgA remain intact.

When whole cells contain the antigens on their surface, the **Z** *potential* (electrical potential produced by the cellular membrane charges) is sometimes strong enough to inhibit the approach of antibody molecules. Salt ions assist in negating this **Z** potential. Sometimes bovine serum albumin (BSA) is added, as in some blood bank procedures, to supply ionic species that associate with and negate cell surface charges so that antibodies can approach and bind to cell surface antigens. Another method used to decrease the **Z** potential is to treat the cells with *pineapple enzyme* or *papain*, which cleaves off the sialic acid residues (negative charges). This enzyme is used in some blood bank procedures.

Most laboratories purchase assay reagents in a kit form and assume that the vendor will have provided solutions of optimum concentration for the assay to be performed. The vendor's directions should be followed very carefully. It is important to dilute the concentrated reagents provided with the kit exactly as directed. A different salt concentration resulting from incorrect dilution could prevent the antigen–antibody reaction or could interfere with enzyme activity. It is also important to collect, process, store, and dilute the specimen according to the vendor's directions. Times and temperatures for incubations and centrifugations must be observed, as any deviation may interfere with the antigen–antibody binding. Vigorous mixing of antibodies or antigens is to be avoided, since bubble formation will cause denaturation.

The remainder of this chapter will describe the principles of immunologic assays and precautions and conditions for optimal results. Interlaced throughout the remainder of this book will be specific assays, precautions for each, reasons for false positives and false negatives, and medical significance of results. Table 4–1 lists the major types of immunologic assays, their end-point criteria, and their average sensitivities.

IMMUNOLOGIC ASSAYS

General Principle

An antigen usually has several different *antigenic determinants*, also called *epitopes*, the exact regions with which antibodies bind. Antibody molecules have two binding sites that are capable of combining with their specific antigenic determinants (Fig. 4–3). One antibody-binding site could bind with an antigenic determinant on one antigen, while the other could bind with a like antigenic determinant on a different antigen.

Antibodies also bind to haptens, which are small molecules usually with only a single antigenic determinant. Figure 4–3 A and B compares a monovalent hapten–antibody complex and a multivalent antigen–antibody complex.

Association of antibody (Ab) and antigen (Ag) is a chemical reaction with kinetics like that of other chemical reactions.

$$Ag + Ab \; \underset{k_2}{\overset{k_1}{\rightleftharpoons}} \; Ag \cdot Ab$$

Stability of the associated versus the disassociated form of the complex is reflected by the equilibrium constant Ka, which is the ratio of the association rate constant over the disassociation rate constant.

$$Ka = \frac{k_1}{k_2} = \frac{[Ag \cdot Ab]}{[Ag]\,[Ab]}$$

As the concentration of either Ag or Ab is increased, the denominator of the Ka equation will be larger, or the Ka will be smaller. Therefore to ensure maximum association of Ag with Ab, the concentrations in the reaction mixture must be in the correct ratio. The optimal Ag : Ab ratio varies with different Ags and Abs.

Some immunologic assays, for example RIAs, may be performed with Ag : Ab ratios distant from that for optimal association because the *end point* (that criterion used for detection of an associated Ag • Ab complex) is detectable under these conditions. The end point is the key to the required Ag : Ab ratios in the reaction mixture and influences the sensitivity of the assay.

Immunologic assays may roughly be divided into two categories (Table 4–1): (1) assays that have lattice formation as the end point, and (2) assays that have other than lattice formation as the end point. Analysis for small molecules or haptens is limited to the second category, because haptens are generally monovalent and therefore incapable of forming lattice networks with antibodies.

Lattice End-Point Assays

A *lattice* is a network of associated antigens and antibodies large enough to be detected by selected criteria, such as precipitation, agglutination or flocculation. Figure 4–4 depicts precipitations resulting in series of mixtures to which a constant amount of antibody has been added to increasing concentrations of antigen. A precipitate is a

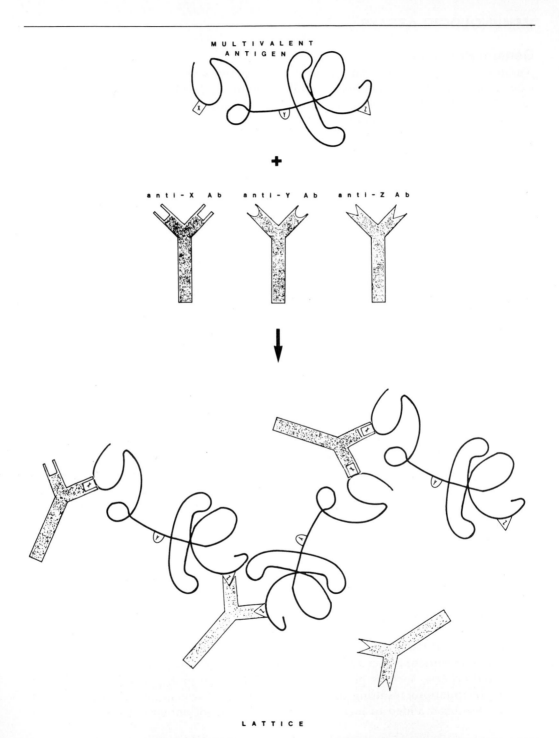

MULTIVALENT
ANTIGEN

+

anti-X Ab   anti-Y Ab   anti-Z Ab

LATTICE

A

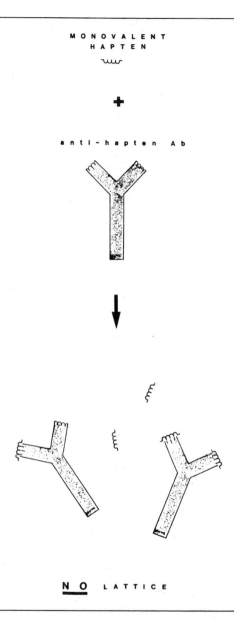

MONOVALENT
HAPTEN

＋

anti - hapten Ab

NO LATTICE

B

Figure 4-3. Antibody Combination with Antigen and Hapten. In (**A**), a multivalent antigen with antigenic determinants x, y, and z are mixed with a pool of antibodies containing anti-x, anti-y, and anti-z to form a lattice. A lattice is many bivalent Abs forming bridges that span two separate Ag molecules. One arm of the Ab combines with its specific determinant, on one Ag and the other arm of the Ab combines with its specific determinant on a different Ag molecule. After the complex of Ags and Abs reaches a large size, it precipitates or falls out of solution. The monovalent hapten (**B**) is incapable of forming a lattice, because the hapten has only one antigenic determinant for Ab association. The Ab bridging is impossible with monovalent haptens.

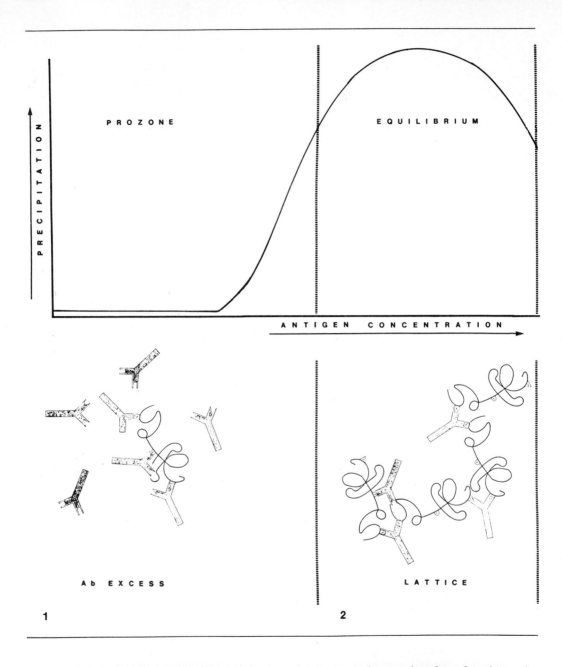

large, insoluble lattice that is formed from stringing together molecules of antigen via antibody bridges. The lattice increases in size and finally falls out of solution. Each antibody molecule has one of its binding sites associated with a different antigen molecule, and each antigen molecule is associated with more than one different antibody molecule. Antigen in a lattice must be multivalent; that is, it must have more than one antigenic determinant to allow bridging with antibody. In the case of a monovalent

POSTZONE

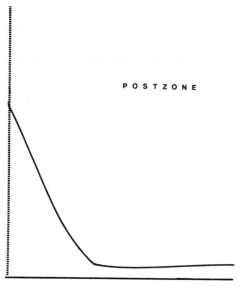

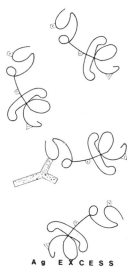

Ag EXCESS

Figure 4–4. Precipitation Curve for Multivalent Antigen and Specific Antibodies. The curve in the upper part of the figure shows precipitation of a series of assays in which a constant amount of Ab is mixed with increasing amounts of Ag. The lower part of the figure depicts what is happening molecularly in the three areas of the precipitation curve. (1) in the *prozone,* Ab is in excess, and result is no precipitation, (2) As the concentration of antigen is increased, an *equilibrium zone* is reached where the ratio of Ab to antigenic determinants is roughly equivalent, and result in maximum formation of lattice that falls out of solution as precipitation, (3) As the concentration of Ag is further increased, a zone of Ag excess occurs *(postzone)* with little lattice formation and no precipitation.

3

hapten that has only one site to bind with antibody, a lattice could never be formed. In the lower Ag concentrations of the series shown in Figure 4–4, antibody excess results in little lattice formation. The condition of no precipitation due to antibody excess is called the *prozone*. Excess antibody molecules either bind with individual antigens or are free and unbound. Either of these conditions results in no bridging. With increasing amounts of Ag, the ratio of Ag to Ab decreases the k_2 or increases the K_1 to increase the Ka until an *equilibrium zone* of maximum lattice formation is seen. As the Ag concentration is further increased, less and less lattice formation occurs. This condition of little precipitation due to antigen excess is called the *postzone*. Some antigen molecules are associated with a single antibody, while many others are free and unassociated. To ensure optimal results in those immunologic assays that use lattice formation as the end point, the reaction ratio of Ag to Ab must be in the equilibrium zone. In fact, even if antibody and complementary antigen are both present in a reaction mixture, there may be no precipitation if the Ag : Ab ratio is not within the equilibrium zone.

Liquid precipitation is an immunologic assay in which soluble antigen and antibody are reacted and the end point of the association is precipitation of large lattice networks. As the lattice grows, it reaches an insoluble size that settles out of solution and is visible to the human eye. This assay was historically one of the original serologic assays; however, it is no longer popular due to its insensitivity and requirement for rather large amounts of antigen and antibody.

Gel precipitation is an immunologic assay in which soluble antigen and antibody are allowed to diffuse through a gel medium. The end point of their association is visual precipitation within the gel. As the antigen or antibody diffuses from the point of application (usually a well cut in the agar) through the gel, its concentration decreases. A gradient is established from greatest concentration at origin to least concentration at the diffusion front. This gel gradient increases the possibility that the equilibrium zone conditions will be met. As discussed later in this chapter, there are many variants of gel precipitation immunoassays that use different strategies for bringing antibodies and antigens together at optimum concentrations for visible precipitation. These include radial immunodiffusion, double diffusion, and a variety of immunoelectrophoresis techniques. Gel precipitation is more sensitive than liquid precipitation and requires much less sample than liquid precipitation.

An important consideration in gel precipitation is the medium. It must allow the reactants to diffuse freely. Commercial agar used in microbiological media is not a good medium because it has surface charges that hinder free diffusion of biological molecules. Pure agarose gel is a better support for gel diffusion because it has fewer associated charges. The selected gel should be suspended in a buffer that provides optimal pH and ionic concentration for antigen–antibody association.

Several physical factors affect diffusion of molecules through gels. The size of the molecule is important. The larger the molecule, the slower its diffusion through the gel. IgM diffuses more slowly than IgG. Large, bacterial cell-wall antigens diffuse even more slowly than IgM. Temperature affects the rate of diffusion and precipitation; the greater the temperature, the more rapid the diffusion. Time of diffusion is important. Precipitation is a slowly reversible reaction. With time the leading edge of the precipitation dissolves and reforms due to the changing position of optimal conditions for equilibrium zone precipitation. Horse antiserum is noted for forming a line of precipitation that dissolves completely within 24 hours. Therefore gel precipitation should be read after a set time. A good rule for gel diffusion assays is to set the physical parameters and to run standards of similar molecular weight and charge as the unknown with each assay.

Radial immunodiffusion assay (RID) (Fig. 4–5) is used in many clinical laboratories.

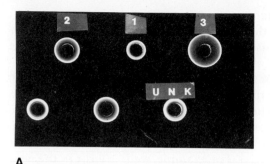

Sample	Ring Diam	Ring Diam^2	IgG mg/dl
STD 1	4.1	16.8	500
STD 2	4.6	21.2	1000
STD 3	5.6	31.4	2000
Unknown	4.3	18.5	760

B

A

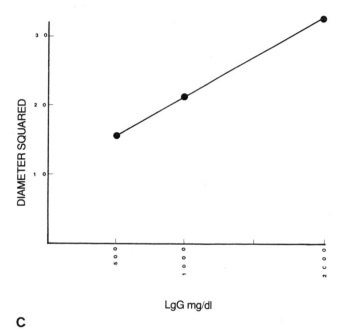

C

Figure 4-5. Radial Immunodiffusion (RID). A. Photograph of precipitation rings of three standard IgG and one unknown samples. **B.** Table of ring diameter, squared diameter, and concentrations. **C.** Standard graph relating squared-ring diameters of standards to their concentration.

Gel, containing antibody, is poured into a plastic dish and allowed to solidify. Specific size wells are cut in the gel, and the gel is removed from the holes. These wells are later filled with antigen to be assayed and allowed to stand for a specific time. As the antigen diffuses out into the gel, it establishes a concentration gradient, and wherever equilibrium zone conditions occur, a circle of precipitation forms. The greater the antigen concentration the farther it must diffuse from its well to drop to equilibrium zone conditions and the larger the circle of precipitation. RID is often used to determine a patient's serum IgG concentration. Each radial immunodiffusion assay includes several antigen standards of increasing concentrations and patient sera or unknowns. After standing for a given time (for example, 24 hours), a micrometer is used to measure the diameter of the circles of precipitation. A standard curve relating the squared diameter of precipitation to the antigen standards is constructed. The squared diameter of each unknown can be compared to the standard curve and a concentration for the unknown determined. This technique is used to quantitate immunoglobulins and some complement factors.

Another variation of gel diffusion is the *double immunodiffusion* technique (Fig. 4–6) in which both antigen and antibody diffuse through the gel toward each other. This process establishes concentration gradients of both antigen and antibody to maximize possibilities for reaching equilibrium conditions. The gel contains neither antigen nor antibody and is made up in a buffer of optimal pH and ionic strength for solubility and charge of the reacting molecules. For example, wells are cut in the agar in a pattern as indicated in Figure 4–6. Antigen is placed into one well, and antibody is placed into the opposite well. After a set time (for example, 24 hours), the agar is examined for precipitation. The distance of the line of precipitation from the antigen well is directly proportional to the antigen concentration. That is, the more concentrated the antigen, the more concentrated the antibody must be for equilibrium zone conditions, and therefore the closer to the Ab well source. As the antibody diffuses from its well, it becomes more dilute. Similar logic applies to the distance of the line of precipitation from the antibody well and the antibody concentration.

When human serum, which is a pool of many proteins, is injected into rabbits, a pool of antibodies is produced. The rabbit antihuman serum contains antibodies specific to various antigenic determinants on the human proteins. This antiserum will react with all of the human proteins. Figure 4–6 A shows the precipitation resulting from placing various purified serum proteins in the outer wells and the rabbit-antihuman-whole-serum antibodies in the center well. Two separate lines of precipitation indicate that at least two different proteins were placed into the antigen well.

Ouchterlony is the designation given to this double gel diffusion when it is used to compare antigens or antibodies for similarity. This comparative technique may be used to identify a purified unknown, to evaluate the purity of a sample, or to compare the antigenicity or antibody specificity of two or more samples. Ouchterlony assays are no longer widely used in clinical laboratories, but an understanding of the precipitation reactions seen in Ouchterlony precipitations gives insight about immunoprecipitation in general. Figure 4–6 B to D depicts the three possible patterns of comparative Ouchterlony precipitation.

The Ouchterlony pattern of *identity* is formed when an antiserum in the center well reacts with two or more wells containing antigens that are identical. Similarly a pattern of identity could be formed when an antigen in the center well reacts with samples of identical antibody specificity in the outer wells. The pattern of identity is characterized by the merging of the lines of precipitation and signifies that the two samples being compared are identical with respect to the presence of the antigen that reacts with the antibody in the center well.

A second pattern of comparative Ouchterlony precipitation is the pattern of *nonidentity,* which is formed when the antigens being compared in the two outer wells have completely different antigenic determinants. For this pattern to occur the antibody well must contain a pool of antibodies that has some antibodies specific for one antigenic species and other antibodies specific for the other antigenic species.

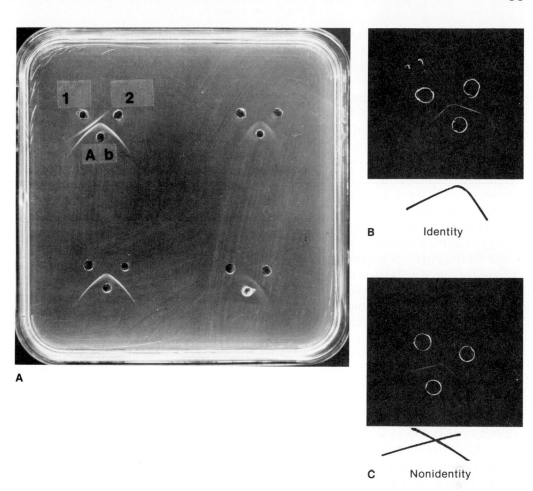

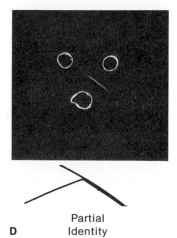

Figure 4-6. Ouchterlony Gel Diffusion Patterns. In all of the three-well series of gel diffusion here, the bottom center well of the three-series well arrangement always contains antiserum, and the other two wells contain Ag. **A.** Antiserum is antiwhole human serum. The labeled series contains two different protein in well 1 and one of the same two proteins in well two. Two lines of precipitation form between well containing the two proteins and the Ab well. **B.** Identity pattern: merging lines of precipitation signify that proteins in the two wells (1 and 2) are identical. **C.** Nonidentity: crossing lines of precipitation signify that Ag in well 1 is antigenically different from Ag in well two. **D.** Partial identity: merging lines of precipitation with a spur continuing off one line signifies that the two Ags have some shared antigenic determinants but that the two Ags are largely antigenetically different. The spur points toward the Ag of least identity with the antibody pool.

The third comparative Ouchterlony pattern of precipitation is that of *partial identity*. This pattern is characterized by two lines of precipitation, with a spur extending from one line. The center well has a pool of antibodies, with one population being specific toward an antigenic determinant that is found on both of the antigens and a second population being specific for antigenic determinants unique to one antigen. As a result a spur pattern forms. The spur points to that antigen that shares some antigenic determinants with the other antigen, or the spur points to the molecular species having the least identity or the fewer specific antigenic determinants to the pool of antibodies in the center well. The thickness or intensity of the lines of precipitation are also different. Precipitation between the antibody pool and the antigen most similar to, or having the most complementary determinants for, the antisera is more dense due to the involvement of more antibodies.

The Ouchterlony assay can be used to identify a particular purified unknown by comparing the unknown to known standards. This gel technique may also be used to examine the purity of an antigen preparation by running it against a pool of antibodies toward the original source from which the purification was begun. Similarly purity of antibody preparations can be evaluated. Antisera used in the clinical laboratory are commonly made by isolating proteins from whole serum. The isolate is then injected into an animal to stimulate antibody production. Resultant antiserum should be specific for that single human serum protein used to stimulate its production. Whole serum would be a good antigen pool for testing the above antibody preparation for a single protein specificity.

Flocculation is a serologic technique that also has lattice formation as its end point. This procedure uses an antigen that is larger and heavier than a single protein. This enlarging of the antigen allows detection of smaller lattices, since the critical size required for a lattice to fall out of solution is much smaller than that for precipitation of soluble protein and specific antibody. The Venereal Disease Research Laboratory (VDRL) assay is a common example of a flocculation method used in the clinical laboratory. The particulate antigen in this assay incorporates cholesterol with cardiolipin antigen to increase the effective antigen size. Flocculation assays are interpreted microscopically. Increased antigen size makes flocculation more sensitive than precipitation, since fewer antigen–antibody bridges are required for detection. Low-power microscopic examination is used to read flocculation assays.

Agglutination has a lattice end point in which the antigen is either a large particle to start with, i.e., bacterium, erythrocyte, or is absorbed onto some large particle (latex or polystyrene beads). Agglutination involving antigen that is an integral part of a bacterium or other cell is *direct agglutination* or *active agglutination*. Agglutination involving erythrocytes is termed *hemagglutination*. Agglutination involving antigen or antibody absorbed or covalently linked to a larger particle is termed *passive agglutination* or *indirect agglutination*. In indirect agglutination the large particle is passively rather than directly involved in the antigen–antibody reaction. Particles commonly used to absorb antigen for agglutination reagent preparation are erythrocytes and inert latex beads. Treating erythrocytes with tannic acid changes the membrane surface to a "sticky" nature that readily absorbs proteins. Antigens may be covalently bound to erythrocyte surfaces with diazotized benzidine, diflurodinitrobenzene, or some other coupling agent. Gluteraldehyde, a preservative, is added to treated erythrocytes to extend their shelf life to months. Passive agglutination using erythrocytes to absorb antigen is termed *passive hemagglutination*. The Monospot or slide agglutination test for infectious mononucleosis antibodies is an example of a hemagglutination assay used in the clinical laboratory (Fig. 4–7). The most common particles used in passive agglutination are latex. In fact, the most common serologic assay is latex agglutination. Recently *liposomes*, synthetically created micelles composed of a bilipid layer, have been used to increase the sensitivity of agglutination assays. During synthesis of liposomes, either antigen or antibody can be incorporated into the bilipid layers. Alternatively, antigen or antibody may be covalently linked to previously synthesized liposomes.

Agglutination inhibition is a variation of agglutination in which patient sample is incubated with antibodies to a given antigen. If the patient has that specific antigen, it will associate with and bind to the antibodies. After incubation particles coated with the given antigen are added. If the patient sample contained the antigen and bound the antibodies, there would be no free antibodies left to bind and agglutinate the particles coated with antigen. No agglutination, resulting from inhibition of agglutination is a positive result. This principle is used in one of the human chorionic-gonadatropin (HCG)–urine assays for pregnancy. If the patient has no HCG, antibodies will be free after incubation to agglutinate the added latex particles. When the particle that is coated with antigen is an erythrocyte, the agglutination inhibition assay is referred to as *hemagglutination inhibition*.

Electrophoresis is the separation of charged molecules in an electrical field. As discussed earlier in this chapter, the charge on antigens and antibodies depends upon their molecular composition and the pH of the solvent in which they are dissolved. When these charged molecules are placed in an electrical field, they will migrate toward the electrical pole of opposite charge. The medium in which the proteins are placed for electrophoresis may be paper, cellulose acetate, agarose, polyacrylamide, starch, or some other supportive material. Both the buffer in the interstices of the supportive medium and the buffer in which the electrophoresis is carried out affect the charge on the protein molecules and their resultant migration.

There are several steps in serum electrophoresis (Fig. 4–8). Sample is applied to

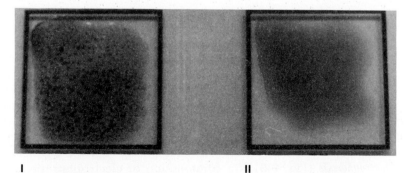

I   II

Figure 4–7. Agglutination. Square I shows agglutination of sheep erythrocytes by infectious mononucleosis heterophile antibodies. Square II has no agglutination.

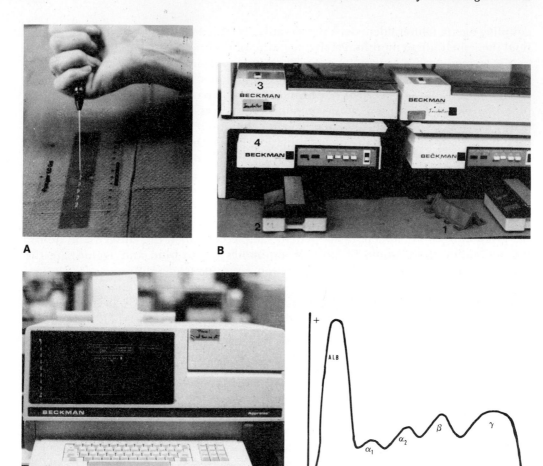

A   B

E   F

electrophoretic medium. Current is applied to establish a negative pole (cathode) and a positive pole (anode). Negative charged molecules (anions) migrate toward the anode, while positively charged molecules (cations) migrate toward the negative pole (cathode). The original pool of proteins is separated into individual proteins, depending upon the charges of the side chains on the proteins. After electrophoresis the medium is stained for protein to identify where the serum proteins are. Figure 4–8 F shows a normal serum electrophoretic pattern with the albumin, α-1, α-2, β, and γ globulin peaks. Serum electrophoresis provides general information concerning concentrations of serum proteins as shown by the examples in Figure 4–8 G.

Immunoelectrophoresis (Fig. 4–9) is a combination of electrophoresis and gel immunodiffusion. First, the patient sample is electrophoresed from a center well as in the above serum electrophoresis. Then antiserum is applied in troughs cut along the outer edge of the electrophoresed medium. As the electrophoresed protein bands dif-

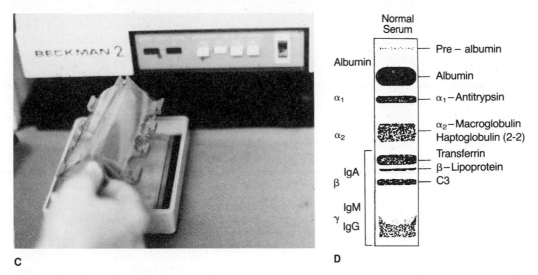

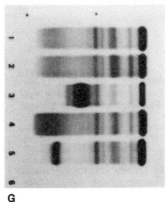

NORMAL

ACUTE INFLAM RESP

IgA MYELOMA

POLYCLONAL INCREASE

IgG MYELOMA

Figure 4-8. Serum Electrophoresis. A. Sample being applied to cellulose acetate sheet. **B.** Electrophoresis apparatus: (1) Frame for acetate sheet; (2) Electrophoresis chamber; (3) Power supply. **C.** Cellulose acetate gel stretched over frame and being placed into the electrophoresis chamber. **D.** Resultant separation of serum proteins after electrophoresis and staining. **E.** Automatic densitometer. **F.** Densitometer scan of normal pattern. **G.** Examples of abnormal serum protein electrophoresis patterns.

fuse out through the medium, the antiserum diffuses out from the trough. The two reactants meet and form a precipitate at the zone of equilibrium. Because the immunoglobulins in the gamma globulin band diffuse out at different rates and because the zone of equilibrium occurs at different distances from the origin, the gamma globulin band can be separated into IgA, IgG, and IgM lines of precipitation. Antiwhole serum is used to screen patient serum for any abnormally high or low protein concentration patterns. If any are seen, antiserum specific for a single protein may be used to identify which protein is responsible for the abnormal electrophoretic pattern.

Immunofixation electrophoresis (Fig. 4-10) is a variation on immunoelectrophoresis. After electrophoresing the sample, instead of applying multispecific or monospecific antisera in a trough, the antisera is spread over the entire gel surface by soaking a thin layer of absorbant material, such as paper, in the antiserum. Then the antiserum-soaked medium is laid on top of the already electrophoresed gel, which is set in a

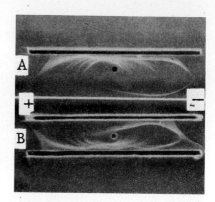

Figure 4-9. Immunoelectrophoresis. IgG myeloma serum (B) compared to that of normal human serum (A). Ab troughs: middle, anti-IgG; top and bottom, antihuman serum.

moist chamber overnight. During this time the antiserum diffuses from the absorbant medium into the gel, the precipitation forms wherever antibody finds its specific serum-protein antigen in equivalent zone conditions. Figure 4–10 shows an immunofixation electrophoresis series that was used to identify an abnormal monoclonal immunoglobulin spike in a patient's serum. The western blot technique which is similar in principle and which is used to confirm a positive enzyme immunoassay for autoimmune deficiency syndrome (AIDS) is discussed in the viral diseases (Chap. 13).

Rocket electrophoresis is a different variation on electrophoresis and gel diffusion. Figure 4–11 shows the final precipitation of a rocket electrophoresis, which is performed by (1) preparing an electrophoretic gel containing antibody; (2) applying patient sample and standards into wells at the end of the medium near the cathode; and (3) applying current and electrophoresing in a buffer of pH 8.6. As the sample mi-

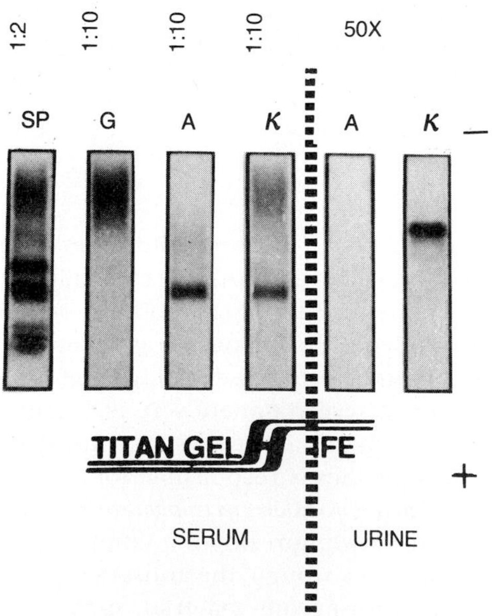

Figure 4-10. Immunofixation Electrophoresis. Protein patterns to the left of the dotted line are serum and to the right are urine. Above the patterns the serum dilution 1 : 2 or 1 : 10 is indicated, and the urine concentration 50X is indicated. Between the dilution and the pattern is the specific antiserum that was used. SP = antiwhole human serum; G = anti-IgG; A = anti IgA, and κ = anti-κ. This sample was a G and A myeloma with κ chains. The κ chains were also in the urine.

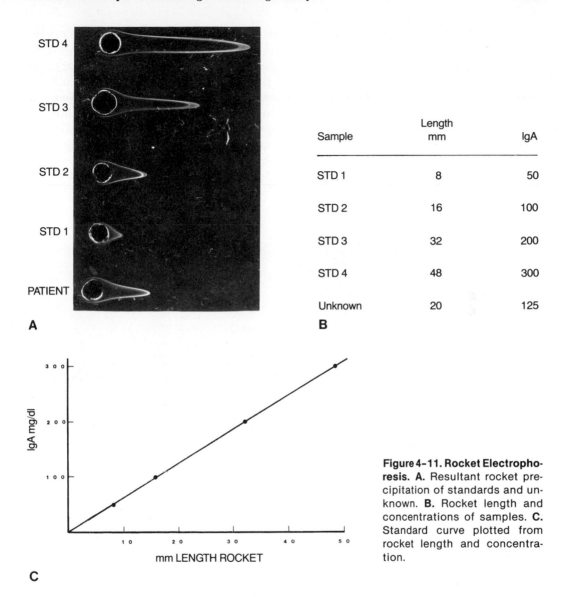

Sample	Length mm	IgA
STD 1	8	50
STD 2	16	100
STD 3	32	200
STD 4	48	300
Unknown	20	125

Figure 4–11. Rocket Electrophoresis. A. Resultant rocket precipitation of standards and unknown. B. Rocket length and concentrations of samples. C. Standard curve plotted from rocket length and concentration.

grates a concentration gradient that diminishes with distance from the point of application is established. Wherever the zone of equilibrium conditions are reached at the leading edge of the migrating rocket, precipitation occurs. From the series of standards, a graph relating concentration to rocket length is drawn. Using this graph, rocket length of an unknown may be converted to protein concentration. The electrophoresis speeds up attainment of equilibrium zone conditions so that this rocket technique yields quantitative results within 1 to 2 hours whereas RID (gel diffusion alone) requires 12 to 24 hours. Some laboratories use this method to quantitate complement components.

Counterimmunoelectrophoresis or *countercurrent immunoelectrophoresis* (Fig. 4–12) is yet another variation on combining electrophoresis and gel diffusion. In this procedure antigen is applied in one well of an electrophoretic medium, and antibody is applied in another well (Fig. 4–12 A). The antigen is placed closest to the cathode, leaving the antibody closest to the anode. The pH of the buffer system must be that which will cause the antigen to be negatively charged and to migrate toward the anode and the antibody to be positively charged and to migrate toward the cathode. When the two meet at equilibrium zone conditions, precipitation will occur (Fig. 4–12 B). This technique was once used to detect antigens in patient serum, especially antigens of the pathogens that cause meningitis. A panel of antibodies to different organisms was run with patient serum. If patient serum contained the antigen of a particular organism,

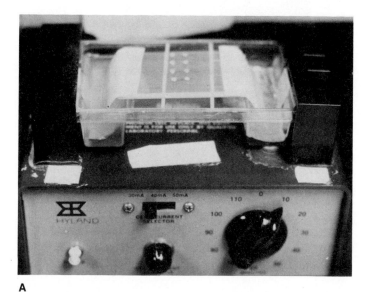

A

Figure 4-12. Countercurrent Immunoelectrophoresis (CIE). Example of stat CIE for meningitis Ags. Patient sample is assayed for presence of Ag. Specific Ab is placed in one well, and patient sample is placed in an opposing well **(A)**. During electrophoresis the two migrate toward one another. If Ab is specific for Ag, a line of precipitation forms **(B)**.

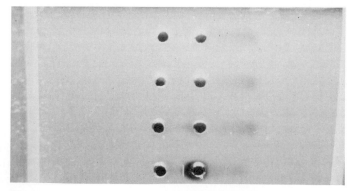

B

a line of precipitation formed with the antibody against that organism. The main advantage over gel diffusion is that the electrophoresis causes the Ag • Ab association to occur much more rapidly. The meningitis-causing organism may be identified within 2 hours versus overnight with the Ouchterlony technique. Major technical factors that must be considered are correct adjustment of electrophoretic buffer pH and ionic strength, correct diluting of the antigen and antiserum to ensure equilibrium zone conditions, correct setting of electrical current, running at the correct temperature and time, and specificity of antisera. This technique is limited to those Ag–Ab systems for which an electrophoretic buffer can be selected to give the Ag and Ab opposite charges.

Complement-Fixation–End-Point Assays

Complement is a group of normal blood proteins that are required for antibody-mediated cell lysis. When antigen and antibody (IgG or IgM) bind together, the complement system is activated. The complement system will be discussed in detail in Chapter 10. Lysis of antibody-coated erythrocytes by complement activation (fixation) can be used as an end point for immunologic assays. Figure 4–13 outlines the complement fixation test, which consists of two steps:

Test System
Step 1.   Patient sample is mixed with a given antigen and complement and incubated. If patient serum contains antibody it will bind to the antigen, and this complex will bind, activate and use complement that is present.

Indicator System
Step 2.   Sheep erythrocytes and antisheep-erythrocyte antiserum (*hemolysin*) is added to the above mixture and incubated. If the complement is consumed in step 1, i.e., patient serum had antibody that related with antigen, in step 2 the antisheep antibody will bind to the sheep erythrocytes, but without complement there will be no hemolysis (Fig. 4–13 A). If the complement in step 1 was not consumed, i.e., patient serum had no antibody against the antigen, in step 2 the sheep erythrocytes will bind hemolysin, and the complement will be activated and will cause hemolysis of the erythrocytes (Fig. 4–13 B).

Thus hemolysis means that the patient had no antibody against the antigen; whereas, lack of hemolysis means that the patient had antibody to the antigen used in the assay. Complement fixation assays are technically difficult to run, because each reagent must be fresh and titered with the other reagents to ensure optimum conditions for hemolysis. Figure 4–13 C is a completed complement fixation that was performed in a microliter dish. The + top row is a positive control, and the sc second row is a negative serum control. Most routine clinical laboratories no longer use complement fixation assays. The Communicable Diseases Center (CDC) and a few other laboratories still use complement fixation assays for some antiviral antibody assays, because there are no good alternative methods.

POSITIVE

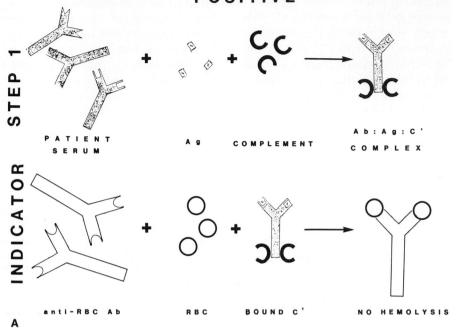

STEP 1

PATIENT SERUM + Ag + COMPLEMENT → Ab : Ag : C' COMPLEX

INDICATOR

anti-RBC Ab + RBC + BOUND C' → NO HEMOLYSIS

A

NEGATIVE

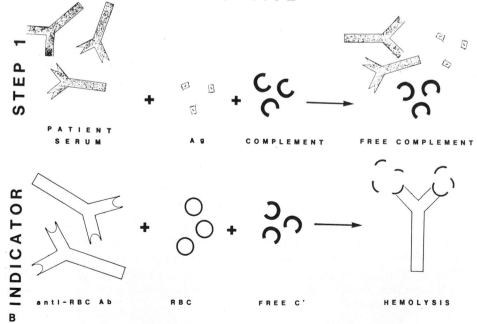

STEP 1

PATIENT SERUM + Ag + COMPLEMENT → FREE COMPLEMENT

INDICATOR

anti-RBC Ab + RBC + FREE C' → HEMOLYSIS

B

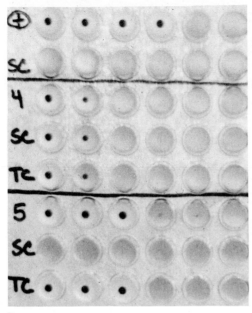

C

Figure 4-13. Complement Assays. A. Positive test. B. Negative Test (see text for description). C. Completed microtiter complement fixation assay with the top (+) row (a positive control) showing no hemolysis and the second (SC) row (a negative control) showing hemolysis.

Light Scattering as End Point (Nephelometry)

When antigen and antibody combine, they form complexes that scatter light. These complexes will gradually become larger and, if allowed to, may finally reach a size that precipitates out of solution. The nephelometer (Fig. 4–14) is an instrument that measures the amount of light scatter. In antibody excess, the rate of Ag • Ab association can be determined by the nephelometric measure of light scatter. A standard curve is made to correlate light scatter readings with antigen concentration (Fig. 4–14 C). Precautions in nephelometry are to use absolutely clean, dust-free glass or plastic ware and to ensure that reaction conditions are kept in antibody excess. Most nephelometers have computers that compare light scatter kinetics of unknowns to that of standards and print out the antigen concentration directly (Fig. 4–14 B). The computer can also distinguish between the kinetics of antibody excess conditions and that of equilibrium or antigen excess conditions. Nephelometry can be used for quantitation of any Ag for which a highly specific antiserum exists. Most frequently, assays for quantitating IgM, IgG, IgA, and C3 and C4 are done by this method.

Labeled Antigens–Antibodies as End Point (Visual Detection)

Labeling the antibody or antigen component of an antigen–antibody assay system can increase the sensitivity. Labels that are used are fluorochromes, enzymes, gold, and radioisotopes. Use of a label allows detection of antibody–antigen associations outside the zone of equilibrium required for lattice formation. These conditions plus the ability to detect the label in low concentrations provide assay methods with much more sensitivity than those previously discussed.

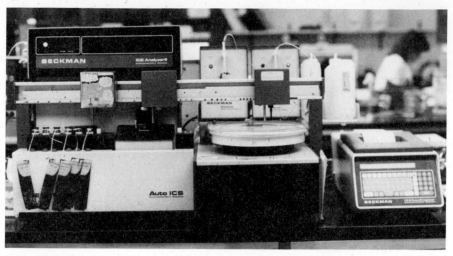

A

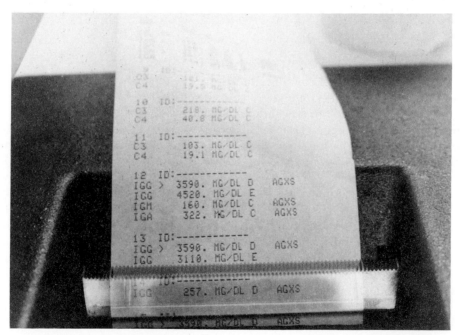

B

Figure 4–14. Nephelometry. A. A Beckman computerized nephelometer. **B.** Direct print-out of computed values. **C.** Graph relating concentration of Ag to extent of light scatter. Assays are performed in Ab excess.

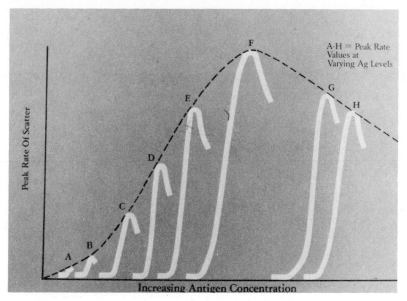

C

Microscopically detected fluorescence is a nonlattice end-point method. The antibody is labeled by covalently linking a fluorochrome to it, and this fluorescing molecule is the detectable end point of Ag • Ab association. Figure 4–15 depicts the two techniques for immunofluorescence staining. In the *direct immunofluorescence stain*, an antigen-containing specimen is reacted with a fluorochrome-conjugated antibody. Excess, unassociated antibody is washed away. The specimen is placed under a fluorescence microscope, which provides an energy source of specific wavelength to excite the fluorochrome. Fluorochromes absorb light at specific wavelengths and in doing so jump to a higher energy state. Each fluorochrome has a specific wavelength at which it is excited, i.e., at which it absorbs energy (Fig. 4–15, top). As the molecule returns to its ground state, this energy is lost by visible light emission at a lesser energy or longer wavelength. The fluorescent *Treponema pallidum* antibody-absorption test (FTA-ABS) is an example of this technique used in the clinical laboratory. Figure 4–16 is a positive FTA-ABS.

A variation of the direct immunofluorescence stain is the *indirect* or *sandwich immunofluorescence stain*. This technique covalently links the fluorochrome to an antiantibody rather than to the antibody specific for the antigen being sought. Figure 4–15 B shows this method. First the specimen is incubated with antigen-specific antibody (primary antibody). The unattached antibody is washed away. Fluorochrome-conjugated antiantibody (secondary antibody) is then applied to the specimen. The secondary antiantibody binds to any primary antibody that has attached to antigen. Fluorescence will be observed only if the specific (primary) antibody has attached to its complementary antigen on the specimen. This method allows using one fluorochrome-labeled reagent (the secondary antiantibody) for any assays using primary antibodies for which

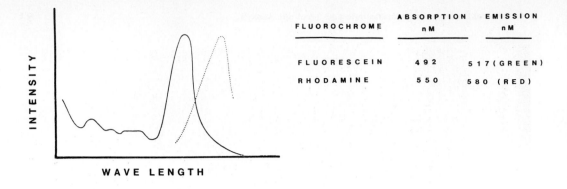

FLUOROCHROME	ABSORPTION nM	EMISSION nM
FLUORESCEIN	492	517 (GREEN)
RHODAMINE	550	580 (RED)

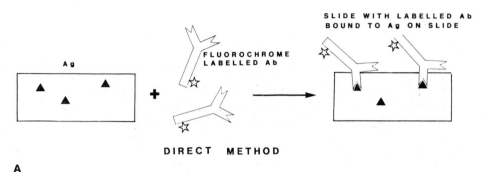

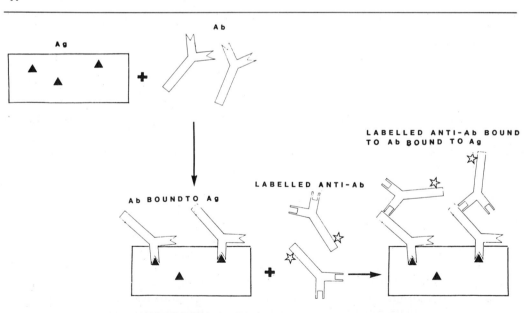

Figure 4–15. Fluorochrome Label. Diagram (*top*) of intensity of energy absorbed or emitted at various wavelengths; ——— is the absorption pattern, · · · · · is the emission pattern. **A.** The direct method of fluorochrome-labeled antibody staining. **B.** The sandwich technique of fluorochrome-labeled antibody staining.

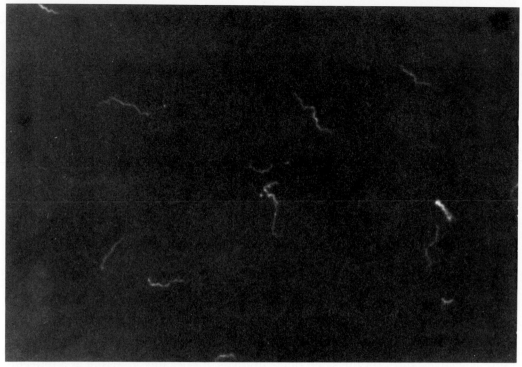

Figure 4-16. Positive Fluorescent Treponemal Antibody-Absorption Stain.

the secondary antibody has specificity. Immunofluorescence microscopy can also be used to detect the binding of fluorochrome-labeled antigens to antibodies in tissue specimens.

Fluorescent microscopes are of two major types: the *transmitted light system*, and the *epi-illumination system* (*incident light system* or *vertical illumination system*). The epi-illumination system is preferred because it allows simultaneous use of normal light and ultraviolet (UV) or excitation light source. This permits focusing of the specimen with a visible light source and enhancing the specimen fluorescence over background fluorescence by using simultaneous darkfield or phase. Major components of a fluorescence microscope and their purpose are shown in Figure 4-17. Beginning with the UV light source and following the beam through the excitation to human visualization, the following components are in order. Excitation light is provided by the UV light source. The heat-exciter filter absorbs heat energy wavelengths and filters out all wavelengths except those desired for exciting the fluorochrome. A *dichroic mirror* reflects the beam down toward the specimen to excite fluorochromes attached to the specimen. Resultant emissions from the fluorochrome are directed upward through the objective and through the dichroic mirror. A barrier filter removes all wavelengths except those selected to be observed. The barrier filter ensures elimination of any extraneous UV waves that would harm the microscopist's eye. An important difference between the transmitted fluorescence microscope system and the epi-illumination system is the dichroic mirror. This component allows using both UV and visible light sources with the

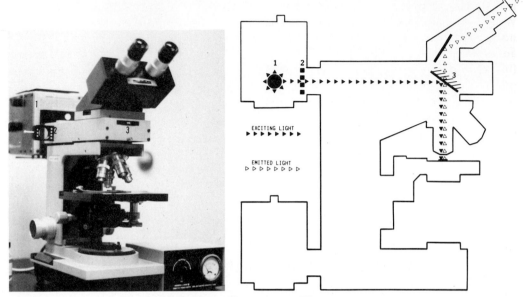

Figure 4-17. Fluorescence Microscope.

same objectives and with the same range of focus. It does this by acting as a reflector for the excitation light while, at the same time, allowing emitted light to pass through it up to the oculars.

Using methods similar to those discussed in visual detection of fluorochrome-labeled antibody or antigen, radioactive isotopes or enzymes can be used as labels in place of fluorochromes in immunostaining procedures. Visual detection of radioisotope labels is limited largely to research laboratories and is accomplished by exposing the specimen with radiolabeled antibodies bound to antigens to photographic film that will be oxidized by rays from the isotope (autoradiography).

Immunoenzyme microscopy is gaining wide use in diagnostic laboratories, especially hematology laboratories. This technique is analogous to immunofluorescence microscopy but uses enzyme-labeled antibodies instead of fluorochrome-labeled. The binding of the enzyme-labeled antibodies to antigens in a specimen is identified by reacting the specimen with a substrate and chromogen. If enzyme-labeled antibody is bound to antigens in the specimen, the substrate reacts with the enzyme and generates products that convert the chromogen to a colored reaction product that can be seen by standard light microscopy. This technique has the advantages over immunofluorescence microscopy of not requiring an expensive fluorescence microscope and of resulting in a permanent preparation that can be re-examined repeatedly if necessary. The most commonly used enzyme lable is peroxidase. Peroxidase can be conjugated to the primary antibody for direct immunoenzyme microscopy or to the secondary antibody for indirect immunoenzyme microscopy. Other sandwich techniques, such as biotin–avidin bridging and antiperoxidase antibody bridging, can be used to link peroxidase to the site of antigen–antibody binding in a specimen.

Labeled Antigens–Antibodies as End Point (Instrument Detection)

With instrument detection these types of end points provide the most sensitive immunoassays available today. All these assays have similar logic in that they utilize labeled antigen or labeled antibody to detect and quantitate Ag–Ab association. Whether a fluorochrome, an isoptope, or an enzyme is used to label antigen or antibody, the purpose of using the label is to provide a means to detect association of that labeled Ag or Ab. Highly specific monoclonal antibodies provide greater specificity. Different instrumentation is used to measure the different physical properties of the three different labels. All three methods allow quantitating Ag–Ab association far outside equilibrium zone conditions, and all require very small sample volume for testing. All three have been adapted to automated processing for large volume sampling and for feeding output directly into computers. Of these three the radioactive and enzyme-labeled methods are the most commonly used.

Flow cell detection of fluorochrome-labeled antibodies is a nonlattice method used to detect cell surface antigens. *Flow cytometry* is a method widely used in larger clinical laboratories for evaluating properties of cells as they are rapidly passed through minute orifices. By keeping track of the volume of sample and the number of cells that possess a particular property in that volume, concentration of those cells may be calculated. The size of the orifice controls which size cells will be passed through. Reduced pressure in the operative tubing causes cells to flow into the orifice when the aperture is immersed in the specimen. Once inside the orifice, cell types may be counted by fluorescence detection or by light scatter. Light scatter detection is most commonly used to count all cells of a particular size, such as in the Coulter counter. Fluorescence detection is used to count only those cells that have a fluorochrome label. Instead of counting all cells, as with light scatter, only those cells with fluorochrome label are counted. For example, fluorochrome-conjugated anti-T lymphocyte monoclonal antibodies are mixed with isolated patient lymphocytes. After incubation and washing away of unbound antibodies, the cells are analyzed on the fluorescence activated flow cytometer. Only those cells labeled with fluorochrome-conjugated antibody will be detected and counted as they pass through the orifice, giving a total T lymphocyte count. By analyzing samples reacted with anti-T helper cell and anti-T suppressor cell antibodies, the ratio of T helper cells to T suppressor cells may be calculated. Figure 4–18 is a picture of the Becton–Dickinson fluorescence-activated flow cytometer, Research Triangle Park, N.C.

The *fluorescence-activated cell sorter* (FACS) is a sophisticated extension of the flow cytometer. It is able to evaluate each cell individually as it passes through the instrument. The droplets containing the evaluated cell can be directed into one of several collecting tubes based on the presence or absence of fluorescence caused by the binding of a fluorochrome-conjugated antibody to the cell surface. Droplets are composed of saline and a cell and are directed by deflection plates producing an electric field to attract the droplet. With the FACS, one may separate, quantitate, and collect a specific type of cell from a general population of cells.

There are some *fluorescence immunoassay* (FIA) procedures available. Either antibody or antigen is labeled with a fluorochrome. The labeled reagent is usually bound to an inert surface such as a plastic test tube or beads. A patient sample that may contain the complementary antigen or antibody is reacted with the fluorochrome-

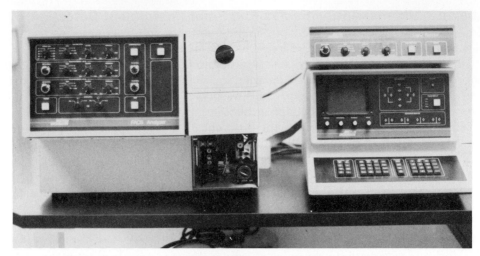

Figure 4–18. Becton–Dickinson Fluorescence-Activated Cell Analyzer.

labeled substrate. Bound products are quantitated with a fluorometer or a spectrofluorometer.

Radioimmunoassay (RIA) uses radioisotopes as labels (Fig. 4–19) for antigens or antibodies. Isotopes commonly used for labeling are iodine-125 and iodine-131 (I-125 and I-131). The most commonly used form of RIA measures competitive binding between labeled antigen and unknown antigen for specific antibody. Such RIA assays incubate labeled antigen, patient sample suspected of containing antigen, and specific antibody. The higher the concentration of antigen in patient serum, the less the binding of labeled antigen to antibody, and therefore the less the radioactivity of the final associated Ag–Ab complex. RIAs require separation of the bound labeled reaction products from the reaction mixture containing nonbound labeled reagents. Some techniques used to accomplish this separation are precipitation with ammonium sulfate, ethanol or polyethyleneglycol, precipitation with an antiantibody, or absorption of unassociated antigen onto particles such as charcoal. Recently methods have been developed to have the antibody immobilized on inert beads or on a plastic tube. Then centrifugation and washing allow easy separation of bound and free radioactive label.

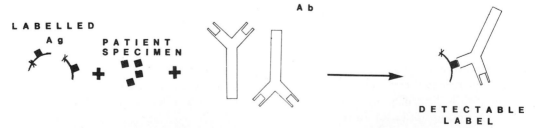

Figure 4–19. Radioimmunoassay (RIA). Isotope-labeled Ag competes with patient Ag for binding to Ab. Soluble patient Ag competes with labeled Ag for binding to Ab. Ab · Ag product is recovered and analyzed for radioactivity. As concentration of patient Ag↑, the concentration of bound radioactive-labeled Ag↓.

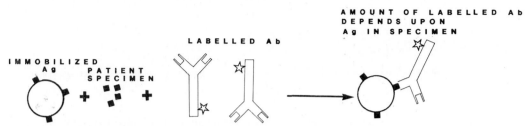

Figure 4-20. Immunoradiometric Assay (IRMA). Immobilized Ag competes with patient Ag for binding to labeled Ab. Unbound patient Ag and unbound labeled Ab are washed away. Immobilized Ag with attached radioactive Ab is quantitated. ↑ Patient Ag = ↓ Radiation from Ab bound to immobilized Ag.

Immunoradiometric assay (IRMA) is a variation of RIA in which the *antibody* is labeled and the reagent antigen is immobilized (Fig. 4-20). Patient sample suspected of containing the antigen is incubated with the immobilized antigen and the labeled antibody. The two antigens compete for binding sites on the antibody. Excess unassociated antibody is washed away, and the immobilized phase is examined for radioactivity from attached antibody.

Enzyme immunoassay (EIA) uses enzymes (e.g., horseradish peroxidase, alkaline phosphatase) as labels. Enzyme-linked immunoabsorbant assay (ELISA) is another term used for EIAs having one of the participants, antigen or antibody, immobilized (Fig. 4-21). Detection of enzyme label is accomplished by addition of specific substrate,

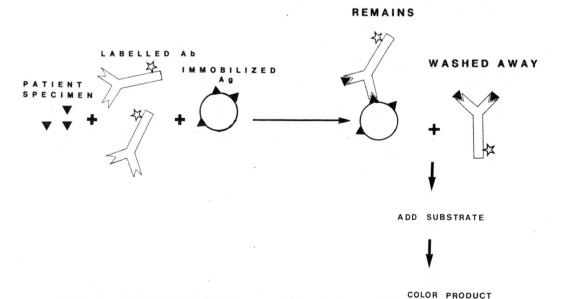

Figure 4-21. Enzyme-Linked Immunosorbent Assay (ELISA). Patient Ag competes with immobilized Ag for binding to enzyme-labeled Ab. Soluble patient Ag · Ab are washed away. Remaining enzyme-labeled Ab bound to immobile Ag is quantitated by adding a substrate that is converted to a color product.

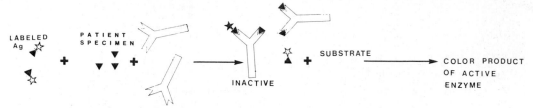

Figure 4-22. Enzyme-Multiplied Immunoassay Technique (EMIT). Patient Ag and enzyme-labeled Ag compete for binding to Ab. When enzyme-labeled Ag binds to Ab, the enzyme is inactivated. Thus color development of substrate is directly related to concentration of active enzyme. The greater the patient's antigen concentration, the greater the enzyme activity or the greater the color product development.

incubation, and quantitation of product. The product is colored and can be spectrophotometrically detected and quantitated.

Enzyme-multiplied immunoassay technique (EMIT) is an EIA in which an enzyme-labeled antigen competes with suspected patient antigen for binding onto specific antibody (Fig. 4-22). There is no need for an immobilized phase or for separating bound and unbound reaction components because binding of antigen to antibody inactivates the enzyme that is labeling the antigen. The higher the patient-antigen concentration, the more antibody that reacts. This leaves less antibody to react with and inactivate enzyme-labeled antigen. Active enzyme remaining after competitive binding is analyzed via conversion of substrate to some colored product. This competitive binding assay promises to become very popular in the future.

NEW TECHNOLOGIES

Several new techniques that are being introduced into laboratory science should be mentioned here. Although these methodologies have not yet received wide acceptance, they promise to increase the sensitivity of certain types of immunologic assays. The immunologic principle underlying each of the methods is the same—amplification of an initial antigen–antibody binding.

The biotin–avidin system is one method used to amplify an antigen–antibody binding. The association constant of antigen to antibody is about 10^5 to 10^{11} mol/L whereas the association constant of biotin to avidin is about 10^{15} mol/L. Specimen that contains antigen is incubated with reagent antibody to which biotin has been covalently linked. Free avidin is also added to the reaction mixture. Ab^{biotin} binds to Ag, and avidin binds to the Ab^{biotin}. Bound avidin binds up to 4 $biotin^{label}$. The label is usually an enzyme. Each avidin binds about 4 biotins so that the initial one antigen-antibody is now multiplied by 4. Antigen–antibody binding is further amplified when the enzyme label converts several times its molar concentration of substrate to quantifiable product. The biotin–avidin system may not be used to assay clinical specimens that contain amounts of natural avidin or biotin, as these would interfere with the results.

$$Ag + Ab^{biotin} + avidin \longrightarrow Ag \cdot Ab^{biotin \cdot avidin}$$
$$+$$
$$4 \text{ biotin*}$$
$$\downarrow$$
$$Ag \cdot Ab^{biotin \cdot avidin \cdot 4biotin*}$$
$$+$$
$$\text{Substrate for enzyme label}$$
$$\downarrow$$
$$\text{Product}$$

Another new methodology for enhancing assay sensitivity for antibody–antigen binding is the use of *liposomes*, which we have mentioned earlier in this chapter. In addition to using liposomes as inert reagents to enlarge antigen area, liposomes have been used in complement systems. Because liposomes are synthetic cells composed of bilipid layers, complement may be activated by binding of antibody to Ag that was incorporated in the liposome membrane. Activated complement damages the membranes to mediate release of materials contained within the micelles. Quantity of released materials is related to concentration of antibody bound to antigen via correlation with antigen standards that are simultaneously run in an assay. Some methods used to quantitate released liposome-contained materials are spectrophotometry, electron spin resonance, and substrate conversion.

$$Liposome^{Ag} + Ab + C' \rightarrow C' \text{activation and liposome degradation}$$
$$\text{with release of intramicelle contents}$$

The third method of amplifying antigen–antigen binding is the *anticomplement immunofluorescent assay* (ACIF). Although this technique has been known for some time, it has recently found renewed interest in assaying for some virus infections. This technique differs from the fluorescent staining immunoassay described earlier in this chapter in that after antibody is allowed to bind to specimen antigen, complement is incubated with the antigen–antibody complex. Each antigen–antibody complex activates several molecules of complement that then bind to the specimen that is being stained. Lastly, fluorescein-labeled anticomplement serum is applied to bind to the complement molecules attached to the specimen. Fluorescence resulting from attached label is then observed under the fluorescence microscope.

Discussion of the Illustrative Case

The presence in this patient of a fever of undetermined origin, lymphadenopathy, splenomegaly, lymphocytosis, and atypical lymphocytes suggested infection by the Epstein–Barr (EBV) virus (infectious mononucleosis), but lymphoma or leukemia were also possible. The negative heterophile test prompted consideration of lymph node and bone marrow biopsy. This would require hospitalization of the patient and cause anxiety and trauma to the patient and family. The alternative that was

---

*Indicates a label is covalently attached. Usually the label is an enzyme.

elected was to have IgG and IgM titers for antibodies to the most common causative agents in fever of undetermined origin (FUO), the cytomegalovirus (CMV), EBV, and toxoplasma. Titers below 1 : 50 are usually not associated with an active disease; therefore the finding of the 1 : 20 IgG titer for CMV was unimportant; however, the 1 : 80 IgM titer for EBV suggested an active infection. A week later the heterophile antibody test was repeated and found to be positive, which confirmed active infectious mononucleosis.

During the course of infectious mononucleosis, IgM antibodies to the viral capsule (viral capsid antigen, VCA) are the first to appear. Later heterophile antibodies appear and are diagnostic of the infection. The heterophile antibodies disappear with resolution of the disease, at which time IgG antibodies for EBV are present. A more detailed discussion of infectious mononucleosis is in Chapter 13 on viral diseases. The point of this illustrative case in this chapter is the usefulness of the serology for IgM antibodies.

QUESTIONS

1. Discuss with diagrams the production of different antibody classes in relation to the course of infection. Relate to your discussion the logic for performing clinical serologic assays for specific antibody class.

2. What physical chemical factors affect antigen–antibody binding?

3. Discuss with diagrams a passive hemagglutination assay.

4. Describe and distinguish the ELISA and the EMIT.

5. Differentiate the direct versus the indirect method for fluorochrome-labeled antibody staining.

6. Define a dichroic mirror as it pertains to the epi-illumination system, and discuss advantages it affords over the transmitted system. Give the purpose of the heat filter and the barrier filter in fluorescence microscopy.

7. Diagram a complement fixation hemolytic assay with a positive result.

8. Differentiate rocket electrophoresis and RID.

9. Differentiate immunoelectrophoresis and immunofixation electrophoresis.

10. Diagram the ACIF assay.

The Lymphoid System and Lymphoid System Diseases

Chapter

5 Lymphocytes and Lymphoid Tissues

OBJECTIVES

1. To discuss the embryonic development of lymphocytes and other leukocytes.
2. To describe the structure of lymphocytes and other leukocytes.
3. To describe the morphology of lymphoid tissues.
4. To comment on the interrelatedness of lymphoid tissue structure and function.

Illustrative Case

A 19-year-old male college student developed fever, headache, sore throat, swollen "glands" in his neck, aching muscles, and easy fatigability. He went to his physician, who confirmed the fever and, on physical examination, noted lymphadenopathy in the neck and splenomegaly. The tonsils were also enlarged, and the overlying mucosa was reddened. The physician obtained blood samples and ordered from the laboratory the following tests: complete blood count (CBC) with differential count of leukocytes, serologic tests for antibodies against streptococcal antigens (i.e., antistreptolysin O and anti-DNAse B), heterophil antibodies, and antibodies against Epstein–Barr virus (EBV). Swabbings of the throat were also sent for bacterial culture.

The antistreptolysin O and anti-DNAse B antibody titers in the serum were not elevated, and only a mixture of normal oral flora grew in the throat cultures. Therefore there was no laboratory support for a diagnosis of streptococcal pharyngitis. The blood count demonstrated a marked leukocytosis, due primarily to lymphocytosis. Microscopic examination of Wright's-stained blood smears revealed the presence of large, "atypical" lymphocytes (Downy cells). Serologic studies demonstrated both heterophil antibodies and antibodies against EBV.

After analysis of the laboratory data, a diagnosis of infectious mononucleosis was made. No specific therapy was instituted. The fever, sore throat, and muscle aches subsided within a week, and the lymphadenopathy and splenomegaly resolved after one month.

EMBRYONIC LEUKOCYTE DEVELOPMENT

Early in mammalian embryonic development, pluripotential stem cells that are the progenitors of blood cells are formed in the yolk sac of the embryo. These hematopoietic stem cells later migrate to the fetal liver and finally, during the second trimester of gestation, to the bone marrow. After birth the bone marrow becomes the major site of hematopoiesis. As will be discussed later in this chapter, many of the blood lymphocytes also arise from cells outside the bone marrow; however, the lineage of these cells can be traced back to the bone marrow.

The developmental lineage of blood cells is depicted in Figure 5–1. Early in devel-

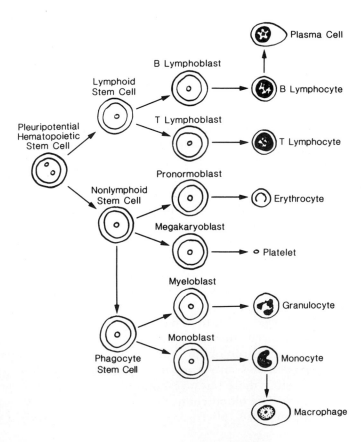

Figure 5–1. Developmental Lineage of Blood Cells.

opment there is a divergence between stem cells destined to produce lymphocytes and those destined to produce erythrocytes, platelets, and phagocytes. Phagocyte stem cells further differentiate into myeloblasts, which give rise to granulocytes, or into monoblasts, which give rise to monocytes capable of maturing into the various types of macrophages.

T Lymphocyte Development

Lymphoid stem cells diverge into two major stem cell pools that produce T lymphocytes (T cells) or B lymphocytes (B cells). T lymphocyte progenitors, called T lymphoblasts, reside in a pyramid-shaped lymphoid organ in the neck, the thymus gland. Immature T lymphocytes in the thymus are called thymocytes. Histologically the thymus contains numerous, small, round cells that are more densely packed in the outer portion of the gland, the cortex, than in the inner portion of the gland, the medulla (Fig. 5–2). There are also epithelial stromal cells in the thymus that are difficult to identify in normal glands. These cells play a major role in inducing thymocyte differentiation to T lymphocytes. Within the thymus progressive maturation of thymocytes to T

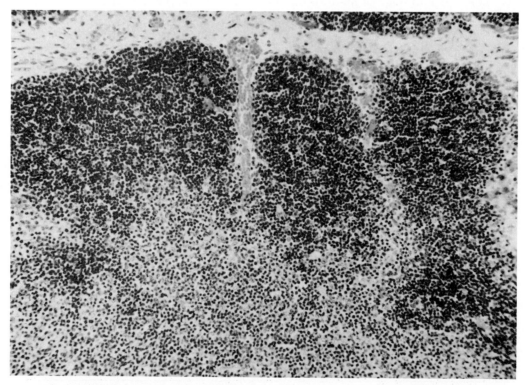

Figure 5–2. Normal Thymus. Photomicrograph of a thymus from a newborn infant showing densely packed thymocytes in the cortex and loosely arranged thymocytes in the medulla (H&E, original magnification ×100).

lymphocytes occurs. Thymocytes in the cortex are less mature than thymocytes in the medulla.

At birth the thymus gland has its greatest weight-to-body weight ratio. Although this ratio diminishes thereafter, the thymus continues to increase in size, in most people, until around puberty. Following puberty the thymus undergoes progressive involution or atrophy and is often difficult to identify in older adults.

During maturation, i.e., differentiation, thymocytes have sequential changes in the protein components of their cell membranes. In addition to receptors for nonself antigens, T lymphocytes develop receptors for two types of self-molecules called class I and class II major histocompatibility (MHC) molecules. As will be discussed in detail in Chapter 8, recognition of MHC molecules is required for T lymphocyte to respond to antigens and to interact with other cells that are participating in immune responses. T lymphocytes with different membrane receptors have different functions. T lymphocytes with class II MHC receptors assist B and T lymphocytes in responding to antigens and are therefore called helper/inducer T lymphocytes. T lymphocytes with class I MHC receptors are called suppressor/cytotoxic T lymphocytes because they suppress lymphocyte responses to antigens and can kill cells that bear antigens for which they have specific antigen receptors.

The type and stage of maturation of lymphocytes can be identified in the laboratory by characterizing lymphocyte cell-surface proteins. Antibodies that specifically react with these proteins are produced in other species that recognize the membrane proteins of human lymphocytes as foreign antigens. Table 5–1 lists some of the many antibodies that are used in clinical laboratories to identify different types of lymphocytes on the basis of surface membrane molecules (antigens).

Using such reagent antibodies, thymocytes are found to have some surface antigens (e.g., T6 and T10) not found on mature T lymphocytes. During thymic differentiation thymocytes diverge into two functionally distinct lines of cells, helper/inducer T lymphocytes and suppressor/cytotoxic T lymphocytes. These can be distinguished in

TABLE 5–1. REPRESENTATIVE LYMPHOCYTE SURFACE-MEMBRANE MOLECULES (ANTIGENS) DETECTED BY COMMERCIALLY AVAILABLE REAGENT ANTIBODIES USED FOR LYMPHOCYTE TYPING

Specificity	CD Number[a]	Commercial Source[b]		
		Coulter	*Ortho*	*BD*
Thymocytes	CD1	T6	OKT6	Leu-6
T cells	CD3	T3	OKT3	Leu-4
Helper T cells	CD4	T4	OKT4	Leu-3a
Suppressor T cells	CD8	T8	OKT8	Leu-2a
Pre-B and B cells	CD19	B4		Leu-12
B cells	CD20	B1		Leu-14

[a]*Cluster of differentiation (CD) numbers have been assigned to leukocyte antigens in an attempt to standardize nomenclature.*
[b]*Coulter Corp., Hialeah, FLA. Ortho Diagnostic Systems, Raritan, NJ. Becton-Dickenson (BD), Mountain View, CA.*

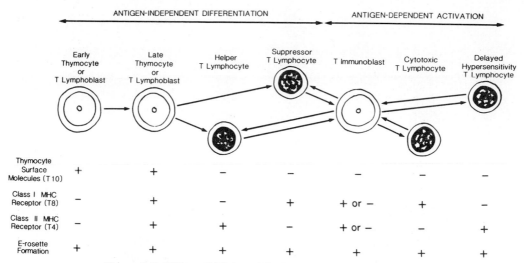

Figure 5-3. Differentiation and Activation of T Lymphocytes.

the laboratory by differences in their cell surface proteins (antigens). For example, helper/inducer T lymphocytes have T4 surface antigens, which are related to class II MHC receptors, while suppressor/cytotoxic T lymphocytes have T8 surface antigens, which are related to class I MHC receptors (Fig. 5–3). All mature T lymphocytes have T3 surface antigen, which is associated with the T lymphocyte antigen receptor. Another laboratory test often used to identify thymocytes and T lymphocytes is the E rosette assay, which is based on the ability of T lymphocytes, but not B lymphocytes, to bind to sheep erythrocytes (E) producing a rosette (Fig. 5–4). This was the first laboratory test used to identify T cells.

Differentiation in the thymus of helper and suppressor T lymphocytes from thymocytes is an antigen-independent event. This means that no foreign substance, i.e., antigen, is required to stimulate the production of T lymphocytes.

As will be discussed in more detail in Chapter 8, mature T lymphocytes can, when stimulated by specific antigen, transform into proliferating stem cell-like T immunoblasts that give rise to a clone of T lymphocyte progeny that will carry out the effects of the cell-mediated immune response.

B Lymphocyte Development

In mammals B lymphocyte differentiation occurs at sites of hematopoiesis. Thus during fetal development, B lymphocyte production initially is predominantly in the fetal liver but subsequently shifts to the bone marrow.

The earliest differentiation from lymphoid stem cells toward B lymphocytes that can be detected in the laboratory is a rearrangement of immunoglobulin genes in the chromosomes in preparation for antibody synthesis. Early in B cell differentiation there are only partial immunoglobulin molecules in the cytoplasm. Such cells with only nascent immunoglobulin-producing capabilities are called pre-B cells.

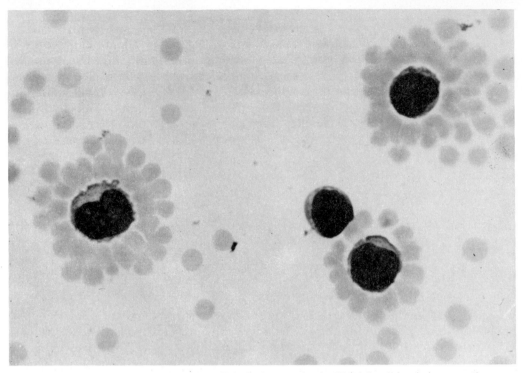

Figure 5-4. Erythocytes Rosettes. Photomicrograph of a Wright's-stained sheep erythrocyte rosette preparation showing three rosetted lymphocytes (i.e., T lymphocytes) and one nonrosetted lymphocyte (original magnification ×2000).

Mature B lymphocytes produce immunoglobulin either for insertion into the membrane to function as antigen receptors or for secretion. Therefore demonstration of immunoglobulin on the surface or in the cytoplasm of a cell is a useful laboratory procedure for identifying B lymphocytes and their precursors. Characterization of the type of immunoglobulin being produced and its site of localization in the cell (i.e., cytoplasmic or surface) is also useful in determining the degree of maturation or activation of B lymphocytes.

As depicted in Figure 5-5, there are progressive changes in immunoglobulin expression during phases of B lymphocyte antigen-independent differentiation and antigen-dependent activation. The earliest expression of complete immunoglobulin molecules is on the membranes of B lymphoblasts. There are different types (called classes) of immunoglobulin molecules, which have different biological functions. The structure and function of these various immunoglobulin classes is discussed in detail in Chapter 9. The designations for the immunoglobulin classes are IgM, IgD, IgG, IgA, and IgE. The first immunoglobulin class manufactured by B lymphocyte precursors is IgM. IgM is present on the surface of B lymphoblasts and mature unactivated B lymphocytes, where it is often also accompanied by IgD.

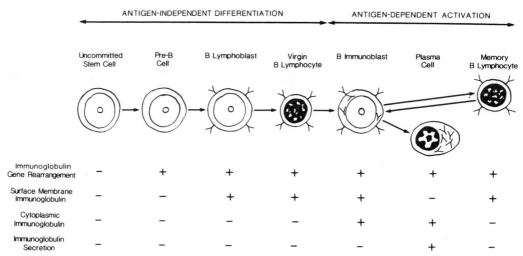

Figure 5-5. Differentiation and Activation of B Lymphocytes.

Once IgM and IgD on the surface of mature B lymphocytes bind the specific antigen that the immunoglobulin is configured to recognize, the lymphocytes transform into stem cell-like B immunoblasts. These cells give rise to immunoglobulin-secreting cells, most notably plasma cells, and memory B cells. During this transformation to plasma cells there is usually a shift in the class of immunoglobulin produced, with most plasma cells producing and secreting IgG. Thus IgG is the most common class of immunoglobulin in the circulation. In adults the serum concentration of IgG is approximately 1200 mg/dl, IgM 100 mg/dl, and IgA 200 mg/dl. The level of immunoglobulin varies with the degree of B lymphocyte activation. For example, someone who is actively combating an infectious pathogen with antibody production may have elevated serum immunoglobulin levels, i.e., hypergammaglobulinemia.

Because antibody production is antigen induced, neonates, who have been sequestered within the mother, manufacture very little immunoglobulin at birth. The major immunoglobulin in the circulation at birth is maternal IgG that has crossed the placenta from the mother's circulation. This maternal IgG is the main antibody de- fense against infection for the newborn infant. By approximately 6 months of age maternal IgG has disappeared and has been replaced by the infants own IgG. In the event that a newborn has suffered an intrauterine infection, IgM will be present in increased levels in the serum at birth. This is because the immature immune system can respond to antigen stimulation with IgM but not with IgG production.

After antigen-dependent B lymphocyte activation, some of the progeny of the proliferating B immunoblasts will develop into B lymphocytes rather than plasma cells. These so-called memory B cells often have IgG as their surface receptor rather than the IgM typical of virgin, unactivated B lymphocytes. Memory B cells are responsible for the rapid production of IgG-secreting cells that produce the accelerated anamnestic response elicited by secondary antigen exposure.

LEUKOCYTE MORPHOLOGY

In stained smears of blood the normal leukocyte cell types that can be readily distinguished morphologically are neutrophilic granulocytes, eosinophilic granulocytes, basophilic granulocytes, lymphocytes, and monocytes. These same cell types, with the addition of macrophages and plasma cells, can be identified in lymphoid tissues and at sites of inflammation, including immune-mediated inflammation. Normally neutrophilic granulocytes are the most numerous leukocyte present in the blood and at sites of antibody-mediated inflammation, while lymphocytes are most numerous in lymphoid tissues and at sites of T cell-mediated inflammation.

Granulocytes are so named because their cytoplasm contains numerous lysosomes that appear in Wright's-stained preparations as clear (neutrophilic), red (eosinophilic), or blue (basophilic) cytoplasmic granules. Mature granulocytes have lobated nuclei and are thus also referred to as polymorphonuclear leukocytes. Monocytes have cytoplasmic lysosomes, but these are less noticeable by light microscopy than are those in granulocytes. Because monocytes, and the macrophages that they mature into, do not have lobulated nuclei, they are called mononuclear phagocytes to distinguish them from polymorphonuclear phagocytes, i.e., granulocytes.

Lymphocytes in the blood have relatively dense, round nuclei and scanty cytoplasm (Fig. 5–4). They range in size from approximately 7 micrometers to around 18 micrometers. In normal adults who are not experiencing extensive lymphocyte activation, approximately 65 to 75% of blood lymphocytes display T cell markets (e.g., E rosette formation, T3 antigen), 15 to 25% B cell markers (e.g., surface membrane immunoglobulin), and the remainder have neither T nor B cell markers and are called null cells. Of the T lymphocytes, approximately twice as many are helper/inducer T cells as are suppressor/cytotoxic T cells. The different functional subtypes of lymphocytes cannot be precisely distinguished on the basis of their morphological appearance. However, there are some lymphocytes that are larger than most and have conspicuous cytoplasmic granules. These are called large granular lymphocytes (LGL). Most of these cells are null cells that are capable of killing other cells without prior exposure to antigens. These natural killer (NK) cells were discussed in Chapter 2. The cytotoxicity of NK cells differs from that of cytotoxic T cells, because the latter require specific activation by antigens.

In tissues lymphocytes can have more varied morphology when they are undergoing antigen-induced transformation into immunoblasts. During this transition transforming lymphocytes become progressively larger, and their nuclear chromatin becomes less dense as the chromosomes unravel in preparation for replication and expression of new genetic information. There is also an increase in the amount of cytoplasm. In tissues monocytes change in morphology as they mature into macrophages, which have much more cytoplasm.

DISTRIBUTION OF LYMPHOID TISSUE

Lymphoid tissue can be divided into central and peripheral lymphoid organs. Central lymphoid organs are responsible for the antigen-independent development of lymphocytes and in mammals include the thymus, fetal liver, and bone marrow. Peripheral lymphoid organs are tissues in which many lymphocytes are present and are available to undergo antigen-dependent activation and proliferation. Peripheral lymphoid organs include lymph nodes, spleen, and masses of lymphoid tissue located in the mucosa, especially that of the respiratory and gastrointestinal tracts.

Lymph nodes are positioned along lymphatic vessels that drain lymph from almost every tissue of the body. The major superficial groups of lymph nodes are the inguinal, axillary, and cervical lymph nodes. These can often be palpated, especially if the tissue from which they are receiving lymph is involved with an inflammatory disease. Major internal groups of lymph nodes include mediastinal and pulmonary hilar lymph node, receiving lymph from tissues in the thorax, and periaortic and gastrointestinal mesenteric lymph nodes, receiving lymph from abdominal tissues. Enlargement of lymph nodes is called lymphadenopathy and inflammation of lymph nodes lymphadenitis.

Mucosal lymphoid tissue is available to respond to antigens contacting the lumenal surfaces of the internal channels that communicate with the external environment, e.g., the gastrointestinal and respiratory tracts. Although there are many small foci of mucosal lymphoid tissue that cannot be identified without the aid of a microscope, there are also masses of mucosal lymphoid tissue large enough to see with the unaided eye, especially if the lymphocytes in this lymphoid tissue have been stimulated by antigen. The largest accumulations of submucosal lymphoid tissue are at the back of the oral cavity and nasopharynx, and are called the palatine tonsils, lingual tonsils, and pharyngeal tonsils (or adenoids). There are also nodules of lymphoid tissue in the small intestine, called Peyer's patches, that are largest in young children. In addition to focal accumulations of lymphoid tissue, the mucosa also has many lymphocytes scattered throughout the connective tissue just below the epithelial covering.

The function of the spleen in the blood circulatory system is similar to that of lymph nodes in the lymph circulatory system. It is a major site of phagocytosis and immune response to antigens in the blood. As such the spleen contains numerous mononuclear phagocytes and many T and B lymphocytes organized so that they come into contact with blood as it percolates through the many sinuses of the spleen.

Because lymphocytes are in the blood and lymph, they are continually circulating throughout all the tissues of the body and are thus available to afford a widespread defense against foreign substances. The number of lymphocytes in a given tissue often dramatically increases when that tissue is intensely or persistently challenged with antigen. When this occurs in lymphoid tissue, e.g., a lymph node, it is called lymphoid hyperplasia, and when it occurs at sites where lymphocytes are normally not numerous, it is called chronic inflammation.

LYMPH NODE STRUCTURE

Lymph nodes are masses of lymphoid tissue with compartmentalization of lymphocytes according to their function (Fig. 5–6). When lymph nodes are examined microscopically, the component parts vary from node to node with respect to proportions and configurations, dictated in large part by the degree of antigen stimulation.

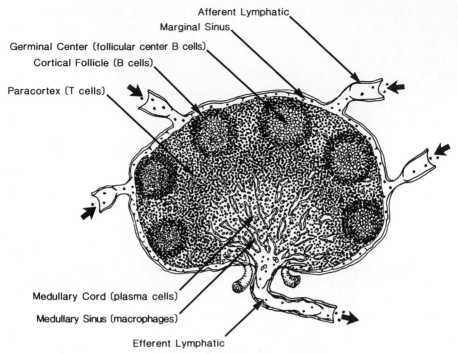

Figure 5-6. Diagram of Lymph Node Architecture.

Lymph from tissue enters lymph nodes through afferent lymphatics that empty into subcapsular or marginal sinuses lined by macrophages. The cortex is the outermost region of a lymph node and contains spherical accumulations of B lymphocytes called follicles (Fig. 5–7).

The location of different types of lymphocytes in tissue can be determined in the laboratory by reacting sections of tissue with labeled antibodies specific for proteins on the surface of lymphocytes. The label can be a fluorochrome that is observed by fluorescence microscopy or an enzyme that produces a colored product that can be observed by light microscopy. Figure 5–8 shows tissue from lymph node cortex that has been reacted with enzyme-labeled antibodies specific for B lymphocyte surface-membrane immunoglobulin (IgM, panel A) or for a T lymphocyte membrane protein (T3 antigen, panel B). This demonstrates that follicles contain predominantly B lymphocytes, while interfollicular tissue contains predominantly T lymphocytes.

Follicles are the sites where B lymphocytes, after antigen stimulation, undergo transformation into immunoblasts. Transformation occurs at the center of a follicle, producing a pale zone called a germinal center (Fig. 5–7). This pale-staining zone is due to the stimulated lymphocytes with enlarged nuclei and less dense chromatin as compared to the unstimulated lymphocytes surrounding them. B lymphocytes within germinal centers are called follicular center cells. Follicular center cells transform into B immunoblasts that in turn produce plasma cells, which secrete immunoglobulin. In

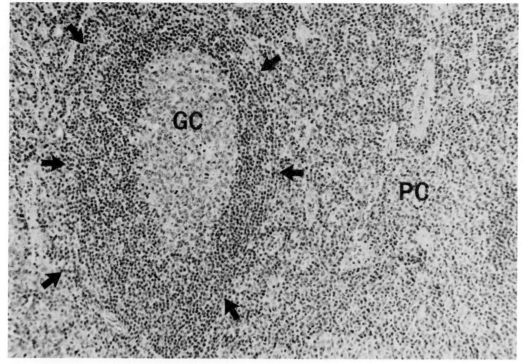

Figure 5-7. Lymph Node Cortex. Photomicrograph of a portion of lymph node cortex showing paracortex on the right (PC) containing T lymphocytes and cortex on the left with a B lymphocyte follicle (*arrows*) having a pale germinal center (GC) (H&E, original magnification × 100).

lymph nodes plasma cells are most numerous in the medulla. The medulla is continuous with the hilum, where the efferent lymphatic vessel receives lymph exiting from the lymph node. Plasma cells are in cords of tissue lying between a network of medullary sinuses lined by macrophages (Fig. 5-9). Plasma cells are therefore in a strategic location for releasing antibodies into the lymph that is exiting the node in route to the systematic circulation.

Between the cortex and medulla is the paracortex (Fig. 5-7), which is particularly rich in T lymphocytes. T lymphocytes are also predominant in the interfollicular areas of the cortex (Fig. 5-8). T lymphocytes can undergo antigen-induced transformation into T immunoblasts, but this occurs throughout the paracortex and not within discrete germinal centers, as is the case for B lymphocyte transformation.

When there has been extensive antigen stimulation of T lymphocytes in a lymph node, for example, due to viral infection, there will be expansion (i.e., hyperplasia) of the paracortical zone. When there has been extensive antigen stimulation of B lymphocytes, for example, due to bacterial infection, there will be marked enlargment (i.e., hyperplasia) of the cortical germinal centers and numerous medullary plasma cells. Stimulation of macrophages will result in expansion of marginal and medullary si-

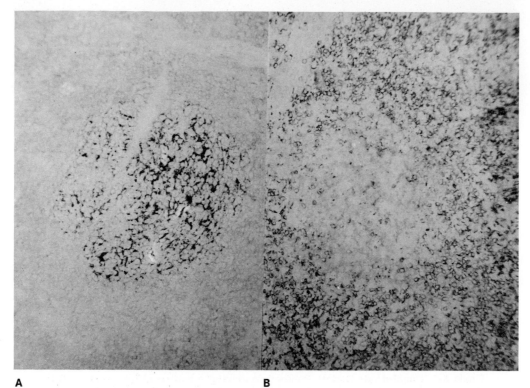

A   B

Figure 5–8. Lymph Node Immunostaining. Sections of lymph node cortex stained with
(A) enzyme-labeled antibodies specific for B lymphocyte surface membrane immunoglobulin (IgM) or, **(B)** a T lymphocyte surface membrane protein (T3 antigen) (immunoperoxidase stain, original magnification ×200). In **A,** B lymphocytes in a follicle are staining
but not interfollicular cells. In **B,** T lymphocytes are staining in the interfollicular area,
but only a minority of the cells in the follicle are staining.

nuses by masses of macrophages, a process called sinus histiocytosis. Lymphoid hyperplasia results in lymphadenopathy.

In addition to macrophages and lymphocytes, lymph nodes also contain another
cell type that is involved in immune responses. These cells are called dendritic cells
and reticulum cells and may be related to macrophages. These cells are named after
the long, narrow extensions of their cytoplasm, dendrites, that extend outward to en-
velop many adjacent lymphocytes. Like macrophages, they participate in the recognition of antigens by B and T lymphocytes, primarily by presenting antigens to lymphocytes in a way that will optimally stimulate lymphocyte activation. Because of this role
macrophages and dendritic cells are called accessory cells of the immune response or
antigen-presenting cells. There are at least two major types of dendritic cells in lymph
nodes, one that acts as accessory cells for B lymphocytes and one for T lymphocytes.
As would be expected, the former, called follicular dendritic reticulum cells, are in

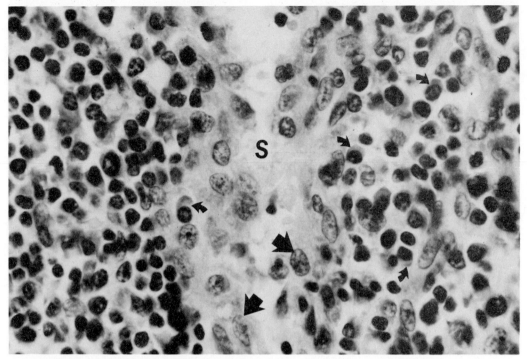

Figure 5-9. Lymph Node Medulla. Photomicrograph of lymph node medulla showing a sinus (S) lined by macrophages (*large arrows*). The medullary cords adjacent to the sinus contain numerous plasma cells (*small arrows*) that secrete antibodies into the lymph exiting the lymph node through the sinus (H&E, original magnification ×1000).

germinal centers, and the latter, called interdigitating reticulum cells, are primarily in the paracortex.

Lymphocytes can enter lymph nodes through both afferent lymphatics and small blood vessels. The blood vessels through which lymphocytes enter are the postcapillary venules. These vessels are lined by a special type of tall endothelial cells for which lymphocytes have a receptor. Thus there is a specific interaction between lymphocytes and lymph node–postcapillary venule–"high" endothelial cells that results in passage of lymphocytes from blood into lymph nodes.

EXTRANODAL LYMPHOID TISSUE STRUCTURE

Extranodal lymphoid tissue often has many of the functional compartments found in lymph nodes. Histologically the palatine, lingual, and pharyngeal tonsils resemble lymph nodes (Fig. 5–10). Because this lymphoid tissue that is immediately beneath the oropharyngeal mucosal epithelium is constantly challenged with environmental

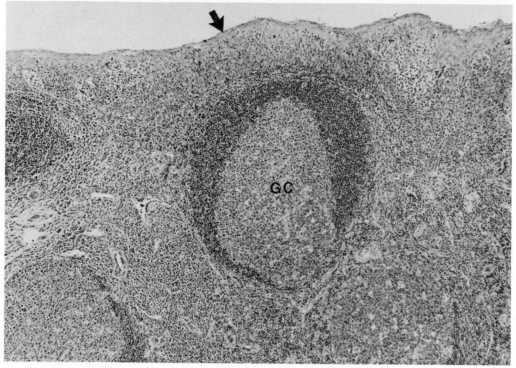

Figure 5-10. Tonsil. Photomicrograph of a tonsil showing lymphoid tissue, including follicles with germinal centers (GC), covered by oropharyngeal mucosa (*arrow*) (H&E, original magnification ×75).

antigens, including many microorganisms, it typically has numerous large germinal centers. When the tonsils are markedly enlarged, especially in association with acute inflammation (tonsillitis), they may interfere with swallowing, breathing, or hearing (because of eustachian tube obstruction).

The Peyer's patches of the small intestine also often have large germinal centers. In general Peyer's patches have a B lymphocyte zone farthest from the intestinal lumen, a T lymphocyte zone nearest the lumen, and a covering of specialized, flattened epithelium that may be specially structured for antigen processing. Peyer's patches are most conspicuous in young children and when there is inflammation of the small intestine, for example, in typhoid fever.

Mucosal and submucosal lymphoid tissue in the lungs rarely contains germinal centers and has a predominance of T lymphocytes.

IgA is the class of immunoglobulins that can be most readily secreted onto mucosal surfaces and is thus also called secretory IgA. Secreted IgA is often synthesized and released by mucosal and submucosal plasma cells, either in lymphoid tissue or in the lamina propria. Secretion is facilitated by the addition to IgA of a polypeptide, secretory piece made by the mucosal epithelial cells. IgA in the mucus acts as a front line of defense against antigens that contact the mucous membranes of the body.

SPLEEN STRUCTURE

The spleen is a relatively oval organ in the left upper quadrant of the abdomen, attached to the tail of the pancreas. In adults it is normally approximately 11 cm long, 7 cm wide, and 4 cm thick and weighs approximately 150 g. Arteries enter and veins exit the spleen in one area, the hilum, adjacent to the pancreas.

The splenic tissue is divided into two major components that can be seen on its cut surfaces, the red pulp and the white pulp. The white pulp, also called malpighian follicles, is composed of masses of lymphoid tissue surrounding arteries (Fig. 5–11). These periarteriolar lymphoid sheaths include a circumferential cuff of T lymphocytes, with intermittent eccentric follicles of B lymphocytes. Upon antigen stimulation

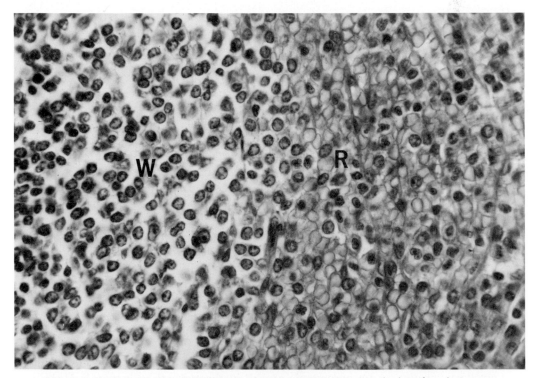

Figure 5–11. Spleen. Photomicrograph of spleen tissue showing the interface between white pulp (W) rich in lymphocytes and red pulp (R) with an admixture of red blood cells, lymphocytes, and macrophages (H&E, original magnification ×900).

T lymphocyte cuffs expand, and B lymphocyte follicles develop germinal centers. The spleen red pulp (Fig. 5–11) is composed of many blood-filled vascular sinusoids lined by discontinuous endothelium and intervening cords (the cords of Billroth) containing numerous macrophages. Much of the substance of the splenic red pulp is occupied by blood that is passing through the sinusoids and cords. As blood passes through the spleen, blood cells and material in the plasma come into intimate contact with many macrophages of the red pulp. The spleen thus serves as a "filter" for the blood, clearing from the circulation, by macrophage phagocytosis, both particulate and cellular debris.

The spleen is a major site for marshalling immune responses to blood-borne and other antigenic stimuli. The marginal zone of periarteriolar sheaths is where most lymphocytes enter and exit and white pulp from the blood and is also where antigen recognition occurs.

Splenic enlargement, splenomegaly, can result from engorgement with blood, for example, secondary to congestive heart failure, or can be due to lymphoid hyperplasia, for example, secondary to the immune response to EBV during infectious mononucleosis or phagocytosis of erythrocytes during autoimmune hemolytic anemia.

LYMPHOID ECOSYSTEMS

Lymphoid tissues contain all of the cellular components necessary to mount immune responses to antigens. Lymphoid tissues are strategically positioned so that they will encounter antigens within the body. For example, lymph nodes straddle lymphatic vessels, splenic lymphoid tissue is in contact with blood percolating through the spleen, and mucosal lymphoid tissue is adjacent to surfaces that are in contact with environmental antigens. Immunocompetent lymphocytes are continually moving throughout the tissues of the body and intermittently returning (homing) to lymphoid tissues where they can "communicate" with other lymphoid cells to amplify immune responses to antigens that have been recognized as foreign.

As described in this chapter, the various functionally distinct types of cells are structurally arranged in lymphoid tissues so that the complex interactions required to mount immune responses are facilitated. For example, in lymph nodes, follicles contain not only B lymphocytes but also follicular dendritic reticulum cells that are accessory cells for antigen recognition. T lymphocytes, which are regulators of B lymphocyte responses, are scattered within follicles and are numerous in the interfollicular areas. Lymph, which contains soluble antigens from the tissues, enters lymph nodes through the marginal sinus and thus contacts both cortical follicular B cells and interfollicular T cells.

The paracortex is particularly suited for T lymphocyte responses. T lymphocytes, which are the major lymphocyte circulating in the blood, enter lymph nodes through postcapillary venules in the paracortex as well as through afferent lymph. Here they can interact with the major T lymphocyte accessory cells, the interdigitating reticulum cells that assist T cells in responding to antigens.

   Macrophages lining the sinuses are in a good position to phagocytose lymph-borne particulate debris and opsonized antigen (i.e., antigens coated with antibodies and/or complement components that facilitate phagocytosis by macrophages). Macrophages within the follicles and paracortex, in addition to assisting in antigen recognition, also phagocytose cell debris generated by the high turnover rate of lymphocytes. Macrophages containing lymphocyte cell debris are particularly conspicuous in areas of lymphocyte hyperplasia.

   Thus rather than being a random admixture of various types of lymphocytes, macrophages, dendritic cells, lymphatic sinuses, and blood vessels, lymphoid tissues are highly organized, functionally compartmentalized organs. Lymphoid tissues are structured for optimum afferent activation of lymphocytes and for efficient efferent delivery to the circulation of the products of lymphocyte activation (e.g., antibodies, lymphokines, specific lymphocytes).

Discussion of the Illustrative Case

The case presented at the beginning of this chapter shows how recognition of lymphoid tissue hyperplasia and serologic identification of the specificity of an immune response can be used to diagnose a disease. This patient was infected with EBV. This virus invaded B lymphocytes and stimulated both a humoral (B lymphocyte) and cell-mediated (T lymphocyte) immune response. B lymphocyte activation resulted in the production of heterophil antibodies and specific antibodies to EBV. T lymphocyte transformation is evidenced by the "atypical" lymphocytes in the blood smear. These were T lymphocytes that had undergone transformation into large blast-like cells after stimulation by viral antigens. The lymphocytosis, tonsillar enlargement, lymphadenopathy, and splenomegaly were due to B and T lymphocyte hyperplasia within lymphoid tissues.

   The diagnosis of infectious mononucleosis led to no specific treatment, since none is known for this typically self-limited disease. However, the specific serologic findings and the absence of evidence for a streptococcal infection, ruled out other diseases in the differential diagnosis, for example, streptococcal pharyngitis and adult toxoplasmosis. This prevented unnecessary antibiotic therapy, which might have produced a hypersensitivity to the drug that would have prevented its use in the future when it could have been beneficial for that individual.

QUESTIONS

1. Detail the antigen-independent embryonic development of T and B lymphocytes.
2. What structural changes take place in lymphocytes after they have been stimulated by antigen in the presence of accessory cells? Why?
3. How would the structure of a lymph node with extensive B lymphocyte activation differ from that of a lymph node with predominantly T lymphocyte activation? Why?

4. The histologic appearance of a tonsil is most like that of what other tissue in the body? Why?

5. Why do patients with infectious mononucleosis have lymphadenopathy, splenomegaly, and tonsillar enlargement?

6. What are two major types of accessory cells in lymph nodes, where are they, and what do they do?

6 Immune Deficiencies and Laboratory Methods for Diagnosis

OBJECTIVES

1. To explain the diagnostic nomenclature system for immune deficiency diseases.
2. To review the laboratory technology used to evaluate immune deficiency diseases.
3. To describe the clinical and laboratory characteristics of the major forms of primary and secondary immune deficiency.

Illustrative Case

A male infant had no problems until about 5 months of age when he developed a fever, cough, and irritability. He was seen by a physician who diagnosed otitis media and bronchitis caused by *Hemophilus influenzae*. The child was treated with appropriate antibiotics and improved. The fever and cough did not completely resolve, however, and within two weeks he developed even worse respiratory problems than before, including much sputum production. Repeat evaluation revealed streptococcal pneumonia in addition to bronchitis and otitis media. These infections improved with antibiotic therapy but did not completely resolve during the subsequent 5 months. At 8 months of age the child developed diarrhea and steatorrhea. The infant's growth rate was noted to have plateaued. *Giardia* trophozoites and cysts were identified in fecal specimens. At 10 months of age, a serum protein electrophoresis showed a virtual absence of gamma globulins. This prompted a more extensive immunologic evaluation. Serum immunoglobulin quantitation demonstrated 75 mg/dl IgG and undetectable levels of IgM, IgA, IgE, and IgD. There were normal numbers of blood T lymphocytes, and these showed normal mitogen stimulation. No B (surface immunoglobulin positive) lymphocytes were identified in the blood.

CLASSIFICATION OF IMMUNE DEFICIENCIES

Defects in the normal development, maturation, or function of the immune system can produce *immune deficiencies*. As a consequence of the great complexity of the immune system, innumerable defects can occur, producing a wide spectrum of immune deficiency diseases. Figure 6–1 depicts a number of sites in lymphocyte development where defects would produce immune deficiencies. The components of the immune system that would be deficient would depend upon the site at which lymphocyte development was disturbed. Depending upon the nature of the defect, the immune deficiency may be so mild that it produces no symptoms and is only identified during screening laboratory testing, or it may be so severe that it leads to multiple uncontrollable infections and death in early infancy.

The multiplicity of immune deficiency syndromes is so great that it defies precise categorization. Although some relatively discrete immune deficiency diseases are recognized, the classification systems that are used to diagnose many immune deficiency states employ categories that encompass related but not identical immune deficiency diseases. The diversity of possible immune defects sometimes gives the impression that no two immune-deficient patients have exactly the same abnormalities. Nevertheless each patient must be diagnostically categorized on the basis of clinical and laboratory data so that medical management based on the experience previously gained with similarly diagnosed patients can proceed.

Classification of immune deficiency diseases is based both on the time when the

Figure 6-1. Immune Deficiencies. Diagram of lymphocyte development and activation showing sites at which defects would produce different types of immune deficiency. A defect at (*1*) would produce reticular dysgenesis, at (*2*) combined immune deficiency, at (*3*) cellular immune deficiency, at (*4*) humoral immune deficiency, at (*5*) selective immunoglobulin deficiency (e.g., IgA deficiency) and at (*6*) selective cellular immune deficiency (e.g., chronic mucocutaneous candidiasis).

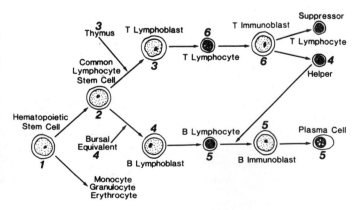

defect develops and on the extent of immune dysfunction (Table 6–1). When the immune system defect develops during gestation and is present at birth, it is called a *congenital* or *primary* immune deficiency. Some congenital immune deficiencies are hereditary, that is, a genetic defect was inherited by the infant from one or both parents. Other congenital immune deficiencies are not inherited. These can result from genetic abnormalities occurring in the gametes or zygote but not present in the genome of the parents. If the affected individual survives to reproductive age, this genetic defect can then be passed on to children. More commonly immune deficiencies that are not inherited develop as a result of some noxious influence in utero that alters the normal ontogeny of the immune system in the embryo or fetus but does not alter the genome and therefore cannot be passed on genetically.

When the immune system is normal at birth and a defect develops at a later time, it is called an *acquired* or *secondary* immune deficiency. Acquired immune deficiencies can be induced by a wide variety of processes, including infections, malignant neoplasms, systemic diseases, irradiation, and certain drugs. The distinction between a secondary (acquired) and a primary (congenital) immune deficiency is sometimes difficult to make because some primary defects do not become apparent until months or even years after birth. For example, *common variable immune deficiency* is currently considered to be a primary immunodeficiency caused by a congenital immune system defect, but the clinical manifestations of this disease do not become apparent until adulthood. Thus the age at onset of symptoms of immune deficiency is not the only criterion for distinguishing primary from secondary immune system defects. A knowledge of the typical time course of each type of primary immune deficiency must also be considered.

TABLE 6-1. CLASSIFICATION OF IMMUNE DEFICIENCY DISEASES

Primary (Congenital)	Secondary (Acquired)
Combined immune deficiencies	Infection associated
Reticular dysgenesis	Malignancy associated
Severe X-linked	Systemic disease associated
Severe autosomal recessive	Drug induced
Partial (Nezelof's syndrome)	Irradiation induced
With enzyme deficiencies	Splenectomy induced
With thymoma	Malnutrition induced
Ataxia–telangiectasia	Excessive antibody and lymphocyte loss
Wiskott–Aldrich syndrome	Nephrotic syndrome
With short-limbed dwarfism	Lymphangiectasia
Cellular immune deficiencies	Gastroenteropathy
Thymic hypoplasia or aplasia	
Chronic mucocutaneous candidiasis	
Humoral immune deficiencies	
Agammaglobulinemia	
Hypogammaglobulinemia	
Selective immunoglobulin deficiencies	
Common variable immune deficiency	

Classification of immune deficiencies is also based on the components of the immune system that are deficient. The designation *combined immune deficiency* indicates that both B lymphocyte function (humoral immunity) and T lymphocyte function (cellular immunity) are impaired. A *cellular immune deficiency* has predominantly T lymphocyte dysfunction, and an *antibody* or *humoral immune deficiency* has mainly impaired B lymphocyte function.

Impairment of cellular immunity results in increased susceptibility primarily to viral and fungal infections, whereas impairment of humoral immunity is most detrimental to defense against bacteria. However, because the components of the immune system function in concert, primary impairment of one component often has secondary effects on other components. For example, deficient helper T lymphocyte function could result in deficient antibody production. Thus laboratory analysis of immune deficiencies often produces evidence of complex defects. Only careful evaluation of the data and a knowledge of the kinds of immune deficiency diseases will result in an appropriate diagnosis.

Before beginning a detailed discussion of the major types of immune deficiencies, another kind of deficient immune defense should be mentioned. This is the impaired immune system function that can result from defects that do not directly effect lymphocyte development but do result in deficiencies of cells or mediators that are required for effective lymphocyte function. For example, impaired macrophage and dendritic cell function will lead to poor antigen recognition and resultant inadequate immune response. Impaired macrophage and granulocyte phagocytic or killing function will result in impaired defense against certain microorganisms, producing, in effect, a deficient immune defense. Deficiencies of components of macromolecular mediator systems can also lead to impaired immune defense. The best known examples of this are complement–component deficiencies. Because complement plays a complementary role in immune elimination of microorganisms, complement deficiencies can lead to impaired defense against infections. Phagocyte defects were discussed in Chapter 2, and complement deficiencies will be discussed in detail in Chapter 10.

LABORATORY TESTS FOR DIAGNOSING IMMUNE DEFICIENCY DISEASES

The laboratory methods required to perform the tests mentioned in this chapter are discussed in greater detail in Chapters 8 and 9. Laboratory tests for identifying and characterizing immune deficiencies can be divided into those that assess B lymphocyte function and those that assess T lymphocyte function (Table 6–2).

Laboratory Tests for B Lymphocyte Function

Because antibody production is a major consequence of normal B lymphocyte functioning, quantitative and qualitative evaluation of antibodies in the serum can be a useful index of B lymphocyte immune competency. Normal immunoglobulin levels vary with age and with the degree of immune stimulation. This is also true of the

TABLE 6-2. LABORATORY TESTS FOR DIAGNOSING IMMUNE DEFICIENCY DISEASES

Evaluating Humoral Immunity	Evaluating Cellular Immunity
Serum protein electrophoresis	Delayed hypersensitivity skin testing
Serum protein immunoelectro-phoresis	Contact hypersensitivity development
	T lymphocyte quantitation
Immunoglobulin class and subclass quantitation	T lymphocyte antigen phenotyping
	T lymphocyte nonspecific mitogen stimulation
Isohemagglutinin quantitation	T lymphocyte specific antigen stimulation
Specific immune antibody quantitation	T lymphocyte allogeneic cell stimulation
B lymphocyte quantitation	
B lymphocyte antigen phenotyping	
B lymphocyte mitogen stimulation	

normal levels of other components of the immune system. Evaluation of the gamma globulin fraction of a serum protein electrophoresis can identify gross abnormalities in immunoglobulin production, such as *agammaglobulinemia* (complete absence of immunoglobulins) are marked *hypogammaglobulinemia* (reduction in the concentration of immunoglobulins). Serum protein immunoelectrophoresis can demonstrate the selective absence or reduction of a specific immunoglobulin class or subclass. More precise quantitation of immunoglobulins is accomplished by techniques such as radial immunodiffusion, nephelometry, radioimmunoassay (RIA), or enzymoimmunoassay. Serum IgG, IgA, and IgM can be quantified by any of these methods, but serum IgE is usually at such a low concentration that only the last two methods have adequate sensitivity to measure it. Quantitation of specific immunoglobulin classes and even subclasses is required to identify selective immunoglobulin deficiencies. Serum levels of IgD, which functions primarily as a B lymphocyte surface receptor, are not routinely determined in clinical immunology laboratories.

The immunoglobulin assays mentioned so far quantify immunoglobulin without regard for the specificity of their antigen-binding sites. When evaluating immune deficiency diseases, it is sometimes important to not only show that antibodies are present but to also document that specific antibodies can be made in response to antigen exposure. A readily available test for specific antibody production is evaluation of isohemagglutinins, for example, anti-A and anti-B blood group antibodies. In most individuals these antibodies are predominantly IgM, thus their evaluation is primarily an assay for IgM-producing capacity. The age and blood group of the patient must be taken into consideration when evaluating isohemagglutinin data. Specific antibody production in response to routine immunizations can also be measured. In children who have been immunized to protect against tetanus and diphtheria, serum antibodies specific for the vaccine antigens can be measured as an index of the ability to mount a humoral immune response to an antigen challenge. Patients can be immunized for the purpose of measuring specific antibody production. Immunization with a live virus, however, should never be attempted in an individual suspected of having an immune deficiency.

Direct quantitative and qualitative analysis of circulating or tissue B lymphocytes can be useful in evaluating some immune deficiency diseases. In addition to a routine total lymphocyte count, B and T lymphocytes can be specifically counted. In the past this was often done by observing the proportion of lymphocytes that formed rosettes with sheep red blood cells (SRBC) or with SRBC coated with IgG, with or without complement. T lymphocytes, but not B lymphocytes, are able to bind and form rosettes with normal uncoated SRBC. B lymphocytes do not have receptors for and do not bind to normal SRBC, but they do have surface receptors for IgG (Fc receptors) and complement (e.g., C3b receptors, CR1). B lymphocytes therefore bind to and form rosettes with SRBC coated with antibody or with antibody and complement. The percentage rosetted cells is determined under a light microscope and the number of B and T lymphocytes calculated.

Rosetting assays are being replaced by assays that evaluate lymphocyte surface antigens that are characteristic for specific lymphocyte types. These assays use antibodies that are specific for the lymphocyte surface antigens. Some of the most frequently used antibodies were discussed in Chapter 5 and were listed in Table 5–1. Many of these reagent antibodies are monoclonal antibodies produced by mouse hybridoma cells. The reagent antibodies are labeled with a fluorochrome or enzyme so that they can be detected on the surface of lymphocytes that bear the antigen for which the antibody has specificity. Lymphocytes with bound antibodies can be counted manually using a microscope or automatically using an automated cell sorter.

The first lymphocyte surface antigen used as a marker was the surface immunoglobulin displayed by B lymphocytes. Lymphocytes bearing endogenously produced immunoglobulin are by definition B lymphocytes. As with serum immunoglobulins, B lymphocyte membrane immunoglobulin class and subclass can be determined and may be abnormal in certain immune deficiency diseases. Analysis of T lymphocyte surface markers is useful not only for counting total numbers of T lymphocytes but also for assessing the proportions of functionally different T lymphocyte subsets.

Laboratory evaluation of in vitro B lymphocyte responses to certain stimuli can also yield useful information about immune deficiencies. Blast transformation or lymphokine production in response to specific antigens or nonspecific mitogens can be measured. Such assays are most often used in clinical immunology laboratories to evaluate T lymphocyte function and will be discussed briefly in the following and also in Chapter 8.

Pathologic evaluation of tissue biopsies can contribute to the diagnostic evaluation of immune deficiency diseases. As was detailed in Chapter 5, the architecture of lymph nodes is determined by the functional status of lymphocytes.

Individuals with B lymphocyte deficiencies often have small or absent cortical follicles. Individuals with T lymphocyte deficiencies have lymphocyte-depleted paracortical and interfollicular regions. As with circulating lymphocytes, the lymphocytes in lymph nodes can be analyzed for surface membrane markers to assess the distribution of lymphocyte subpopulations.

Biopsy of other tissues can also be useful. The mucosa of the gut normally contains antibody-producing plasma cells, but these may be absent in an individual with a humoral immune deficiency. This is detected by a small bowel biopsy.

Laboratory Tests for T Lymphocyte Function

The most readily available and technically simple assay of cellular immunity is the *delayed type hypersensitivity (DTH) skin test*. This is a measure of T lymphocyte response to an intradermally injected antigen. If T lymphocytes recognize the antigen, they recruit lymphocytes and macrophages to the injection site, producing, after approximately 24 to 48 hours, a hard knot in the skin that is called an area of *induration*. Induration greater than 5 mm in diameter is generally considered to be positive evidence for cellular immunity against the injected antigen. A humoral immune response to the injected antigen may also occur, resulting in vascular alterations that produce a reddened area in the skin called *erythema*. The extent of erythema is not a measure of cellular immunity. Delayed hypersensitivity skin testing is not effective in children under 1 year old.

There are certain antigens that most adults and many children will have been exposed to, normally resulting in the development of cellular immunity. These antigens usually come from common microorganisms, such as mumps virus, Candida, trichophyton, histoplasma and mycobacteria, and tetanus toxoid. Such antigens are used for DTH skin testing. Individuals with cellular immune deficiencies will not develop (primary defect) or will lose (acquired defect) the ability to mount a cellular immune response to challenge with these antigens and thus will have negative DTH skin tests. Failure to respond to antigen challenge is called *anergy*.

Evaluation of the development of cutaneous contact hypersensitivity following the first exposure to an antigen is a measure of the primary cellular immune response. A commonly used substance is the chemical dinitrochlorobenzene (DNCB). DNCB is a hapten and becomes immunogenic when it complexes with proteins in the skin. In immunologically intact individuals, re-exposure to DNCB two or more weeks after an initial exposure will result in dermal inflammation at the site of application. As with other forms of contact dermatitis, such as that induced by poison ivy or jewelry, erythema, vesicles (small blisters), and slight induration occur at the application site.

T lymphocytes have a great deal of functional heterogeneity that is reflected in the expression of different surface antigens by different functional subsets. For instance, helper T lymphocytes and suppressor T lymphocytes can be distinguished by their unique surface antigens (see Table 5–1). The repertoire of antigens on the surface of a cell is called its *antigen phenotype*, and the process of identifying the antigens that are present is called *antigen phenotyping*. As will be discussed later in this chapter, antigen phenotyping is important in the laboratory evaluation of some cellular immune deficiency diseases, for example, AIDS.

Functional status of T lymphocytes can also be tested in vitro. The most widely used in vitro tests for T lymphocyte function evaluate blast transformation in response to specific antigens or, more commonly, nonspecific mitogens. After recognition of antigen, lymphocytes with small, dense nuclei undergo transformation into blasts with large nuclei having loosely arranged chromatin. This blast transformation prepares the lymphocyte for expression of additional genetic information and for replication, both of which will be required for an effective immune response. In addition to spe-cific antigen recognition, there are substances that can induce polyclonal lymphocyte blast transformation and proliferation independent of the antigen-recognition proc-ess. Such substances are called *mitogens*.

The mitogens most commonly used for in vitro lymphocyte stimulation tests are phytohemagglutinin (PHA), concanavilin A (Con A) and pokeweed mitogen (PWM). PHA and Con A preferentially stimulate T lymphocytes, while PWM stimulates both T and B lymphocytes. Antigen-specific in vitro T lymphocyte blastogenesis can be stim-ulated using the same antigens as those employed for delayed hypersensitivity skin testing. Extracts of the common fungus *Candida albicans* is an antigen frequently used in T lymphycyte in vitro stimulation studies. Response to in vitro exposure of lympho-cytes to antigens or mitogens can be measured by a variety of techniques. The simplest but least accurate is to count the proportion of blasts that appear in a population of lymphocytes after exposure to the stimulus. Currently most laboratory procedures as-sess blastogenesis by measuring the incorporation of radiolabeled thymidine into lymphocyte DNA. Blasts actively synthesize DNA and thus incorporate radiolabeled thymidine into their nuclei.

COMBINED IMMUNE DEFICIENCY DISEASES

The most profound deficiency of leukocytes is *reticular dysgenesis*. Individuals with this congenital defect are deficient in lymphocytes, granulocytes, and mononuclear phago-cytes. Blood smears show marked leukopenia. This disease appears to result from a developmental defect at the differentiation level of the hematopoietic stem cell that gives rise to all types to leukocytes (Fig. 6–1). This disease is not compatible with ex-trauterine survival.

Other forms of combined immune deficiency have defects in T and B lympho-cytes but normal phagocyte populations. There are two genetically distinct forms of *severe combined immune deficiency* (SCID), one inherited by an X-linked pattern and the other by an autosomal recessive pattern (Swiss type). SCID can also occur in patients with no family history of immune deficiency. The developmental defect causing SCID is putatively in the common lymphoid stem cell that gives rise to both T and B lympho-cytes (Fig. 6–1). Histologic examination of the thymus reveals a marked reduction in thymocytes (Figs. 6–2 and 6–3), presumably due to lack of bone marrow generation of precursor cells that normally would have gone to the thymus to take up residence as proliferating thymocytes. This morphological abnormality is called *thymic dysplasia*.

Because of severe impairment of both cellular and humoral immunity, untreated SCID patients almost always die of overwhelming infections within the first year of life. They are susceptible to infections with all types of pathogens, but oral infection with Candida, pneumonia due to *Pneumocystis carinii*, and systemic cytomegalovirus infection are particularly common. Persistent diarrhea and otitis media are also char-acteristic. The greatest threat from bacteria occurs after the first few months of life, when maternal IgG that crossed the placenta during gestation has dwindled away. The therapy most often used in SCID patients is bone marrow transplantation in an at-

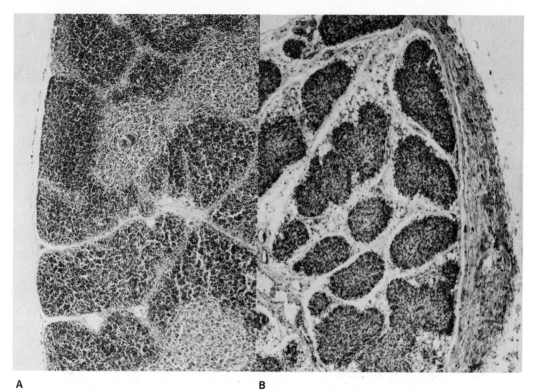

A   B

Figure 6-2. Thymic Dysplasia. Low magnification photomicrographs of a normal (**A**) and dysplastic (**B**) thymus. Note the demarcation between cortex and medulla in the normal but not the dysplastic thymus. The lobules of the dysplastic thymus are much smaller because of the paucity of thymocytes (H&E, original magnification ×100).

tempt to supply the absent lymphoid stem cells. A major complication that can arise from this therapy is a *graft versus host* (GVH) reaction, in which the transplanted immunocompetent lymphoid cells attack the tissues of the immunodeficient recipient.

SCID patients are sometimes said to have *lymphopenic agammaglobulinemia* because laboratory evaluation usually reveals a marked reduction in numbers of blood lymphocytes and a virtual absence of immunoglobulins (once maternal IgG is lost). When lymphocytes can be identified in the blood, they have abnormal antigen phenotypes, often expressing immature rather than mature surface markers.

PARTIAL COMBINED IMMUNE DEFICIENCY (NEZELOF'S SYNDROME)

Some individuals with combined immune deficiency have more severe T lymphocyte than B lymphocyte defects. A number of terms are used to designate this deficiency,

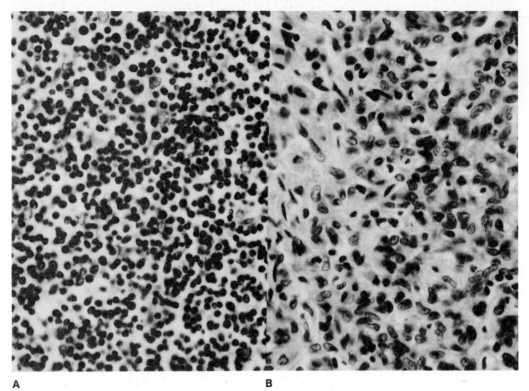

A   B

Figure 6-3. Thymic Dysplasia. High magnification photomicrograph of a normal (**A**) and dysplastic (**B**) thymus. Note the paucity of thymocytes and predominance of stromal cells in the dysplastic compared to the normal thymus (H&E, original magnification ×550).

including *Nezelof's syndrome*. The T lymphocyte defects are variable in these individuals, ranging from moderate to as severe as those in SCID patients. They have thymic dysplasia, suggesting an abnormality in bone marrow-derived thymocyte precursors. The number of T lymphocytes in the blood is usually reduced. In vitro stimulation of T lymphocytes by antigens and mitogens is depressed. There is a less severe B lymphocyte defect. The number of blood and tissue B lymphocytes is normal. Serum immunoglobulins can be normal, decreased, or increased. The distribution of immunoglobulin classes may be abnormal. Specific antibody production to antigen challenge is defective. Some patients lack isohemagglutinins. Nezelof's patients are susceptible to overwhelming infections with all types of microorganisms but to a lesser degree than SCID patients. It is not uncommon for Nezelof's patients to survive into later childhood. Long-term survival in this and many other forms of immune deficiency disease is associated with the development of malignant neoplasms, especially lymphoid neoplasms.

COMBINED IMMUNE DEFICIENCY ASSOCIATED WITH OTHER ABNORMALITIES

A minority of patients with combined immune deficiency have identifiable enzyme defects. Approximately half the patients with autosomal recessive SCID have *adenosine deaminase deficiency*. Their clinical laboratory features are similar to other SCID patients. Other enzyme defects are associated with more selective immune deficiencies. *Purine nucleoside phosphorylase* deficiency is associated with severe T lymphocyte defects but relatively normal B lymphocyte function. Most patients with this disease die of overwhelming viral infections. Low levels of *5'-nucleotidase* have been reported in some patients with B lymphocyte deficiencies. This enzyme is produced by B lymphocytes, and the low levels most likely result from the reduced number of B lymphocytes.

Immune deficiency can occur in association with a benign or, less commonly, malignant neoplasm of the thymus called a *thymoma*. The cause-and-effect relationship between the thymoma and immune deficiency is not completely understood. If the development of immune deficiency is induced by the thymoma, this would best be considered a secondary or acquired immune defect. Surgical removal of the thymoma does not correct the immune deficiency. Laboratory evaluation demonstrates varying degrees of combined or predominantly humoral immune defects in patients with thymoma-associated immune deficiency.

Ataxia–telangiectasia is associated with an autosomal recessive form of variable combined immune deficiency. In these individuals, ataxia, a loss of muscular coordination, begins in early childhood. Also in early childhood, telangiectasia (dilation of small blood vessels) develops, especially in the conjuctiva of the eyes and the skin of the nose and ears. Although often not becoming a major problem until later childhood, these individuals are susceptible to many infectious processes, particularly recurrent and chronic infections of the sinuses and respiratory tract. This may be due to the reduction or absence of IgA and IgE observed in over half the patients. Other immunoglobulin abnormalities may also be present. The numbers of circulating B lymphocytes is typically normal, but T lymphocytes may be reduced in number and frequently yield abnormal results in in vitro functional tests. Abnormalities in the chromosomes containing the genes that code for T lymphocyte antigen receptors have been found in ataxia–telangiectasia patients. In this immune deficiency disease T lymphocyte defects become more severe over time.

Wiskott–Aldrich syndrome is a disease characterized by eczema and thrombocytopenia associated with an X-linked partial-combined immune deficiency. Reduced numbers of platelets in the blood, *thrombocytopenia*, is present at birth. Platelets are also smaller than normal and give abnormal results in functional laboratory tests such as adenosine diphosphate (ADP)-induced aggregation. Quantitatively and qualitatively abnormal platelets predispose to bleeding complications, the most severe of which is intracranial hemorrhage. *Eczema*, a form of dermatitis, typically develops within the first year of life. Recurrent infections become a problem after several months of age and become progressively more severe in parallel with worsening immune defects over time. The earliest problems are usually pyogenic bacterial infections, including pneumonia, meningitis, and otitis media. Ultimately fatal infection with bacteria, viruses, and fungi can occur.

A small minority of individuals with *short-limbed dwarfism* have immune deficiency that ranges from combined to predominantly T lymphocytic to predominantly B lymphocytic. Laboratory evaluation is required to define the category of the defect in an individual dwarf. The severity of infectious complications is dependent upon the degree of immune deficiency. Some patients with selective immune defects survive to adulthood, but patients with combined immune deficiency die in early childhood.

All forms of partial combined immune deficiency as well as other immune deficiencies that allow years of survival are associated with a higher than normal frequency of malignant neoplasms, especially lymphoid neoplasms such as lymphomas.

CELLULAR (T LYMPHOCYTE) IMMUNE DEFICIENCIES

The best known T lymphocyte immune deficiency, called DiGeorge's syndrome is associated with thymic *aplasia* or *hypoplasia*. This disease is caused by abnormal development in the embryo of the third and fourth pharyngeal pouches. These embryonic pharyngeal pouches normally give rise to structures in the mediastinum, neck, and face, including the thymus, parathyroid glands, great vessels of the heart, external ears, and jaw. Therefore DiGeorge's syndrome patients have T lymphocyte immune deficiency due to inadequate thymic tissue, hypocalcemia due to hypoparathyroidism, cardiac dysfunction due to malformation of cardiac vessels, and low-set, misshapen ears, small jaw, and abnormally positioned eyes due to aberrant facial development. Except in rare cases, this disease is not familial. It is most likely caused by some damaging intrauterine influence on the developing embryo during the sixth to eighth week of gestation. Most patients die in infancy from heart failure or uncontrollable hypocalcemia. In addition to hypocalcemia, laboratory evidence of hypoparathyroidism includes hyperphosphatemia and absent parathyroid hormone.

All of the manifestations of DiGeorge's syndrome are heterogeneous among different individuals, including the immune deficiency. T lymphocyte number and function are characteristically deficient but to varying degrees. The impairment may improve with time. The number of blood B lymphocytes and the amount of serum immunoglobulin are normal. The degree of T lymphocyte deficiency may relate to the developmental status of the thymus. A small amount of thymic tissue development, hypoplasia, would be expected to support more T lymphocyte production than no thymic development, aplasia. When hypoplastic thymic tissue is found in the mediastinum of autopsied DiGeorge's syndrome patients, it is small in amount but histologically normal. Lymph nodes have small cortical regions with inactive B lymphocyte follicles and markedly depleted T lymphocyte paracortical regions (Fig. 6–4). DiGeorge's patients appear to have normal bone marrow production of thymocyte precursors but absent or too little thymic tissue in which these precursors can take up residency, proliferate, and differentiate into T lymphocytes. The defective T lymphocyte production can be corrected by fetal thymus transplantation.

As mentioned above, selective T lymphocyte deficiency can be associated with

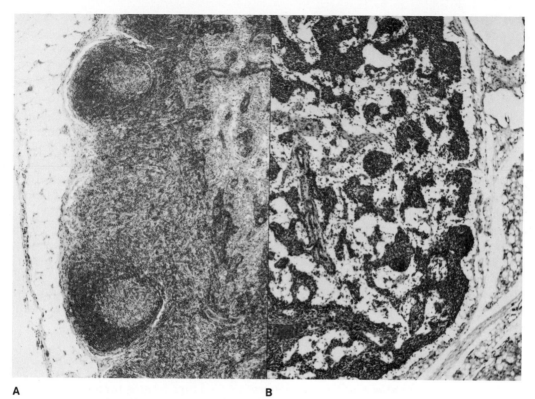

Figure 6-4. DiGeorge's Syndrome. Normal lymph node (**A**) and hypoplastic lymph node (**B**) from a patient with DiGeorge's syndrome. Note the thick cortex with active follicular germinal centers in (**A**) compared to the thin islands of lymphoid tissue in (**B**) (H&E, original magnification ×100).

purine nucleoside phosphorylase deficiency, an autosomal recessive trait. Some patients with short-limbed dwarfism have selective cellular immune deficiency.

Patients with *chronic mucocutaneous candidiasis* have a heterogeneous form of immune deficiency, but a unifying feature is a predominantly T lymphocyte immune defect. The Candida infections in these patients are extremely refractory to the treatment that is effective in individuals with normal immune systems. Patients make antibodies specific for Candida but have negative DTH skin tests and negative in vitro T lymphocyte stimulation tests against Candida antigens. The total number of blood T lymphocytes and mitogen stimulation of T lymphocytes is normal. The specific defect in anti-Candida cellular immunity distinguishes this syndrome from other forms of immune deficiency, which can also have chronic candidal infections. Chronic mucocutaneous candidiasis can be associated with a variety of endocrine deficiencies, most commonly hypoparathyroidism and adrenal insufficiency. Autoantibodies reactive with the diseased endocrine gland tissue can often be identified in the circulation.

ANTIBODY (B LYMPHOCYTE) IMMUNE DEFICIENCIES

Transient Hypogammaglobulinemia of Infancy

At birth infants normally have IgG obtained transplacentally from the mother during gestation but no IgA, IgM, IgE, or IgD, which cannot cross the placenta. Presence of IgM and IgA at birth indicates that there has been an intrauterine infection. Maternal IgG disappears during the first 6 months of life. By this time the infant has begun its own immunoglobulin production, but this is still at a relatively low, although increasing, rate. In virtually all normal individuals, serum immunoglobulin levels are at their lowest point at approximately 5 to 6 months of age. This *physiologic* or *transient hypogammaglobulinemia* is of variable degree, dependent upon the temporal relationship between the loss of maternal IgG and the active production of immunoglobulins by the infant. During the period of hypogammaglobulinemia, infants are more susceptible to recurrent respiratory tract infections. In the most severely affected children, gamma globulin administration is necessary. Unlike the more severe immunoglobulin deficiencies discussed below, infants with physiologic hypogammaglobulinemia have normal numbers of blood B cells and a rise in immunoglobulin levels once the low point is past. An increase in antibody levels can usually be seen within 2 months. A few children have persistent hypogammaglobulinemia beyond 1 year of age but eventually attain normal immunoglobulin levels.

Congenital Agammaglobulinemia or Hypogammaglobulinemia

The best known congenital severe deficiency of B lymphocytes is called *X-linked agammaglobulinemia* or *X-linked hypogammaglobulinemia*. The latter term is preferred by some because there may be small amounts of IgG in individuals with this disease. Another designation sometimes used is *Bruton's agammaglobulinemia*, in honor of the person who first recognized severe hypogammaglobulinemia in a child, although his patient probably had common variable immune deficiency. Male infants with this immune deficiency typically become symptomatic at around 5 or 6 months of age, when transplacentally acquired maternal IgG disappears. The immune deficiency predisposes to recurrent and chronic pyogenic infections, especially with streptococci, staphylococci, and *Hemophilus influenzae*. The most frequent infectious diseases are pneumonia, bronchitis, sinusitis, otitis, meningitis, and pyoderma. Sepsis is a serious complication. Pneumonia may also be caused by *Pneumocystis carinii*. Chronic diarrhea can result from persistent Giardia or rotavirus infections. Infections in patients with X-linked agammaglobulinemia often cannot be controlled with antibiotic therapy alone. The appropriate therapy for this deficiency is regular injection of immune gamma globulin preparations. With immune gamma globulin and antibiotic therapy, individuals with X-linked agammaglobulinemia can survive into the third decade of life but usually eventually die of chronic lung disease.

Individuals with X-linked agammaglobulinemia have normal cellular immunity. Laboratory evaluation of the number, antigen phenotype, and function of blood T lymphocytes demonstrates no abnormality. Blood B lymphocytes are characteristically absent. Serum immunoglobulin levels are profoundly depressed. IgM, IgA, IgD, and IgE are usually undetectable in routine assays. IgG may be absent or present at markedly reduced concentration. Rarely patients will have normal IgE levels. Isohemagglutinins and other specific antibodies are absent. Bone marrow cell–antigen phenotyping demonstrates pre-B cells but no B lymphocytes. Pre-B cells are not capable of whole immunoglobulin production, either for insertion into their membrane as a receptor or for secretion. Putatively there is a block of differentiation at the level of the pre-B cell, thus resulting in the absence of immunoglobulin-bearing B lymphocytes and serum immunoglobulins. Plasma cells are absent from the gut mucosa and other lymphoid tissue sites.

In addition to X-linked agammaglobulinemia, there is a very rare disease called *autosomal recessive agammaglobulinemia.* This disease is similar to X-linked agammaglobulinemia but affects females as well as males.

Selective Immunoglobulin Abnormalities

Some individuals have absence or marked depression of one or more, but not all, immunoglobulin classes or subclasses. The most common defect of this type is *selective IgA deficiency,* occurring in more than 1 in 1000 individuals. This deficiency may be symptom free, or it may cause recurrent sinusitis and respiratory tract infections. Selective IgA deficiency is also associated with an increased incidence of allergic and autoimmune diseases. Some cases of IgA deficiency appear to be primary, including autosomal recessive and dominant hereditary forms. Other cases appear to be acquired, including cases secondary to anticonvulsant drug therapy. Laboratory evaluation of patients with selective IgA deficiency demonstrates very low serum IgA levels but usually normal or elevated levels of IgG, IgM, IgE, and IgD. Some patients will have, in addition to depressed IgA, a reduction in IgE or the IgG subclasses IgG2 and IgG4. Both subclasses of IgA, IgA1, and IgA2 are almost always deficient, but rare patients have a selective absence of IgA1, which is the major IgA subclass found in the serum. There are normal numbers of blood B lymphocytes, including IgA-bearing B lymphocytes. T lymphocytes are quantitatively and qualitatively normal.

Selective deficiency of other immunoglobulin classes or subclasses is very rare. *Selective IgM deficiency* and *selective IgG subclass deficiency* have been identified. These individuals are susceptible to recurrent and chronic bacterial infections. Rare instances of *immunoglobulin light chain deficiency* have also been reported. These individuals have an absence of one of the two light chains, more often κ light chains. In these patients, other immunoglobulin defects are also present, most often, reduced IgA.

Hyper-IgM Immune Deficiency Syndrome

Hyper-IgM immune deficiency syndrome is a rare disease in which there is an absence of IgG and IgA production but increased IgM, and occasionally IgD, production. Even when stimulated in vitro, B lymphocytes from these individuals are unable to produce IgG and IgA. There appears to be a defect in B lymphocyte switching from IgM to IgG, IgA, or IgE synthesis. T lymphocyte numbers and function are normal. Individuals with this disease have recurrent pyogenic bacterial infections, especially of the respiratory tract.

COMMON VARIABLE IMMUNE DEFICIENCY

As the name implies, *common variable immune deficiency* is a relatively common, immunologically and pathogenetically diverse group of immune defects. Symptoms of immune deficiency can begin at any age but usually begin in late childhood or early adulthood, and the severity of the deficiency frequently varies with time. The symptoms are similar to those in patients with X-linked agammaglobulinemia, although usually less severe. Chronic respiratory and gastrointestinal tract infections are most frequent. Depending upon the severity and time of onset of the immune defect, individuals with common variable immune deficiency can have a normal life span. Chronic lung disease is a frequent cause of death. Some individuals with common variable immune deficiency have a primary inherited lymphocyte defect, while others have acquired lymphocyte abnormalities, for example, depletion of lymphocytes by anti-lymphocyte autoantibodies. Serum immunoglobulin is characteristically very low. IgG is markedly depressed, while IgM and IgA are variably reduced. Blood B lymphocytes are reduced or normal. Even when normal in number, B lymphocytes may not function normally. Specific antibody production in response to antigen exposure is deficient. Cellular immunity usually is impaired also, and this often becomes progressively more severe with time. Some patients have an imbalance of immunoregulatory T lymphocytes, in particular, a greater than normal proportion of suppressor cells. An oversupply of suppression or an undersupply of help could be responsible for deficient B lymphocyte responses in some patients. A variety of autoimmune disease can occur in association with common variable immune deficiency. In addition, a rare minority of patients appear to have developed the immune defect as a result of formation of autoantibodies directed against B or T lymphocytes.

ACQUIRED IMMUNE DEFICIENCIES

Acquired or secondary immune deficiencies are far more common than congenital or primary immune deficiencies. The severity of secondary immune deficiencies is extremely variable, ranging from asymptomatic laboratory abnormalities to fatal immune compromise. Secondary immune deficiencies are important to recognize because they must be taken into consideration for optimum medical management of the primary disease process that induced the immune defect. In particular, infectious complications must be guarded against. Most secondary immune deficiencies will resolve when the primary disease is brought under control, but sometimes there is permanent damage to the immune system. The kinds of diseases capable of inducing secondary immune deficiencies are quite diverse, as shown in Table 6–1 and discussed below.

Infection-Associated Acquired Immune Deficiencies
Viral infections are the most common infectious cause for acquired immune deficiencies. Many common viral infections induce a transient immune defect, especially of T lymphocyte function. This is most often documented by a loss of delayed hypersensitiv-

ity responsiveness to intradermal antigen challenge. This anergy can occur during measles, rubella, varicella, mumps, influenza, and Epstein–Barr (infectious mono-nucleosis) viral infections. In addition to skin test anergy, laboratory evidence for viral infection-induced T lymphocyte dysfunction includes frequent reduction in T lymphocyte mitogen stimulation and occasional reduction in the helper/suppressor T lymphocyte ratio. The impaired cellular immunity accompanying most viral infections is usually not a cause of major complications. In individuals infected with certain vi-ruses or with particular genetic predisposition, however, lethal complications can arise.

X-linked lymphoproliferative syndrome is an unusual form of infectious mononucleosis occurring in individuals with a genetically determined abnormal response to Epstein–Barr virus (EBV) infection. When infected with EBV these males either develop an acute fulminant fatal infectious mononucleosis or more slowly evolving processes such as hypogammaglobulinemia, B lymphocyte neoplasms (e.g., Burkitt's lymphoma), and aplastic anemia. The acquired hypogammaglobulinemia may be the result of viral rep-lication within B lymphocytes leading to cytotoxicity.

The designation *AIDS* (acquired immune deficiency syndrome) denotes a form of immune deficiency induced by *HTLV-III* (*human T lymphocyte leukemia virus type III*) infection. This retrovirus is also called *HIV* (*human immunodeficiency virus*) and *LAV* (*lymphadenopathy-associated virus*). AIDS is transmitted by intimate sexual contact and injection of blood products. In addition to a life-threatening immune deficiency, AIDS patients have lymphadenopathy and increased susceptibility to malignant neo-plasms, especially Kaposi's sarcoma. Recurrent and chronic infections with many dif-ferent microorganisms are a major complication and the most frequent cause of death. Many patients are simultaneously infected with a number of bacterial, fungal, and viral pathogens, including some that normally have a low pathogenic potential. *Pneumocystis carinii* is a frequent cause of pneumonia in AIDS patients (Fig. 6–5) and other immune deficiency patients but is an uncommon cause for pneumonia in the general popula-tion. Cytomegalovirus infections are also common. Laboratory evaluation of AIDS pa-tients typically demonstrates lymphopenia, selective depletion of T lymphocytes, and a marked reduction in the ratio of helper/suppressor T lymphocytes (from a normal of approximately 1.8 to less than 0.5). There is impaired T and B lymphocyte in vitro stimulation by mitogens and specific antigens. Serum immunoglobulin levels are often elevated, but specific antibody production in response to antigen challenge is defi-cient.

Immune deficiency can accompany mycobacterial infections, such as tuberculosis. As with viral infections, T lymphocyte function is more impaired than B lymphocyte function. Anergy is recognized when previously positive DTH skin tests to mycobacte-rial antigens (e.g., PPD) become negative.

Malignancy-Associated Immune Deficiency

Leukemias and lymphomas are the neoplasms most often associated with acquired immune deficiencies. These neoplasms can induce immune defects independent of concomitant drug therapy. These immune deficiencies are worsened by drugs that are

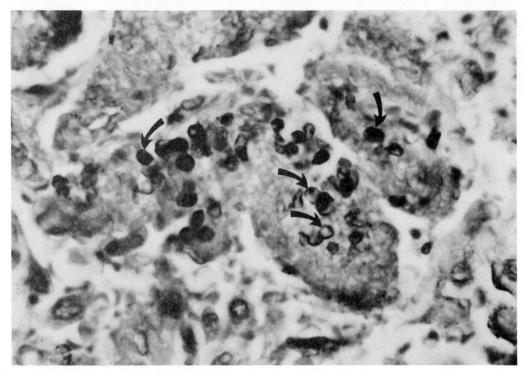

Figure 6-5. Pneumocystis Pneumonia. Photomicrograph of the lung of an AIDS patient with *Pneumocystis carinii* pneumonia. The tissue is stained with a silver stain to reveal the round *Pneumocystis carinii* organisms (*arrows*) (silver methenamine stain, original magnification ×1400).

used to treat the neoplasms and that also impair immune function as an adverse side effect.

Neoplasms of B lymphocyte lineage are associated with predominantly humoral immune defects. Chronic B lymphocytic leukemia, multiple myeloma, and B cell lymphomas can all inhibit specific antibody production. Some of these neoplasms may produce large amounts of monoclonal (produced by one clone of cells) immunoglobulins, resulting in an elevation in the total serum immunoglobulins; however, the amount of normal serum immunoglobulins is reduced. Impairment of specific antibody production can be documented by evaluating the response to antigen challenge. Patients with B lymphocyte lineage neoplasms are at risk for developing serious bacterial infections, and this is a frequent cause of death.

Hodgkin's disease is a neoplasm of poorly understood origin. Current theory suggests that the neoplastic cell is derived from an immune system accessory cell. Patients with Hodgkin's disease develop a predominantly cellular immune defect. Laboratory tests often reveal lymphopenia, reduced cutaneous delayed hypersensitivity, and impaired in vitro mitogen and specific antigen stimulation. As would be predicted from these data, patients with Hodgkin's disease are particularly susceptible to severe, life-threatening fungal, viral, and mycobacterial, infections.

A wide variety of other neoplasms, including some carcinomas, can be associated with acquired immune deficiency, usually primarily cellular immune defects. In addition to the direct effects of the neoplasms, accompanying malnutrition and anti-tumor therapy also impair immune function.

Systemic Disease-Associated Immune Deficiency

Secondary immune defects of varying severity are produced by systemic diseases for example, sarcoidosis, diabetes mellitus, Down's syndrome, rheumatoid arthritis, and systemic lupus erythematosus. Individuals with hyperfunctioning of the adrenal glands, Cushing's syndrome, develop immune deficiency. This results from the immunosuppressive effects of increased levels of corticosteroid hormones produced by the adrenal glands. Patients with severe liver or kidney failure have immune deficiency, probably caused by the accumulation of waste products that are toxic to the immune system. Severe burns, malnutrition, and aging are also associated with acquired immune deficiency.

Iatrogenic Immune Deficiency

Iatrogenic means caused by the physician. Iatrogenic immune deficiency can be produced purposefully or can be an unwanted complication. Purposefully produced immune deficiency may be induced to reverse an immune-mediated disease process. For example, steroids or cytotoxic drugs are sometimes administered to patients to ameliorate autoimmune tissue injury. *Immunosuppressive therapy* is also used to prolong the survival of organ transplants, such as kidney and heart allografts. Unwanted immune suppression is a frequent complication of anticancer chemotherapy or irradiation therapy. This therapy is designed to kill the rapidly proliferating cancer cells, but it also kills the similarly rapidly proliferating lymphoid cells of the immune system. Fulminant infection caused by therapy-induced immune deficiency is a frequent cause of death in cancer patients.

Immune deficiency resulting from surgical removal of the spleen, *splenectomy*, is another example of iatrogenic immune deficiency. Splenectomy may be required because of traumatic rupture of the spleen or anemia mediated by splenic lysis of erythrocytes. The impaired immune defense secondary to splenectomy is due more to deficient phagocytosis and mediator production than to lymphocyte dysfunction. These individuals have a greater risk of developing fulminant fatal bacterial septicemia.

Excessive Antibody and Lymphocyte Loss

Another mechanism for acquiring an immune deficiency is to lose components of the immune system from the body, usually via the gastrointestinal or urinary tract. Although the losses can be great enough to produce laboratory abnormalities, the immune impairment is usually not severe enough to cause major problems. Inflammation of the stomach and intestine can cause leakage of plasma proteins into the gut. This is called *protein-losing gastroenteropathy*. Among the proteins lost are immunoglobulins. The *nephrotic syndrome* is a condition in which the kidney allows passage of large amounts of plasma proteins, including IgG, into the urine, which normally contains only minute amounts of plasma proteins. Patients with protein-losing gastroenteropathy and the nephrotic syndrome have acquired hypogammaglobulinemia.

An uncommon disease called *intestinal lymphangiectasia* leads to the loss of both immunoglobulins and lymphocytes into the gut. This is caused by leakage from large dilated abnormal lymphatics in the intestinal mucosa. Laboratory evaluation demonstrates cellular and humoral immune system abnormalities.

Discussion of the Illustrative Case

The patient described at the beginning of this chapter had X-linked agammaglobulinemia. Infectious complications did not begin until 5 months of age, when transplacentally acquired IgG had declined. Thereafter the patient had recurrent and persistent bacterial otitis, bronchitis, and pneumonia, in spite of appropriate antibiotic therapy. The antibiotic therapy was suppressing the infections to a degree and probably saved the child's life, but without an intact immune defense the pathogens could not be totally eradicated. The giardiasis produced malabsorption and growth retardation. The persistent pulmonary infections also contributed to this failure to thrive. Once the diagnosis was made by laboratory evaluation, the child was treated with bimonthly intramuscular injections of gamma globulin, and the respiratory and gastrointestinal tract infections were brought under control.

QUESTIONS

1. Define primary (congenital) and secondary (acquired) immune deficiency.

2. What laboratory tests are useful for evaluating B lymphocyte function?

3. What laboratory tests are useful for evaluating T lymphocyte function?

4. Why are many congenital immune deficiencies not recognizable until after 5 to 6 months of age?

5. In general, what symptoms suggest the presence of an immune deficiency?

6. What laboratory abnormalities would you expect with severe combined immune deficiency, Wiskott–Aldrich syndrome, DiGeorge's syndrome, transient hypogammaglobulinemia of childhood, and AIDS?

Chapter

7 Lymphocytic Leukemias and Lymphomas

OBJECTIVES

1. To describe the neoplasms arising from cells of the immune system (lymphocytic leukemias and lymphomas) and to briefly discuss neoplasms of other leukocytes and immune system accessory cells.
2. To show that laboratory studies are required for precise diagnostic classification of leukemias and lymphomas.
3. To relate current trends in nomenclature of leukemias and lymphomas to current knowledge about the normal development and activation of lymphocytes.
4. To describe the clinical, histologic, and laboratory characteristics of the major types of lymphocytic leukemias and lymphomas.

Illustrative Case

A 65-year-old woman developed recurrent, moderately severe pain in her mid-back and progressive weight loss. When lifting her 2-year-old grandchild, she experienced very severe midback pain that persisted. She went to a local emergency department where a physician noted marked tenderness and swelling in the region of the fourth thoracic vertebra. A radiograph of the vertebral column demonstrated a fracture of the fourth thoracic vertebra in addition to multiple, radiolucent oval defects in other vertebrae and ribs. Skull radiographs also demonstrated lytic defects in the calvarium. The patient was found to be anemic. The technologist performing a blood group determination and a crossmatch test in preparation for transfusion therapy noted extensive rouleaux formation (stacking of erythrocytes), which made evaluation of true agglutination difficult. A serum protein electrophoresis showed an abnormal spike in the gamma globulin region and a depression of the normal gamma globulins. Immunoelectrophoresis demonstrated that the abnormal gamma globulin contained immunoglobulin γ heavy chains and κ light chains. Laboratory tests on the urine identified Bence Jones proteins composed of κ immunoglobulin light chains.

DIAGNOSTIC CLASSIFICATION OF LEUKEMIAS AND LYMPHOMAS

A *leukemia* is a neoplasm arising from bone marrow cells. Because of this origin the neoplastic marrow cells, which resemble some normal type of leukocyte, usually spill into the blood in large numbers. This massive leukocytosis is the basis for the designation leukemia. Leukemias are further classified on the basis of the normal cell type that the neoplastic cells most closely resemble and from which the neoplastic cells are presumably derived. The cells of *lymphocytic leukemia* resemble lymphocytes, while those of *lymphoblastic leukemia* resemble the immature blastic stem cells of lymphocytes. Leukemias derived from nonlymphoid bone marrow cells include *myelogenous leukemia,* composed of neoplastic granulocytes; *monocytic leukemia,* composed of neoplastic monocytes; and *erythroleukemia,* composed of neoplastic erythrocyte precursors.

Both lymphoid and myelogenous leukemias have *acute* and *chronic* variants. Acute leukemias are composed of immature neoplastic cells with a morphology resembling primitive blast cells with large nuclei and prominent nucleoli. If untreated acute leukemias typically have a very aggressive, rapidly fatal course. Chronic leukemias are composed of neoplastic cells that closely resemble mature leukocytes and often have a more indolent, slowly progressive course.

The discussions on leukemias in this chapter will focus on immunologic features and relationships to normal lymphocytes. Nonlymphocytic leukemias will not be discussed in detail. The reader should turn to a hematology text for more information on these leukemias.

Lymphomas are solid neoplasms arising from cells in lymphoid tissues, usually within lymph nodes. The vast majority of lymphomas are derived from lymphocytes, but a few arise from mononuclear phagocytes. Lymphomas often produce massive enlargement of lymph nodes (lymphadenopathy). Other processes, including lymphoid hyperplasia, can also produce lymphadenopathy. Pathologic evaluation of abnormal lymphoid tissue is required to diagnose a lymphoma. Pathologic classification of lymphomas utilizes both morphological and immunohistochemical characteristics of the abnormal lymphoid tissue.

LYMPHOMA NOMENCLATURE

Prior to the 1970s lymphomas were diagnosed exclusively on the basis of their light microscopic morphology. *Hodgkin's disease* is a major form of cancer arising in lymph nodes. As will be discussed later in this chapter, its cell of origin is still unproven, but Hodgkin's disease has a distinctive morphology. Based on this morphology, lymphomas are classified as either Hodgkin's disease or *non-Hodgkin lymphomas*. For the remainder of this chapter the term lymphoma will be used to refer to non-Hodgkin lymphomas.

Until recently the most commonly used nomenclature system for lymphomas was the Rappaport classification. According to this system lymphomas that resembled small, round, "mature" lymphocytes were called *well-differentiated lymphocytic lymphomas*. Those composed of slightly larger, more irregular cells were called *poorly differentiated lymphocytic lymphomas*. Lymphoid tissue neoplasms composed of large round to oval cells with loose nuclear chromatin and moderate amounts of cytoplasm were called *histiocytic lymphomas* because the neoplastic cells looked more like histiocytes (a synonym for macrophages) than lymphocytes. *Mixed lymphocytic and histiocytic lymphomas* were also recognized. The final category of *undifferentiated (stem cell) lymphomas* was for neoplasms composed of cells that resembled primitive stem cells.

This morphological classification of lymphomas is still widely used to diagnose lymphomas. However, the marked expansion of knowledge about normal lymphocytes that has occurred over the past two decades has resulted in the development of new approaches to the pathologic classification of lymphomas. The realization that there are lymphomas and leukemias corresponding to virtually every functional subtype of lymphocyte has provided the impetus for change in the nomenclature system. Figure 7–1 depicts the normal development and activation of lymphocytes and lists the lymphoid neoplasms that correspond morphologically and functionally to each normal cell type. The diagnostic and clinical features of each of these neoplasms will be discussed in this chapter.

Lymphomas need to be classified not only on the basis of morphology but also on the basis of functional characteristics. In vitro tests of functional capabilities are not practical laboratory methods for analyzing lymphomas. Surface membrane antigens of the neoplastic lymphocytes can be analyzed more conveniently. The expression of surface antigens correlates with the functional characteristics of the cells. Based on the surface membrane antigens identified in a particular lymphoid neoplasm (called the *antigen phenotype* or *immunophenotype*), the neoplastic lymphoid cells, just like normal

TABLE 7-1. REPRESENTATIVE ANTIGEN MARKERS COMMONLY USED TO IDENTIFY THE LINEAGE OF LYMPHOMAS

| Lymphoma Lineage | SIg | Marker | | | | | | | |
		CD20 B1	DC19 B4	CD2 T11	CD3 T3	CD4 T4	CD8 T8	CD13 MY7	CD14 Mo2
B cell	+	+	+	−	−	−	−	−	−
T cell	−	−	−	+	+	+	+	−	−
Histiocyte (macro-phage)	−	−	−	−	−	−	−	+	+

Abbreviations: CD (cluster of differentiation) numbers refer to the international nomenclature for leukocyte markers; SIg = surface membrane immunoglobulin; B1, B4, T11, T3, T4, T8, MY7, and Mo2 = monoclonal antibodies marketed by Coulter Corp., Hialeah, FLA.

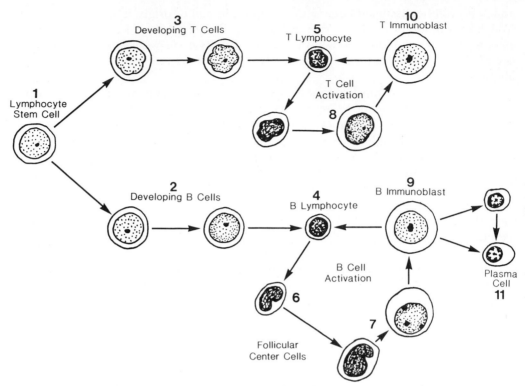

Figure 7–1. Lineage of Lymphocytic Lymphomas. The numbers on the diagram of normal lymphocyte differentiation and activation indicate the cell type most analogous morphologically and functionally to the lymphoid neoplasms listed after those numbers in the following: *(1)* null-acute lymphoblastic leukemia (ALL); *(2)* common-ALL, pre-B-ALL, B-ALL, small noncleaved cell (Burkitt's) lymphoma; *(3)* T-ALL, T lymphoblastic lymphoma; *(4)* B-chronic lymphocytic leukemia (CLL), B-small lymphocytic lymphoma; *(5)* T-CLL, T-small lymphocytic lymphoma; *(6)* small-cleaved cell lymphoma; *(7)* B-large cell lymphoma; *(8)* T-large cell lymphoma; *(9)* B-immunoblastic lymphoma; *(10)* T-immunoblastic lymphoma; *(11)* multiple myeloma.

lymphoid cells, can be categorized into many types (Table 7–1). For example, neoplastic T lymphocytes can be distinguished from neoplastic B lymphocytes on the basis of markers such as T3 (CD3) in the former and B1 (CD20) in the latter. Neoplastic helper T lymphocytes, which have the antigen phenotype T3+, T4+, T8−, B1−, can be distinguished from neoplastic suppressor T lymphocytes, which have the antigen phenotype T3+, T4−, T8+, B1−. Leukemias can similarly be characterized by antigen phenotyping (Table 7–2). The methodology and interpretation of lymphoma and leukemia antigen phenotyping will be discussed in greater detail later in this chapter.

The functional and antigenic characterization of lymphomas has led to a better

TABLE 7-2. MARKER DISTRIBUTION IN LEUKEMIAS

Type of Leukemia	Marker									
	CALLA CD10	RIg	SIg	4 CD19	B1 CD20	TdT	DR	ER	T3 CD3	MY7 CD13
N-ALL	−	−	−	−	−	+	+	−	−	−
C-ALL	+	+	−	+	−	+	+	−	−	−
pre-B-ALL	+	+	−	+	−	+	+	−	−	−
B-ALL	+	+	+	+	+	−	+	−	−	−
T-ALL	−/+	−	−	−	−	+	−	+	+	−
AML	−	−	−	−	−	−	−	−	−	+
B-CLL	−	+	+	+	+	−	+	−	−	−
T-CLL	−	−	−	−	−	−	−	+	+	−
CML	−	−	−	−	−	−	−	−	−	+

Abbreviations: ALL = acute lymphoblastic leukemia; N = null; C = common; B = B cell; T = T cell; AML = acute myelogenous leukemia; CLL = chronic lymphocytic leukemia; CML = chronic myelogenous leukemia; CALLA = C-ALL antigen; RIg = rearranged immunoglobulin genes; SIg = surface immunoglobulin; TdT = terminal deoxynucleotidyl transferase; DR = membrane HLA-DR antigens; ER = sheep erythrocyte rosette formation; B1, B4, T3, and MY7 = monoclonal antibodies marketed by Coulter Corp., Hialeah, FLA.

appreciation of morphological categories. This prompted the development of a new nomenclature system, called the National Cancer Institute (NCI) Working Formulation (Table 7–3), that is being used in addition to or instead of the Rappaport system. This nomenclature system divides lymphomas into three groups based on the usual degree of clinical aggressiveness, with low-grade lymphomas being least aggressive and high-grade most aggressive. When antigen phenotyping is performed, the T or B cell lineage of the neoplasm is also indicated in the diagnosis.

The presence or absence of a nodular growth pattern in a lymphoma relates to prognosis. In general, among lymphomas having morphologically similar cells, a nodular growth pattern (Fig. 7–2) correlates with a better prognosis than a diffuse growth pattern. The Rappaport nomenclature divides lymphomas into "diffuse" and "nodu-

TABLE 7-3. NATIONAL CANCER INSTITUTE WORKING FORMULATION FOR LYMPHOMA NOMENCLATURE

Low Grade	Intermediate Grade	High Grade
Small lymphocytic	Follicular large cell	Large cell immunoblastic
Follicular small-cleaved cell	Diffuse small-cleaved cell	Lymphoblastic
Follicular, mixed small and large cell	Diffuse, mixed small and large cell	Small noncleaved cell
	Diffuse large cell	

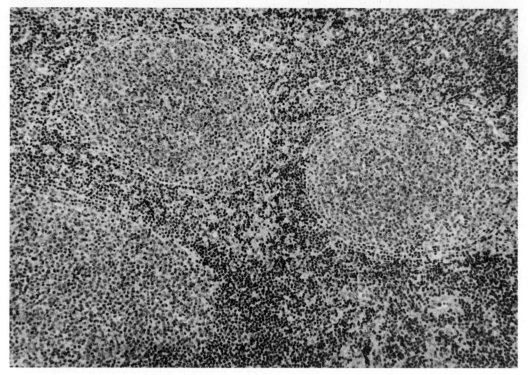

Figure 7-2. Follicular Lymphoma. A follicular (nodular) growth pattern in a follicular center cell lymphoma (H&E, original magnification ×200).

lar" types, while the Working Formulation uses the designation "follicular" to indicate
nodularity. The nodular pattern of growth is a facsimile of lymphoid follicle formation
that normally takes place in the B lymphocyte regions of lymph nodes. Nodular lymphomas are B cell in lineage, as would be expected from their capacity to form follicles.

Antigen phenotyping of lymphomas and leukemias has shown that morphologically indistinguishable neoplasms can have different surface membrane antigens, and
morphologically dissimilar neoplasms can have similar surface antigens. For example,
two patients with morphologically identical well-differentiated (small) lymphocytic
lymphomas could be found to have totally different neoplastic populations by antigen
phenotyping, one having a B lymphocyte lymphoma and the other a T lymphocyte
lymphoma. Conversely, two patients with morphologically very dissimilar lymphomas,
one composed of small round cells and the other of large irregular cells, could be
found to have neoplasms that both have surface membrane immunoglobulin μ and λ
chains. Both the morphology and the antigen phenotype of lymphomas and leukemias
can be important in predicting the natural history and response to therapy of the
neoplasm. Therefore laboratory evaluation should include analysis of morphology as
well as antigen expression.

LABORATORY METHODS FOR EVALUATING LYMPHOMAS AND LEUKEMIAS

Morphological evaluation is still essential for the laboratory diagnosis of leukemias and lymphomas. Lymph nodes and bone marrow are biopsied and examined microscopically for the presence of neoplastic cells. The morphological features of specific lymphomas and lymphocytic leukemias will be described later in this chapter.

Very high white blood cell (WBC) counts are sometimes the first indication of leukemia. Neoplastic leukemic cells are usually first identified in Wright's- or Giemsa-stained blood smears or marrow aspirate smears. Special histochemical stains for cytoplasmic enzymes can be used to further characterize certain leukemias, especially myelocytic and monocytic leukemias that have neoplastic cells containing enzyme-laden lysosomal granules. Antigen phenotyping is performed on leukemic cells from blood or bone marrow aspirates. Immunofluorescence microscopy, immunoenzyme microscopy, or flow cytometry are used to identify the antigens expressed by the neoplastic cells of lymphomas and leukemias.

Antigen phenotyping of lymphocytic leukemias is usually done on viable cells suspended in physiologic buffer. In larger medical centers the antigen phenotyping is analyzed by automated fluorescence flow cytometry. Lymphoma tissue can be mechanically disrupted to yield viable cell suspensions that can also be analyzed by flow cytometry. At the present time, however, most antigen phenotyping of lymphomas is done by immunoenzyme microscopy on thin sections of frozen tissue. A series of sections of tissue are first overlaid with different primary antibodies, each specific for a lymphocyte antigen. Unbound antibody is washed off. Next, the tissue sections are overlaid with a secondary antibody that is specific for the first antibody. This second antibody is linked to an enzyme, such as peroxidase, that produces a colored product when exposed to the proper substrate. After substrate is added, cells will show surface staining if they have an antigen for which the reagent antibody has specificity (Fig. 7–3).

Antigen phenotyping of lymphomas by immunoenzyme microscopy on frozen sections of tissue has advantages over antigen phenotyping of lymphoma cells brought into suspension by mechanical disruption. The disruption of tissue required to produce cell suspensions can result in preferential loss of some cell populations, making the final cell typing not representative of the cell population in the original tissue specimen. Examining tissue sections allows the relationship of the suspected lymphoma to the surrounding tissue to be observed (Fig. 7–4). If there is only a small focus of lymphoma in the tissue, this can be identified better in tissue sections than in cell suspensions that contain the minor population of abnormal cells admixed with the more numerous non-neoplastic cells.

Tables 7–1 and 7–2 list some of the many markers analyzed in clinical immunology laboratories to assist with the diagnosis and categorization of lymphomas and leukemias.

Some laboratory abnormalities observed in patients with leukemias and lymphomas are caused by the infiltration and destruction of normal tissues by the neoplastic

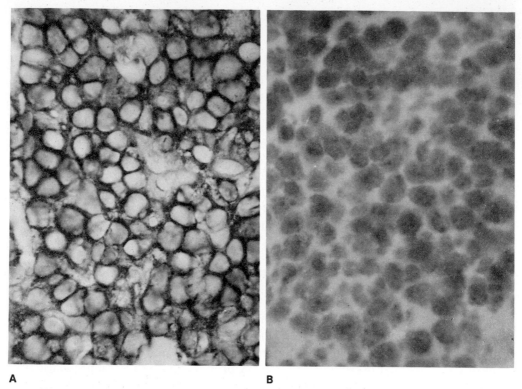

A   B

Figure 7–3. B Cell Lymphoma. Immunoenzyme staining of a large-B cell lymphoma that was expressing surface membrane IgM λ. **(A)** was stained using anti-λ light chain antibodies and is positive, whereas **(B)** was stained using anti-κ light chain antibodies and is negative (Immunoperoxidase, original magnification ×750).

cells. Replacement of bone marrow by neoplastic cells can produce anemia, thrombocytopenia, and reduction in non-neoplastic blood leukocytes. Destruction of bone predisposes to fractures in weight-bearing bones, such as the vertebrae. Extensive infiltration of organs can lead to abnormal laboratory values, for example, abnormal liver function test values in patients with liver involvement.

ACUTE LYMPHOBLASTIC LEUKEMIAS

Acute leukemias occur more often in children, while chronic leukemias are more frequent in adults. Acute leukemias are characterized by increased numbers of immature blast cells in the bone marrow, usually accompanied by numerous blasts in the blood. *Aleukemic leukemia* has leukemic blast cells in the marrow but not in the blood. The optimum treatment and the prognosis differ among different types of acute leukemia. Acute leukemias are classified on the basis of morphology, enzyme histochemistry, and antigen phenotype. The first major division is into acute *lymphoblastic* (or lymphocytic)

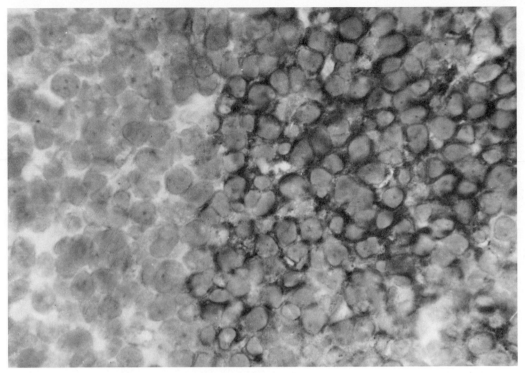

Figure 7–4. B Cell Lymphoma. Immunoenzyme microscopy (using anti-κ light chain antibodies) of a lymph node showing, on the left, immunostaining of non-neoplastic T lymphocytes; and, on the right, positive staining of a focus of B cell lymphoma with surface membrane IgM κ (I&E, original magnification ×750).

leukemia (ALL) and *acute nonlymphoblastic leukemia (ANLL)*. ANLL is further subdivided into acute myelogenous leukemia, acute promyelocytic leukemia, acute myelomonocytic leukemia, acute monoblastic leukemia, erythroleukemia, and acute megakaryocytic leukemia. This subdivision often requires the use of special histochemical stains, most of which demonstrate cytoplasmic enzymes that have restricted distributions in the various types of ANLL. ANLL cells lack the membrane antigens that are characteristic of lymphocyte-derived leukemias. For example, as shown in Table 7–2, acute myelogenous leukemia cells are negative for the lymphocyte markers B4 (CD19), B1 (CD20), and T3 (CD3) but are positive for MY7 (CD13). Because it is not a neoplasm of the immune system, ANLL will not be discussed in detail in this book.

ALL is the most frequent childhood malignant neoplasm. The peak incidence is in the middle of the first decade of life, but the disease can occur at any age, and there is a second smaller peak in incidence during the eighth decade. If untreated, ALL is typically rapidly fatal, usually leading to death within a few months of diagnosis. Chemotherapy using a combination of drugs markedly improves survival and in some patients may lead to a permanent cure. Approximately 90% of children with ALL will have remission of the leukemia when treated with combinations of vincristine, prednisone, and L-asparaginase. Injections of methotrexate into the cerebrospinal fluid and cranial irradiation are used to prevent central nervous system involvement. Adults and children under 2 years old respond less well to therapy. In a given individual the optimum combination of drugs and the prognosis are dependent upon the type of ALL.

The major types of ALL are *common ALL (C-ALL). T cell ALL (T-ALL).* B *cell ALL (B-ALL), pre-B cell ALL (pre-B-All),* and *null cell ALL (N-ALL).*C-ALL accounts for 50 to 60% of ALL, while the approximate frequency of T-ALL is 20%, N-ALL 10%, pre-B-ALL 10%, and B-ALL 2%. Laboratory findings other than morphology alone are required to identify the types of ALL. Table 7–2 lists some of the laboratory markers used to type ALL. Each type of ALL has a specific reaction pattern with this panel of tests.

B-ALL and T-ALL share markers, respectively, with B lymphocytes and T lymphocytes. B-ALL bears surface membrane immunoglobulin. Since neoplasms are monoclonal proliferations, all of the cells in a B-ALL make the same type of antibody with respect to the antigen-binding region. Thus the membrane immunoglobulin on all of the leukemic cells will have the same light chain and idiotype (the antigenic composition of the antigen-binding site). The heavy chain, usually μ is also often the same. This monotypic production of immunoglobulin that is typical of B cell neoplasms differs from the polytypic immunoglobulin production by polyclonal proliferations of normal B lymphocytes reacting to an antigen challenge.

Pre-B-ALL has not developed the capacity to manufacture whole immunoglobulin molecules and to insert them in the membrane but can produce μ light chains in the cytoplasm. This indicates less differentiation toward B lymphocytes than in B-ALL. An even more primitive stage of B lymphocyte differentiation is the rearrangement of genes that must precede the synthesis of immunoglobulin molecules. This will be discussed in detail in Chapter 9. This gene rearrangement can be detected in the laboratory using DNA *hybridization* techniques. B-ALL and pre-B-ALL have immunoglobulin gene arrangement. C-ALL also has immunoglobulin gene rearrangement but no evidence for immunoglobulin synthesis. C-ALL thus shows even more primitive B cell differentiation than pre-B-ALL. C-ALL, B-ALL, pre-B-ALL, and a minority of T-ALL have a membrane antigen called C-ALL antigen, *CALLA* (CD10). The monoclonal antibody B4 (CD19), which reacts with immature and mature B cells, also immunostains C-ALL, pre-B-ALL, and B-ALL, whereas B1 (CD20), which reacts with mature but not immature B cells, immunostains B-ALL but not C-ALL or pre-B-ALL.

T-ALL cells form rosettes with sheep erythrocytes, as do normal T lymphocytes. T-ALL cells also express some of the T cell membrane antigens found on immature and mature T lymphocytes. Monoclonal antibodies that immunostain T-ALL include T11 (CD2), which is specific for determinants on T cell sheep erythrocyte receptors, and T3 (CD3), which is specific for determinants on a protein associated with the antigen receptor of T cells.

N-ALL does not show evidence for differentiation into either T or B lymphocytes and therefore could also be considered an undifferentiated ALL (U-ALL). N-ALL cells have membrane HLA-DR antigens and contain terminal deoxynucleotidyl transferase (TdT), which is detected immunohistologically. These are not specific markers, since they are shared by other types of ALL. These markers do differentiate between T-ALL and B-ALL, the former having TdT and the latter HLA-DR.

LYMPHOBLASTIC AND SMALL-NONCLEAVED CELL LYMPHOMAS

Lymphoblastic and small-noncleaved cell lymphomas are morphologically and antigenically similar to ALL. These aggressive lymphomas are in the high-grade category of the NCI Working Formulation. By definition, at the time of diagnosis these neoplasms are proliferating predominantly in tissues other than the bone marrow. Later in the course of the disease, however, these neoplasms can invade the marrow and produce all the features of ALL. Patients with ALL can develop masses of neoplastic cells in tissues other than the marrow. Thus the distinction between ALL and lymphomas of similar morphology can be difficult in some patients, especially those with advanced disease.

Lymphoblastic and small-noncleaved cell lymphomas are also called undifferentiated or stem cell lymphomas because of their primitive blastic appearance and expression of markers shared by immature T or B cells. Morphologically these lymphomas have cells with a high nuclear-to-cytoplasmic ratio and finely dispersed nuclear chromatin (Fig. 7–5). Lymphoblastic lymphomas arise from T cells and small-noncleaved cell lymphomas from B cells.

Lymphoblastic lymphomas are most frequent in older children and young adults. Approximately half the patients have mediastinal masses, possibly indicating a thymic origin for these T cell neoplasms. The neoplasm can involve any lymphoid tissue of the body and often invades the central nervous system. An overlap with T-ALL manifestations can develop. The antigen phenotype of T lymphoblastic lymphoma is similar to that of T-ALL. The neoplastic cells are characteristically T3 (CD3) and T11 (CD2) positive. The treatment is similar to that for T-ALL, but the prognosis is worse.

As the name implies, small-noncleaved cell lymphomas have round nuclear contours. They must be distinguished morphologically from large, noncleaved cell lymphomas, which will be discussed later. Small-noncleaved cell lymphomas are also called Burkitt's lymphoma. This neoplasm was first recognized in Africa, where it is endemic. In Africa Burkitt's lymphoma usually begins as a mass in the jaw of a child. In the United States an abdominal mass is the most common initial finding. Epstein–Barr virus (EBV) infection is incriminated in the pathogenesis of Burkitt's lymphoma. Patients with Burkitt's lymphoma often will have serologic evidence for EBV infection. This is a B cell neoplasm that has membrane monoclonal immunoglobulin and is B4 (CD19) and B1 (CD20) positive. Cytogenic studies show abnormalities in chromosomes involved with immunoglobulin synthesis.

CHRONIC LYMPHOCYTIC LEUKEMIA

Chronic lymphocytic leukemia (CLL) is a slowly progressive neoplasm that increases in frequency with age. CLL is rare in individuals under 30 years old. The median age at diagnosis is 65. Patients survive an average of 7 years after diagnosis. The earliest

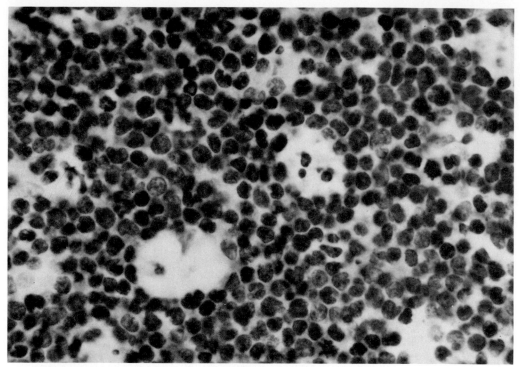

Figure 7-5. Small-Noncleaved Cell (Burkitt's) Lymphoma. Note the relatively round nuclei, less dense chromatin than in the cells shown in Figure 7-6, and scant cytoplasm. The scattered cells with abundant clear cytoplasm are macrophages phagocytosing dead neoplastic cells (H&E, original magnification ×1100).

symptoms of the disease, such as malaise and fatigue, are nonspecific. The diagnosis is often first diagnosed when a complete blood count (CBC) reveals a lymphocyte count of 15,000/mm³ or more. Death usually results from impaired immune defense or replacement of bone marrow leading to anemia and thrombocytopenia. Laboratory evaluation of CLL patients at diagnosis and during the course of the disease is important in prognostication and directing therapy. The degree of blood lymphocytosis, anemia, thrombocytopenia, lymphadenopathy, hepatomegaly, and splenomegaly correlate with the prognosis. The median survival of patients with leukemic lymphocytosis alone at the time of diagnosis is greater than 10 years, whereas that of patients with lymphocytosis, lymphadenopathy, and anemia or thrombocytopenia is less than 2 years.

CLL cells resemble normal blood lymphocytes. Laboratory evaluation shows blood and bone marrow lymphocytosis. Greater than 90% of CLL patients have neoplastic cells with B lymphocyte markers, including surface membrane monoclonal immunoglobulin, typically IgM, and immunostaining with B4 (CD19) and B1 (CD20). Most of the remaining cases show T lymphocyte markers. Leukemic cells can infiltrate many tissues of the body, especially lymph nodes, liver, and spleen. CLL infiltrates in tissue are morphologically and antigenically indistinguishable from small cell (well-differentiated) lymphocytic lymphoma.

SMALL-CELL (WELL-DIFFERENTIATED) LYMPHOCYTIC LYMPHOMA

As in CLL, the neoplastic cells of small *lymphocytic lymphoma* resemble normal blood lymphocytes (Fig. 7–6). This was the basis for the synonymous Rappaport system designation of *well-differentiated lymphocytic lymphoma (WDLL)*. The difference between WDLL and CLL is that CLL begins the bone marrow and characteristically produces a blood lymphocytosis, whereas at the time of diagnosis WDLL is characterized by predominantly extramyeloid (outside the marrow) neoplastic cell proliferation, especially in lymph nodes. The diagnosis is made by histologic and immunohistologic examination of biopsy specimens from involved tissue, usually a lymph node. Most patients with WDLL will have a minor degree of bone marrow involvement, and during the course of their disease approximately 15% will develop blood lymphocytosis comparable to that of CLL. Therefore WDLL and CLL are pathologically very closely

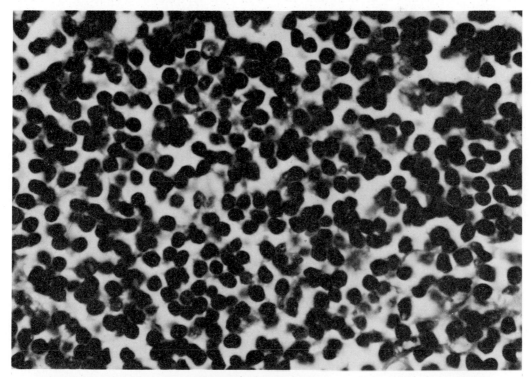

Figure 7–6. Small-Cell (Well-Differentiated Lymphocytic) Lymphoma. Note the uniformity, round nuclei, dense chromatin, and resemblance to normal, unstimulated lymphocytes (H&E, original magnification ×1100).

related diseases. This is also true immunologically and clinically. Greater than 90% of WDLL is of B cell lineage. The disease is most frequent in older adults and typically has a slowly progressive course. The prognosis is based on the extent of involvement at the time of diagnosis.

FOLLICULAR CENTER-CELL LYMPHOMAS

The neoplastic counterparts to the germinal centers in B lymphocyte follicles are called *follicular center-cell* (FCC) *lymphomas.* In normal follicle germinal centers, small B lymphocytes undergo transformation into large blast cells after antigen stimulation. There are a number of morphological phases in this transformation (Fig. 7–1). Small cells with irregular nuclei and moderately dense chromatin are called small-cleaved FCC; large cells with irregular nuclei and loose chromatin are called large-cleaved FCC; and large cells with round to oval nuclei, loose chromatin, and multiple nucleoli are called large-noncleaved FCC. Lymphomas can have cells resembling all of these FCC types. Often there is an admixture of various FCC types in a FCC lymphoma. The lymphoma is named on the basis of the predominant cell type. If there are approximately equal numbers of small and large FCC, the lymphoma is called mixed. FCC lymphomas have either a diffuse or follicular growth pattern. FCC lymphoma cells express B lymphocyte markers, including large amounts of surface membrane monclonal immunoglobulin. This feature can be useful in differentiating neoplastic FCC follicles from hyperplastic follicles. By immunoenzyme microscopy, the membrane immunoglobulin on the former would be monoclonal, while that on the latter would be polyclonal.

Because of their irregular nuclei (Fig. 7–7), *small-cleaved cell lymphomas* are called *poorly differentiated lymphocytic lymphomas* in the Rappaport nomenclature system. Of all the follicular center cell lymphomas, small-cleaved cell lymphomas are most likely to have a follicular growth pattern (Fig. 7–2). When the follicular growth pattern is present, small-cleaved cell lymphomas have a low grade aggressiveness; but when it is absent, that is, when there is a diffuse growth pattern, these lymphomas have an intermediate aggressiveness.

FCC lymphomas composed of large cells are called *large-cell lymphomas* by the Working Formulation and *histiocytic lymphomas* by the Rappaport system (Fig. 7–8). The latter term is a misnomer, since the vast majority of neoplasms having this morphology are of lymphocytic and not histiocytic (macrophage) lineage. Most large cell lymphomas are of B cell type and display surface membrane monoclonal immunoglobulin and immunostain with B4 (CD19) and B1 (CD20). These neoplastic cells are analogous to completely transformed FCC. Only a minority of B-lineage cell lymphomas will have a follicular growth pattern. Not all large-cell lymphomas are of B cell origin; a small proportion are of T cell type, as determined in the laboratory by rosetting with sheep erythrocytes or immunostaining with monoclonal antibodies such as T11 (CD2) and T3 (CD3). A few will not have specific markers for T or B lymphocytes. All large cell lymphomas have an intermediate grade of aggressiveness. Even with combination chemotherapy, survival of patients with large cell lymphomas average less than 3 years. A

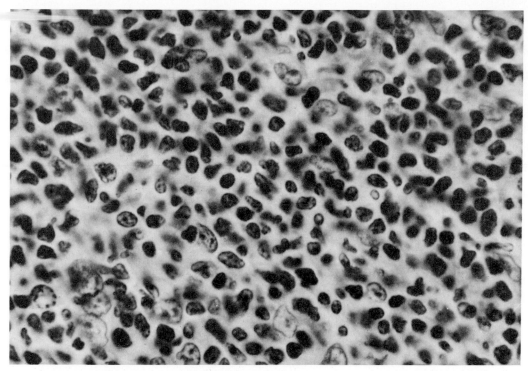

Figure 7-7. Small-Cleaved Cell (Poorly Differentiated Lymphocytic) Lymphoma. Note the irregularity of nuclei compared with Figure 7-6 and smaller size compared with the cells in Figure 7-8 (H&E, original magnification ×1100).

special variant of even more aggressive large cell lymphomas, called immunoblastic lymphomas, will be discussed later.

FCC lymphomas can have a relatively equal proportion of small and large cells. These neoplasms are called *mixed small and large cell lymphomas* by the Working Formulation and *mixed lymphocytic and histiocytic lymphoma* by the Rappaport system. These neoplastic cells are analogous to lymphocytes in various stages of blast transformation. As with large cell lymphomas, mixed lymphomas are usually, but not always, of B cell type. These tumors can be either diffuse or follicular. The latter virtually always have B lymphocyte markers typical of FCC. The growth pattern has prognostic importance, because follicular mixed lymphomas have low-grade aggressiveness, whereas diffuse, mixed lymphomas have intermediate aggressiveness.

T CELL LYMPHOMAS

As stated in the previous sections, T cell lymphomas account for a minority of the diffuse small-cell, large-cell, and mixed lymphomas. T cell lymphomas never have true follicle formation and thus are not in the follicular diagnostic categories. T cell lym-

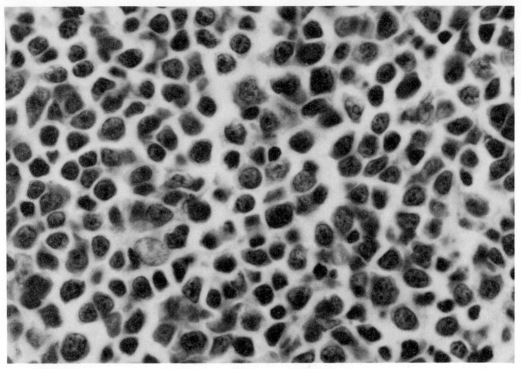

Figure 7-8. Large-Cell (Histiocytic) Lymphoma. Note the large nuclei with loose chromatin, resembling those in lymphocytes that have undergone antigen-induced blast transformation (H&E, original magnification ×1100).

phomas often have a mixed small-and large-cell composition. In addition to the neoplastic T lymphocytes, non-neoplastic eosinophils and mononuclear phagocytes often are present. These may have been drawn to the neoplasm by lymphokines released by the neoplastic T lymphocytes.

Some T cell lymphomas have a predilection for the skin. These neoplasms arise in the skin but eventually spread to involve other tissues, especially lymph nodes. Involvement of the skin produces reddened inflamed lesions, raised plaques, or tumor nodules. Marker studies of neoplastic cells infiltrating the skin show a T cell origin. Most cutaneous T cell lymphomas have a helper T lymphocyte antigen phenotype, that is, they are T4 (CD4) positive and T8 (CD8) negative. *Mycosis fungoides* and *Seźary syndrome* are the two most common types of cutaneous T cell lymphoma. The major difference between these two diseases is the presence of abnormal neoplastic T lymphocytes in the blood of Seźary syndrome patients. These cells are of moderate to large size and have very irregular, so-called cerebriform, nuclei. Mycosis fungoides and Seźary syndrome are probably variants of the same basic neoplastic process.

IMMUNOBLASTIC LYMPHOMAS

Immunoblastic lymphomas are a very aggressive variant of large-cell lymphoma. The analogous normal cell type is the totally transformed blast cell that is the precursor to effector T cells or immunoglobulin-producing B cells, including plasma cells (Fig. 7–1).

Since the neoplastic cells of B immunoblastic lymphoma are analogous to plasma cell precursors, they frequently contain cytoplasmic immunoglobulin. Many B immunoblastic lymphomas have a minor population of cells with plasmacytic differentiation. These neoplastic plasma cells have arisen from the same clone as the immunoblasts and contain the same cytoplasmic immunoglobulin. A minority of patients with B immunoblastic lymphoma will have an identifiable monoclonal immunoglobulin in their plasma.

T immunoblastic lymphomas do not have cytoplasmic or surface membrane immunoglobulin and do not contain cells with plasmacytic features. They form rosettes with sheep erythrocytes and express a T lymphocyte–antigen phenotype.

PLASMA CELL DYSCRASIAS

A variety of B cell neoplasms secrete whole or partial monoclonal immunoglobulin molecules into the blood. These abnormal proteins are detected by a number of laboratory procedures, including serum protein electrophoresis, immunoelectrophoresis, and specific immunoglobulin quantitation. Monoclonal immunoglobulins can be found in the blood of individuals with B cell lymphomas, B cell leukemias, lymphoplasmacytic lymphomas, plasma cell neoplasms, or no identifiable neoplasm.

Less than 5% of patients with B cell lymphomas or leukemias have detectable plasma monoclonal immunoglobulins. The frequency of secreted immunoglobulin correlates with the differentiation of the neoplasm. Thus a B immunoblastic lymphoma would be more likely to secrete monoclonal immunoglobulin than a small, noncleaved B cell lymphoma. Greater than 90% of plasma cell neoplasms have an accompanying monoclonal immunoglobulin in the blood. The most common type of immunoglobulin secreted is influenced by the type of B cell neoplasm producing it. B cell lymphomas and leukemias most often produce IgM, followed in order by IgG and IgA. Plasma cell neoplasms most often produce IgG, followed in order by IgA, IgD, IgM, and IgE. A small proportion of B cell neoplasms will secrete incomplete immunoglobulin molecules, that is, light chains or heavy chains alone. When only incomplete immunoglobulin molecules are produced, heavy chains are most often secreted by lymphomas and light chains by plasma cell neoplasms.

Multiple myeloma is a plasma cell neoplasm characterized by extensive infiltration of the bone marrow by the neoplastic cells (Fig. 7–9). The disease typically occurs in older individuals, usually during the seventh or eighth decade of life. The neoplastic infiltrates in the bone marrow can erode bone and produce bone pain, fractures, and lucent defects seen on radiographs. Replacement of marrow tissue produces reduced

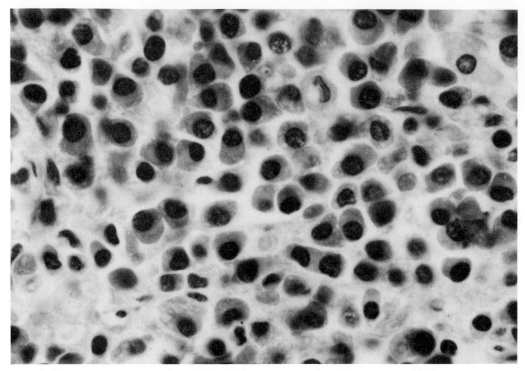

Figure 7-9. Multiple Myeloma. Note the abundant eccentric cytoplasm that contains a large amount of immunoglobulin molecules (H&E, original magnification ×1100).

hematopoiesis that can lead to anemia and other cytopenias. The most specific laboratory abnormalities in patients with multiple myeloma result from the production of large amounts of monoclonal immunoglobulin molecules by the neoplastic plasma cells. Approximately 99% of multiple myeloma secrete immunoglobulin molecules. These molecules are almost always of one immunoglobulin type. IgG accounts for over half of the immunoglobulins produced by multiple myelomas and IgA for about 20%. Approximately 20% of multiple myelomas produce an immunoglobulin light chain only. IgD, IgE, and IgM account for less than 2% of the multiple myeloma secretory products. When IgM is seen as a monoclonal immunoglobulin in the blood, it is most often the product of a B cell neoplasm other than multiple myeloma. A frequent source is a lymphoma with neoplastic cells having intermediate differentiation between lymphocytes and plasma cells, so-called lymphoplasmacytic cells. The presence of large amounts of monoclonal IgM in the blood is called *Waldenström's macroglobulinemia.*

Diagnosis of multiple myeloma is dependent upon radiographic bone examination and evaluation of blood, bone marrow, or other tissues. Most criteria for diagnosis require combinations of findings to confirm the diagnosis. In a bone marrow specimen the percentage of plasma cells that is considered to be consistent with multiple myeloma depends upon how many other diagnostic features are present in the patient. Marrow involvement is focal, so a biopsy or aspiration specimen may not contain large numbers of neoplastic plasma cells even though the marrow has extensive disease. The diagnostic utility of a specimen containing only a small proportion of plasma cells can be increased by using immunofluorescence or immunoenzyme microscopy to determine the presence or absence of cytoplasmic monoclonal immunoglobulin in the plasma cells. Confluent masses of plasma cells (Fig. 7–9) in the biopsies of marrow or other tissues is strong support for a plasma cell neoplasm.

Identification of monoclonal immunoglobulin in the blood is important in making the diagnosis. By serum protein electrophoresis, approximately 85% of patients with multiple myeloma will have a well-defined dense band of monoclonal immunoglobulin in the γ- or β-globulin region. A densitometer graph will show a sharp spike corresponding to the dense band. This is called an *M spike* (monoclonal spike). Serum immunoelectrophoresis is not only a sensitive means of detecting monoclonal immunoglobulin but is very specific, since it demonstrates the monoclonal nature of the immunoglobulin by defining its monotypic heavy-and light-chain composition. Specific serum immunoglobulin quantitation showing greater than 3.5 g/dl IgG or greater than 2 g/dl IgA is strong evidence for multiple myeloma. Serum protein electrophoresis and specific quantitation characteristically reveal a reduction in normal immunoglobulins in patients with multiple myeloma. This deficiency of normal antibody production results in increased susceptibility to infections, and this is the most common cause of death in myeloma patients.

In patients with multiple myeloma, monoclonal immunoglobulins can also spill into the urine and be detected by immunoelectrophoresis or specific quantitation. The urine may contain free monoclonal immunoglobulin light chains, called *Bence Jones proteins.* Urine protein measurement by dipstick or sulfosalisylic acid precipitation is insensitive for detecting immunoglobulin light chains.

There are other laboratory findings in patients with multiple myeloma. Most patients have a normochromic and normocytic anemia caused by replacement of marrow by the neoplastic plasma cells. Leukopenia and thrombocytopenia are less common. Rarely, abnormal plasma cells are found in blood smears. Bone destruction results in hypercalcemia. The high protein content of the plasma leads to rouleaux formation by erythrocytes. This is seen by technologists in the hematology laboratory or blood bank when blood is examined microscopically. The high protein content can lead to a *hyperviscosity syndrome,* in which there is poor perfusion of the microvasculature, usually causing central nervous system abnormalities. This problem is most frequent with Waldenström's macroglobulinemia.

Most patients with monoclonal immunoglobulins in the blood have no identifiable B cell neoplasms. Such patients are said to have a *benign monoclonal gammopathy.* Unlike multiple myeloma patients, patients with benign monoclonal gammopathy typically do not have a reduction in normal immunoglobulins. This process increases in frequency with age and may be associated with another disease process, such as infection, autoimmune disease, or cancer. Approximately 5% of patients with what is thought to be a benign monoclonal gammopathy will eventually develop multiple myeloma.

NEOPLASMS OF TRUE HISTIOCYTES AND DENDRITIC CELLS

Recognized malignant neoplasms of immune accessory cells (macrophages and dendritic cells), are less common than lymphomas of lymphocytic lineage. Approximately 98% of lymph node neoplasms that have the morphology of a large cell lymphoma (histiocytic lymphoma by Rappaport system) are of lymphocyte lineage, and only 2% are of histiocyte (macrophage) lineage. Antigen phenotyping is required to determine the lymphocytic or histiocytic origin of such large cell neoplasms (Table 7-1). True histiocytic lymphomas lack lymphocyte antigen markers and express macrophage markers, such as reactivity with the monoclonal antibodies MY7 (CD13) and Mo2 (CD14). The histochemical demonstration of certain cytoplasmic enzymes, such as non-specific esterase, is also used as a marker of macrophage differentiation. Some true histiocytic neoplasms have morphologies that differ from those of lymphocytic lymphomas, including some with conspicuous phagocytosis of erythrocytes.

There are neoplasms having cells with features in common with dendritic cells. A group of diseases known as *histiocytosis X* (Fig. 7–10) have antigenic and ultrastructural

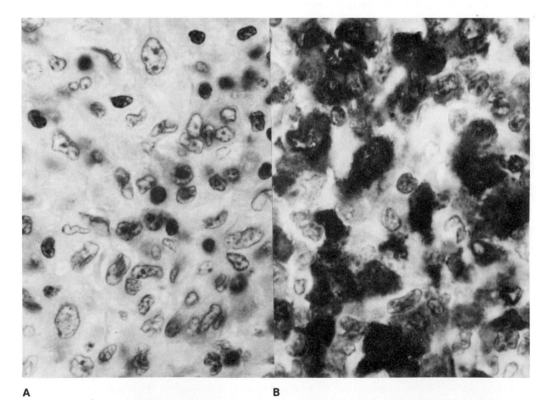

A   **B**

Figure 7-10. Histiocytosis X. (A) is a hematoxylin and eosin stained section showing elongated nuclei, loose chromatin and abundant pale cytoplasm. **(B)** is stained by an immunoenzyme method using an antibody specific for an antigen (S100 protein) found in Langerhan's cells (original magnification ×1100).

similarities to a dendritic cell of the skin called a Langerhans' cell. These neoplastic cells immunostain with antibodies specific for S100 protein. These neoplasms often contain an admixture of eosinophils, especially the variant called eosinophilic granuloma.

HODGKIN'S DISEASE

Hodgkin's disease is a neoplastic disease with extensive lymphoid tissue involvement. The neoplastic cell is a large irregular cell that is either binuclear (Reed–Sternberg cell, (Fig. 7–11) or mononuclear (Hodgkin's cell). The nuclei often are multilobated and characteristically have very large nucleoli. The presence of Reed–Sternberg cells in biopsy tissue is required for the diagnosis, but these cells are not completely specific for Hodgkin's disease. Reed–Sternberg cells can be seen in marrow aspirates as well as in biopsies of bone marrow, lymph nodes, and other involved tissues. In addition to the neoplastic cells, the lesions of Hodgkin's disease contain a polymorphous admixture of other non-neoplastic cell types, including lymphocytes, plasma cells, eosinophils, and macrophages. The proportions of these cell types is the basis for the classi-

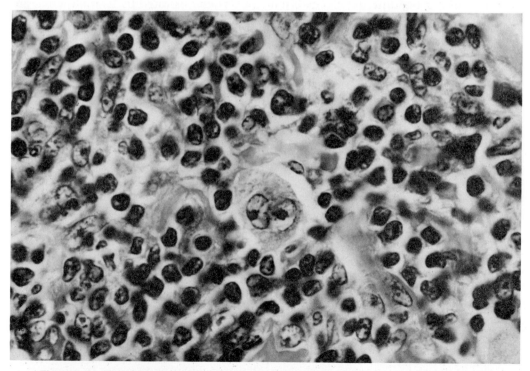

Figure 7-11. Hodgkin's Disease. Note the binucleated Reed-Sternberg cell at the center of the photograph and the surrounding polymorphous infiltrate of predominantly non-neoplastic leukocytes (H&E, original magnification ×1100).

fication of Hodgkin's disease into lymphocyte predominance, mixed cellularity, or lymphocyte-depletion types. This classification system has prognostic importance. Lymphocyte-predominance Hodgkin's disease has a 5-year survival of approximately 90%, mixed cellularity 70%, and lymphocyte-depleted 50%. A fourth type of Hodgkin's disease, called nodular sclerosis, is characterized by dense bands of collagen and a special cell type. Nodular sclerosis Hodgkin's disease has a prognosis similar to mixed cellularity.

The origin of the neoplastic cells of Hodgkin's disease is unknown. The evidence for derivation from the mononuclear phagocyte or dendritic cell systems is stronger than that for lymphocytic lineage. If the neoplastic cells are derived from immune accessory cells functionally analogous to macrophages or dendritic cells, they may produce chemical mediators (monokines) that call in the non-neoplastic leukocytes that often predominate in Hodgkin's disease lesions. This would be an abnormal facsimile of the interaction between accessory cells and leukocytes that takes place during an immune response.

Hodgkin's disease can occur at any age but is most frequent in young adults and in the elderly. Individuals usually become aware of the disease because of swelling of the neck caused by cervical lymphadenopathy. Less common symptoms are weight loss, pruritis, fever, and night sweats. There are no specific laboratory tests for Hodgkin's disease. Cellular immune deficiency often can be demonstrated by lymphopenia, absence of delayed cutaneous hypersensitivity, and reduced in vitro T lymphocyte stimulation by mitogens and specific antigens. This acquired immune deficiency can result in fatal viral, fungal, or mycobacterial infections.

Combination chemotherapy and radiation therapy markedly improve survival and in some patients apparently eradicate the disease. The extent of the disease throughout the body has a major effect on the prognosis and optimum therapy. Therefore patients undergo careful clinical and pathologic evaluation to determine the distribution of the neoplasm. This may require microscopic examination of tissue from lymph nodes, bone marrow, liver, and spleen. Patients are then categorized on the basis of the extent of disease into stages that will determine the choice of therapy and prognosis. With appropriate therapy greater than 90% of patients with the less extensive involvement (stage I) will be cured, while less than 60% of those with the most extensive disease (stage IV) are cured.

Discussion of the Illustrative Case

The woman described in the case report has radiographic and laboratory findings indicative of multiple myeloma. She is in the high-risk age group for this disease and has the most frequent initial symptom, i.e., bone pain. She developed a vertebral fracture while lifting a child. This was the result of weakening of the vertebra by destruction of bone by the neoplastic process. The problem the technologist experienced with rouleaux formation was caused by the high protein content of the blood. Addition of a small amount of saline to the reaction mixture usually eliminates the erythrocyte stacking so that true agglutination can be seen.

QUESTIONS

1. What is the difference between a lymphoma and a leukemia?
2. In general, what characteristics are used to classify leukemias and lymphomas?
3. What is antigen phenotyping, and how does it help in classifying leukemias and lymphomas?
4. Can leukemias that look alike or lymphomas that look alike have different antigen phenotypes?
5. Why is it important to classify leukemias and lymphomas into so many categories?
6. What is an M spike, and what laboratory procedures are useful in analyzing it?

Section IV

Immune Responses and Immune-Mediated Diseases

Chapter

8

T Lymphocyte Immune Responses and T Cell-Mediated Inflammation

OBJECTIVES

1. To describe the antigen-specific activation of T lymphocytes, including the requirements for accessory cells and histocompatibility antigens.
2. To detail the participation of T lymphocytes in chronic inflammation and delayed hypersensitivity.
3. To discuss the importance of lymphokines in the activation of lymphocytes and the induction of chronic inflammation.
4. To discuss cell-mediated cytotoxicity carried out by T lymphocytes, macrophages, natural killer (NK) cells, and K cells, particularly against virus-infected and tumor cells.
5. To describe laboratory methods for evaluating T lymphocytes and T lymphocyte function.

Illustrative Case

A 60-year-old man with a 10-year history of alcohol abuse developed progressive weight loss, night sweats, and hemoptysis. Medical evaluation included a chest radiograph that showed opacities and cavities in the apex of the right lung. Examination of sputum smears by technologists in the microbiology laboratory revealed acid-fast bacilli. Intradermal injection of intermediate-strength–tuberculin-purified protein derivation (PPD) resulted in the development after 48 hours of an erythematous, indurated area at the injection site. *Mycogbacterium tuberculosis* was cultured from sputum specimens.

ANTIGEN RECOGNITION BY T LYMPHOCYTES

T lymphocytes have membrane receptors for antigens. These receptors are functionally analogous to the membrane-bound immunoglobulin molecules used by B lymphocytes as antigen receptors. T lymphocyte antigen receptors are involved in activation of T lymphocytes and in the effector functions of some T lymphocytes. Specific recognition of an antigen by a T lymphocyte receptor, when accompanied by the appropriate accessory events, leads to induction of blast transformation, resulting in the production of *T immunoblasts*. This is analogous to the antigen-stimulated transformation of B lymphocytes into B immunoblasts, which will be discussed in Chapter 9. *T immunoblasts* give rise to clones of T lymphocytes having the same antigen specificity (i.e., antigen receptors) as the initially transformed lymphocytes. The accessory events required for T lymphocyte activation are (1) antigen presentation to the T lymphocyte by an accessory cell, (2) stimulation of the T lymphocyte by soluble mediators released by accessory cells, and (3) interaction of the T lymphocyte with cell-surface molecules (histocompatibility antigens) of the accessory cell (Fig. 8–1).

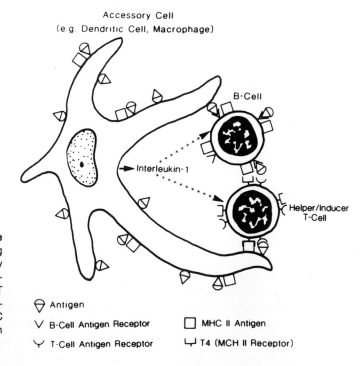

Figure 8-1. Immune Response Initiation. Diagram depicting the interaction of accessory cell, B lymphocytes, and T lymphocytes. To proliferate, the T lymphocyte requires three signals: antigen recognition, MHC class II molecule recognition and interleukin 1.

Accessory Cells

T lymphocytes, like B lymphocytes, require the assistance of *accessory cells* to respond optimally to antigens. The most important accessory cells for both B and T lymphocytes are macrophages and *dendritic cells*. The exact ontogenetic relationship between macrophages and dendritic cells is not known. They both may be components of the mononuclear phagocyte system and thus derived from monocytes. They are, however, functionally different and display different surface membrane protein markers. Macrophages are efficient phagocytic cells, whereas dendritic cells are not. Both cell types function well as *antigen-presenting cells* (APC) for lymphocytes. There are distinct types of dendritic cells that function as accessory cells for T lymphocytes and others for B lymphocytes.

Antigen-specific T lymphocyte proliferation requires physical contact with an antigen-presenting accessory cell. For presentation to lymphocytes, macrophages can bind antigens nonspecifically, or they can bind antigens using the specificity of immunoglobulin held to the macrophage surface by Fc receptors.

In addition to antigen presentation, accessory cells provide two more factors required for T lymphocyte activation: a secretory product called *interleukin 1* and surface membrane interactions between histocompatibility molecules and receptors for these molecules (Fig. 8–1).

Interleukin 1

Interleukin 1 (IL 1) is a monokine, that is, a secretory product of macrophages. It stimulates T lymphocyte activation and proliferation. IL 1 is required for maximal DNA synthesis in T lymphocytes that have interacted with antigen-presenting cells. IL 1 stimulates the production by T lymphocytes of the lymphokine *interleukin 2* (IL 2), which stimulates T lymphocyte proliferation. IL 1 also mediates the development of fever and increased numbers of polymorphonuclear leukocytes in the blood (leukocytosis). Fever and leukocytosis are frequent signs of inflammatory diseases resulting from the activation of macrophages and T lymphocytes.

Histocompatibility Antigens

Interaction between accessory cells and lymphocytes is modulated in part by proteins on the surfaces of the cells. These proteins were first recognized because of their role in immune-mediated transplant rejection. When tissue is transplanted between different species or between two genetically different members of the same species, the transplanted tissue is not antigenically compatible with that of the recipient and is rejected by the immune system. A series of closely linked genetic loci, called the *major histocompatibility complex* (MHC), have the greatest control over tissue compatibility. The protein gene products of these loci are called *MHC antigens or molecules*. The MHC in man is called the *human leukocyte antigen (HLA) system*.

The HLA system has four major loci, A, B, C, and D. There is extensive polymorphism at each of these loci, that is, any one of many alleles can be present at a locus in a given individual. Loci A, B, and C encode what are called *class I antigens or molecules* while D encodes *class II antigens or molecules*. The latter are also called *DR* (D-related) antigens or molecules. Class I and II molecules, and receptors for these molecules, play important roles in T and B lymphocyte immune responses. A third region of the MHC encodes class III molecules, mostly proteins of the complement system, which will be discussed in Chapter 10.

Class I molecules are present on the surfaces of almost all cells of the body. Class II molecules are restricted to B lymphocytes, some accessory cells, and a subpopulation of activated T lymphocytes. As will be discussed below, both class I and II HLA molecules are involved in T and B lymphocyte immune responses.

Laboratory evaluation of the HLA molecules present on an individual's cells, *HLA typing*, can yield clinically important data. HLA typing is essential when trying to identify the most compatible organ for transplantation. Certain diseases are more common in individuals with particular HLA phenotypes. Thus HLA typing indicates the relative risk of developing one of these HLA-associated diseases. The best known association is between HLA-B27 and a form of arthritis called ankylosing spondylitis. HLA-B27 is 90 times more frequent in persons with this disease than in the general population.

Class I HLA molecules are usually identified by serologic assays performed on lymphocytes isolated from anticoagulated whole blood. The assay end point is often a cytotoxic reaction, or lack thereof, between sample lymphocytes and reagent antibodies of known reactivity against HLA class I molecules. Class II molecules have classically been identified by lymphocyte blast transformation assays, *mixed lymphocyte reactions (MLR),* but technically easier serologic assays are now available.

Antigen Receptors on T Lymphocytes

A T lymphocyte has surface membrane receptors that recognize the specific antigen that will stimulate that lymphocyte. The T lymphocyte antigen receptor is functionally analogous to B lymphocyte surface membrane immunoglobulin. Like immunoglobulin molecules, T lymphocyte receptors for antigens have a variable and constant region and have two protein chains, the alpha and beta chain. As in B lymphocytes prior to immunoglobulin synthesis, in T lymphocytes there is rearrangement of the genes that code for antigen receptors prior to synthesis of these receptors. There are structural homologies among T lymphocyte antigen receptors, B lymphocyte antigen receptors (i.e., immunoglobulins), and MHC antigens, suggesting that these molecules required for antigen recognition and lymphocyte interactions arose by gene duplication from a common ancestral gene.

Antigen stimulation of T lymphocytes is *MHC restricted.* That is, T lymphocytes will respond only to foreign antigens that are displayed on cells that have the same MHC phenotype as the T lymphocyte. This indicates that T lymphocytes have receptors for both foreign antigen and MHC molecules, either on the same molecule or on separate molecules.

The class of MHC molecule that is recognized in conjunction with foreign antigen differs among T lymphocyte functional subsets. For specific immune activation, cytotoxic/suppressor T lymphocytes must recognize the appropriate foreign antigen along with the compatible class I MHC molecules. Therefore a T lymphocyte specific for a *Herpes simplex* viral antigen will attack only *Herpes simplex*-infected cells of the same class I MHC phenotype. Helper/inducer T lymphocytes must recognize foreign antigen in conjunction with compatible class II MHC molecules Class II molecules are intimately involved in the production of both humoral and cell-mediated immune responses. Therefore cytotoxic/suppressor T lymphocytes have receptors for class I MHC molecules, and helper/inducer T lymphocytes have receptors for class II molecules.

These MHC receptors are themselves antigenic and are recognized by the lymphocyte-typing mouse monoclonal antibodies T8 and T4 respectively. The proportions of suppressor and helper T lymphocytes in blood or other specimens can be determined with T8 and T4 antibodies. The ratio in the blood of T4 to T8 T lymphocytes is normally approximately 2. Another monoclonal antibody, T3, reacts with all T lymphocytes, since it recognizes determinants associated with the antigen receptor of T lymphocytes. Many additional monoclonal antibodies are available for lymphocyte typing. Table 8–1 lists some of the monoclonal antibodies that are used to identify T lymphocyte surface markers.

T LYMPHOCYTE SUBSET FUNCTION AND INTERACTION

T lymphocytes can carry out many different functions, including (1) helping B and T lymphocytes respond to antigens, (2) inducing activation, migration, and proliferation of macrophages, (3) suppressing B and T lymphocyte function, and (4) killing cells. Different subsets of T lymphocytes are responsible for different functions. As stated above, distinct functional subsets of T lymphocytes display distinct surface-membrane molecules that can be identified in the clinical laboratory using mouse monoclonal antibodies specific for these T lymphocyte surface antigens.

Helper T lymphocytes are required for optimum immune responses to foreign antigens. Helper T lymphocytes are activated by the simultaneous recognition of specific antigen and class II molecules on the surface of an antigen-presenting cell, such as a

TABLE 8–1. SURFACE MARKER MOLECULES AND MONOCLONAL ANTIBODIES USED TO IDENTIFY T LYMPHOCYTES

Population Identified	CD Number	Commercial Antibody[a]			Associated Function
		Coult	*Ortho*	*BD*	
Thymocytes	CD1	T6	OKT6	Leu-6	
All T cells	CD2	T11	OKT11	Leu-5	E rosette receptor
All T cells	CD3	T3	OKT3	Leu-4	Antigen receptor
Helper T cells	CD4	T4	OKT4	Leu-3a	MHC II receptor
All T cells	CD5	T1	OKT1	Leu-1	
All T cells	CD6		OKT12		
All T cells	CD7			Leu-9	
Suppressor T cells	CD8	T8	OKT8	Leu-2a	MHC I receptor
Activated T cells	CD25			IL 2R	IL 2 receptor

[a]*Abbreviations:* Coult = Coulter Corp., Hialeah, FLA; Ortho = Ortho Diagnostic Systems, Raritan, NJ; BD = Becton-Dickenson, Mountain View, CA.

macrophage. These cells then help B lymphocytes that have recognized specific anti-gen via membrane immunoglobulin to proliferate and differentiate into antibody-secreting cells (Fig. 8–2). This is discussed in greater detail in Chapter 9. The effects of T helper cells on B cells are probably mediated by lymphokines that act as growth factors to stimulate proliferation and differentiation factors to stimulate development into plasma cells. Thus B lymphocyte activation, except under rare conditions, involves three major events: (1) antigen presentation by an accessory cell, (2) antigen recognition by membrane immunoglobulin, and (3) MHC-restricted T lymphocyte help. Helper T lymphocytes also assist T lymphocyte immune responses.

Suppressor T lymphocytes down-regulate immune responses, primarily suppressing helper T lymphocytes (Fig. 8–2). Paradoxically, suppressor T lymphocytes may need the help of *inducer T lymphocytes* to become activated. Inducer and helper T lymphocytes share some surface membrane markers for example, both express the T4 antigen. In addition to suppressor T lymphocytes, a major mechanism for down-regulating anti-body production is the synthesis of antibodies directed against the antigen-binding site of the antibodies being suppressed. These anti-idiotypic antibodies will be discussed in Chapter 9.

Cytotoxic T lymphocytes can produce direct lysis of cells. Cells are selected for lysis on the basis of foreign MHC antigens (especially class I) or the coexpression of foreign

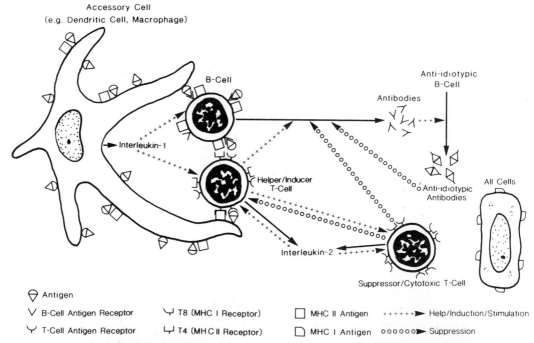

Figure 8-2. Immune Response Regulation. Diagram depicting the regulatory interactions between accessory cells, T lymphocytes, and B lymphocytes. Also shown are anti-idiotypic antibodies that act as a negative feedback for antibody production.

antigens and self-MHC. An example of the former is rejection of an incompatible graft; an example of the latter is the destruction of a virus-infected cell. Activation of helper T lymphocytes requires corecognition of antigen and compatible class II molecules, whereas activation of cytotoxic T lymphocytes requires corecognition of antigen and compatible class I molecules. Lysis is accomplished by the release from cytotoxic T lymphocytes of the lytic contents of cytoplasmic granules. This lytic substance is a pore-forming protein, *perforin,* that produces holes in the target cell membrane, leading to cytolysis. Cytotoxic and suppressor T lymphocytes express some of the same membrane markers, for example, both have the T8 antigen. T cells can also release a soluble *lymphocytotoxic factor* that will kill cells other than lymphocytes.

LYMPHOKINES

Activated T lymphocytes release many soluble mediators, called *lymphokines,* that modulate immune responses and inflammation (Table 8–2). Interleukin 2 (IL 2), which stimulates T lymphocyte proliferation, has already been mentioned. T lymphocytes express membrane receptors for IL 2 once they have been activated, for example, by binding of antigen to antigen receptors. The binding of IL 2 to IL 2 receptors stimulates clonal proliferation. IL 2 also stimulates proliferation and maturation of B lymphocytes and NK cells (discussed below). Activated T lymphocytes can be identified in the laboratory with anti-IL 2 receptor antibodies. Activated T lymphocytes also release IL 2 receptors into the circulation where it can be detected with immunologic assays. Another lymphokine, γ *interferon,* enhances class II molecule expression on po-

TABLE 8–2. LYMPHOKINE NOMENCLATURE AND FUNCTIONS.

Name[a]	Action
Interleukin 2 (IL 2)	Stimulates T cell proliferation
	Stimulates B cell proliferation
	Stimulates B cell differentiation
	Activates NK cells
Interleukin 3 (IL 3)	Stimulates myeloid cell growth
	Stimulates mast cell proliferation
γ interferon (IF)	Inhibits viral replication
	Activates macrophages
	Activates NK and K cells
Macrophage chemotactic factor (MCF)	Attracts macrophages
Macrophage migration inhibitory factor (MIF)	Immobilizes macrophages
Macrophage activating factor (MAF)	Activates macrophages
Leukocyte migration inhibitory factor (LIF)	Immobilizes neutrophils
B cell growth factor (BCGF)	Stimulates B cell growth
B cell differentiation factor (BCDF)	Stimulates B cell differentiation
Lymphocytotoxic factor (lymphotoxin, LTF)	Kills nonlymphocytic cells

[a]Individual lymphokines may have more than one functional name.

tential antigen-presenting cells. γ Interferon also stimulates T cells, activates macrophages and NK cells, and suppresses viral replication in cells.

Other lymphokines are promoters of B lymphocyte growth and differentiation into antibody-producing cells. As will be discussed below, lymphokines recruit T lymphocytes and macrophages to sites of cell-mediated immune responses, producing chronic inflammation. Lymphokines cause the accumulation of macrophages at sites of T cell activation by chemoattraction of macrophages and inhibition of migration of macrophages away from the area. Lymphokines enhance the activity of many cells involved in defense, including macrophages, NK cells, and K cells.

MEDIATION OF INFLAMMATION BY T LYMPHOCYTES

Inflammation is the responses of a tissue to injury. Inflammatory responses are complex interactions of humoral, vascular, cellular and neural events that lead to a variety of tissue changes. The two major types of inflammation are acute and chronic. *Acute inflammation* typically develops quickly, in a matter of seconds to a few hours. It is characterized histologically by the influx of predominantly neutrophilic polymorphonuclear leukocytes into the site of injury. *Chronic inflammation* develops more slowly, requiring days to produce the characteristic tissue infiltration of predominantly lymphocytes and macrophages. It sometimes persists for months or years if the injurious stimulus remains. Most causes of tissue injury can induce inflammation. Some agents, such as thermal extremes, toxic chemicals, and trauma, cause direct injury to tissue and resultant inflammation. The immune system can also cause tissue injury.

Immune-mediated tissue injury results from the specific recognition of antigens by B lymphocytes, antibodies, or T lymphocytes, followed by the activation of inflammatory mediator systems and the recruitment of leukocytes to the site of the immune response. Interaction of antibodies with antigens in tissues recruits predominantly neutrophilic polymorphonuclear leukocytes, leading to acute inflammation. Antibody-mediated tissue injury will be discussed in detail in Chapter 11. T lymphocyte stimulation by antigens in tissues recruits predominantly T lymphocytes and macrophages, leading to chronic inflammation (Fig. 8–3).

A variant of chronic inflammation, called *granulomatous inflammation,* is characterized by a marked predominance of macrophages. Granulomatous inflammation can be either immune-mediated or nonimmune-mediated. An example of the latter is the granulomatous inflammation stimulated by the presence of a synthetic suture material at a site of prior surgery. Immune-mediated granulomatous inflammation is initiated by specific antigen recognition by T lymphocytes. This results in the release of lymphokines that mediate the accumulation and activation of macrophages.

Immune-mediated granulomatous inflammation is frequently caused by mycobacterial or fungal infections. Immune responses to viral infections typically induce lymphocyte-rich chronic inflammation, whereas immune responses to most bacterial infections usually cause neutrophil-rich acute inflammation.

Viral hepatitis caused by hepatitis B virus is an example of cell-mediated immune injury to the liver. Viral antigens expressed by infected hepatocytes are corecognized,

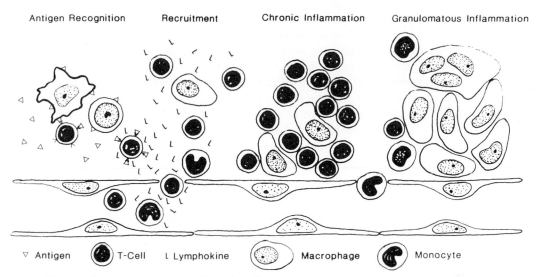

Antigen Recognition   Recruitment   Chronic Inflammation   Granulomatous Inflammation

▽ Antigen   T-Cell   ʟ Lymphokine   Macrophage   Monocyte

Figure 8-3. Immune-Mediated Chronic Inflammation. Diagram depicting the sequential events leading from antigen recognition by T lymphocytes to induction of chronic tissue inflammation.

along with HLA antigens, by T lymphocytes with specific receptors for the viral antigens. These T lymphocytes are activated, undergo blast transformation, proliferate, and secrete lymphokines. More lymphocytes and macrophages are recruited by lymphokines to the site of antigen recognition and are activated. Cytotoxic T lymphocytes and macrophages destroy infected hepatocytes and some innocent bystander hepatocytes. Although injurious to the liver, this chronic inflammatory response is required to prevent uncontrolled destruction of the liver by the virus. If the immune attack can control the viral infection without destroying too much liver tissue, the individual will survive. If the cytopathic effects of the virus or the destruction wrought by the immune response result in an inadequate amount of functioning liver tissue, the individual dies of hepatic failure.

Delayed Type Hypersensitivity

Delayed type hypersensitivity (DTH) is the enhanced secondary or anamnestic T lymphocyte-mediated response to antigens that have previously stimulated a primary cellular immune response. A classic example of delayed type hypersensitivity is the tissue response to tuberculin in a person who has had an infection with *Mycobacterium tuberculosis*. Tuberculin is an antigenic mycobacterial derivative. When injected intradermally into an individual who has had prior exposure to *M tuberculosis*, mycobacterial antigens are recognized by specific T lymphocytes, with the assistance of accessory cells. These T lymphocytes are activated, undergo blast transformation, and proliferate. Lymphokines are released and recruit more T lymphocytes, macrophages, and lesser numbers of other leukocytes to the site of antigen recognition. The majority of these recruited inflammatory cells do not have specific receptors for the antigens, but they can be activated by lymphokines to participate in the inflammatory process. The end result of the dermal DTH response is the development of a focus of chronic inflammation containing numerous lymphocytes and macrophages. This can be identified on the skin as a raised, erythematous, indurated area that reaches its maximum size approximately 24 to 48 hours after injection of tuberculin (Fig. 8–4).

In contrast to delayed hypersensitivity is *immediate hypersensitivity*. This form of inflammation is induced in the skin of an individual who has preformed antibodies, especially IgE, because of earlier exposure to the antigen. Intradermal injection of antigen results in the almost immediate development of acute inflammation that peaks in a matter of minutes to hours. This form of hypersensitivity will be discussed in detail in Chapter 11.

CELL-MEDIATED IMMUNE RESPONSES TO TUMORS

The body can mount humoral and cell-mediated immune responses to malignant neoplasms (cancers). Currently cell-mediated immune and nonimmune lysis of tumor cells

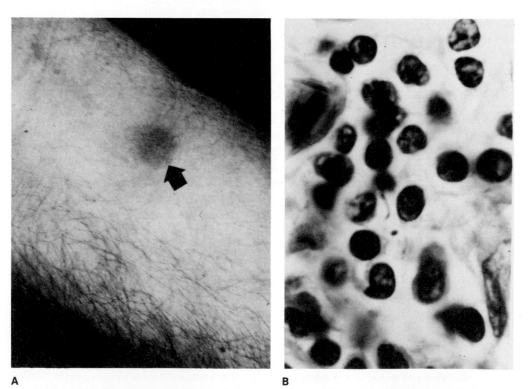

A   B

Figure 8–4. Tuberculin Skin Test. Positive tuberculin delayed hypersensitivity skin test showing the zone of erythema and induration *(arrow)* **(A)** and the histologic appearance of a focus of T cell-mediated inflammation containing numerous lymphocytes and macrophages **(B)**.

is considered to be more important than humoral immunity in defending against neoplasms. Cell-mediated attacks could provide protection against the development of cancer by destroying neoplasms before they attain significant size. Cytotoxic T lymphocytes, macrophages, NK cells, and K cells are all capable of destroying neoplastic cells.

A variety of leukocytes (Table 8–3) are capable of destroying certain target cells, such as virus-infected cells and tumor cells. Cytotoxic T lymphocytes are able to mediate antigen-specific lysis of tumor cells by the mechanisms described earlier in this chapter. This involves specific recognition of antigens on the surface of tumor cells. One category of antigen recognized on neoplastic cells is tumor *neoantigens.* These are molecular structures displayed by the abnormal neoplastic cells but not by normal cells *Oncofetal antigens* are molecules normally expressed predominantly by fetal cells during ontogeny. These antigens can also be produced by neoplasms, which often have many characteristics resembling immature cells. Immune system recognition of oncofetal antigens is probably not of major importance in immune defense against neoplasms but can be detected in blood by immunologic assays and used as laboratory markers for certain neoplasms. Two oncofetal tumor markers that are assayed for in clinical laboratories are carcinoembryonic antigen and alphafetoprotein.

NK cells are a subset of lymphocytes that can, without prior sensitization, mediate cytotoxicity against tumor cells and virus-infected cells. NK cells release a pore-forming protein from cytoplasmic granules. This protein forms channels in target cell membranes, resulting in lysis. NK cells may provide an early means of attacking neoplastic and virus-infected cells that is operational prior to the development of specific immunity. NK cells have membrane receptors for the non-antigen-binding portion (Fc region) of immunoglobulin. Because NK cells are relatively large and have conspicuous cytoplasmic granules, they are in the cell population called *large granular lymphocytes.*

In addition to NK cells, the large granular lymphocyte population contains *K cells* that carry out *antibody-dependent–cell-mediated cytotoxicity* (ADCC). ADCC can be accomplished by a variety of cell types, including polymorphonuclear leukocytes and macrophages. A feature that all cells capable of producing ADCC share is the presence of surface membrane receptors for the Fc region of IgG. The IgG serves as a link between the target cell to be lysed and the ADCC effector cell. The IgG binds to specific antigen on the target cell and to Fc receptors on the ADCC effector cell (Fig. 8–5). The effector cell then causes lysis of the target cell.

Macrophages can produce tumor cell lysis by ADCC and also by direct attack.

TABLE 8-3. LEUKOCYTES THAT CAN DESTROY TARGET CELLS

Cell Type	Mechanism of Attack
Cytotoxic T lymphocyte	Specific immune recognition
NK Cell	Nonimmune recognition
K cell	Antibody-dependent recognition
Macrophage	Antibody-dependent recognition and activation-induced attack
Polymorphonuclear leukocyte	Antibody-dependent recognition

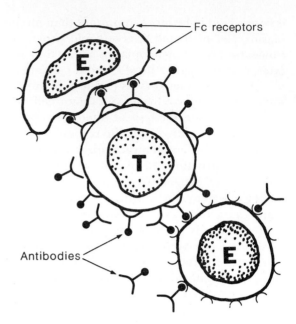

Figure 8–5. Antibody-Dependent Cell-Mediated Cytotoxicity. Diagram depicting antibody-dependent–cell-mediated cytotoxicity showing linkage between target cell *(T)* and effector cells *(E)* via antigen-antibody–Fc receptor.

Direct attack requires that the macrophage be in an activated or stimulated state. Macrophages can be activated, for example, by factors (lymphokines) released by antigen-stimulated T lymphocytes.

LABORATORY EVALUATION OF T LYMPHOCYTES

Clinical laboratory evaluation of T lymphocytes can be divided into methods for enumeration of T cells and T cell subsets and methods for in vitro and in vivo functional analysis of T cells. Enumeration methods are used most often in clinical laboratories; however, since different T cell subsets have different functions, determination of the proportions of different subsets in an individual sheds some light on the functional status of T cells in that individual. Table 8–4 lists some of the laboratory tests used to evaluate T lymphocytes.

T Lymphocyte Enumeration

All T cells have membrane receptors that bind sheep erythrocytes. These receptors are the basis for the first method used to identify T lymphocytes, the *sheep erythrocyte rosette technique* (Fig. 8–6 A). To perform this test mononuclear leukocytes are first isolated from blood by one of the density-gradient centrifugation procedures described in Chapter 3. These cells are mixed with sheep erythrocytes, incubated, and then examined microscopically. Lymphocytes with three or more attached erythrocytes are counted as rosettes and the % rosetted lymphocytes determined. From this value and the total lymphocyte count, the total T cells per mm³ of blood is calculated.

TABLE 8-4. LABORATORY TESTS FOR EVALUATING T LYMPHOCYTES

Laboratory Test	Purpose of Test
Sheep RBC rosetting	Enumerating all T cells
IgM-ox RBC rosetting	Enumerating helper T cells
IgG-ox RBC rosetting	Enumerating suppressor T cells
CD2 or CD3 immunostaining	Enumerating all T cells
CD4 immunostaining	Enumerating helper T cells
CD8 immunostaining	Enumerating suppressor T cells
DR and IL 2R immunostaining	Enumerating activated T cells
PPD and Candida skin test	Testing secondary T cell response
DNCB skin test	Testing primary T cell response
Mitogen stimulation	Testing proliferation capacity
Mixed lymphocyte culture	Testing allogeneic recognition
Migration inhibition test	Testing lymphokine production
Chromium release essay	Testing cytotoxic activity

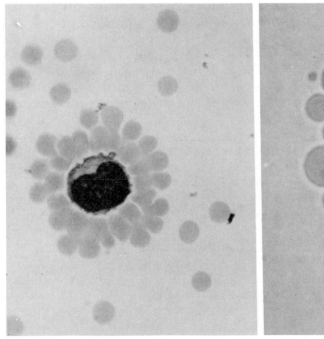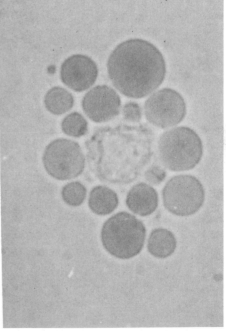

A   B

Figure 8-6. T Lymphocyte Rosettes. A. T lymphocytes rosetted with sheep erythrocytes (Wright's stain, original magnification ×2000). **B.** T lymphocytes rosetted with colored beads coated with CD4 monoclonal antibodies (phase contrast, original magnification ×2000).

Additional rosetting assays that have been used for the laboratory analysis of T cells are the *antibody-coated ox erythrocyte rosette assays*. These assays, however, are no longer used in clinical laboratories. They are based on the presence of a membrane receptor for the Fc portion of IgM on most helper T cells and a receptor for the Fc portion of IgG on most suppressor T cells. Ox cells are used in the assay because they are not bound by sheep erythrocyte receptors. In preparation for these assays, separate aliquots of ox erythrocytes are incubated with either anti-ox erythrocyte IgM or anti-ox erythrocyte IgG. The IgM-coated ox erythrocytes are then incubated with isolated mononuclear leukocytes and the % rosetted cells determined. The percentage of these T μ cells is an approximation of the percentage of helper T cells. Similarly, IgG-coated ox erythrocytes are incubated with mononuclear leukocytes and the % rosetted cells counted. The percentage of these T γ cells is an approximation of suppressor T cells.

Most current clinical laboratory techniques for enumeration of T cells and T cell subsets are based on the identification of T cell membrane antigens using monoclonal antibodies such as those listed in Table 8–1. The reaction of these antibodies with T cells is identified microscopically or by flow cytometry. The antibodies can be labeled with fluorochromes, enzymes, gold, or colored beads. The binding of antibodies with the last three labels is identified by light microscopy. For example, one commercially available assay uses red beads coated with T4 antibodies and yellow beads coated with T8 antibodies (Fig. 8–6 B). After these beads have been incubated with leukocytes, the total number of T lymphocytes and the proportion of T4 positive (helper) T cells and T8 positive (suppressor) T cells can be determined by counting the lymphocytes with attached red or yellow beads. Differently colored beads can also be coated with antibodies to B cells or T cells to enumerate total B cells versus total T cells. Binding of fluorochrome-labeled antibodies to lymphocytes is identified by fluorescence microscopy or fluorescence flow cytometry. The latter method is the method of choice in a laboratory with high specimen volume. Dual staining can be performed using different fluorochromes conjugated to different antibodies.

Determination by any of these methods of the T4/T8 ratio (CD4/CD8 or helper/suppressor ratio), which is normally approximately 2, is a useful laboratory finding in the diagnosis and evaluation of a number of diseases. For example, many viral diseases, especially AIDS, have a reduced T4/T8 ratio. Other diseases, for example multiple sclerosis and rheumatoid arthritis, have an increased T4/T8 ratio.

Evaluation of Activation-Induced T Cell Antigens

In addition to enumerating T cells and T cell subsets, antibodies are used to evaluate T cell activation. This is done by identifying antigens on T cells that are present on activated but not on unactivated T cells. The most commonly identified activation antigens are IL 2 receptors and DR antigens (MHC class II molecules). Antibodies to activation antigens are used to analyze T cells immediately after they are isolated from blood. This gives a measure of the degree of in vivo T cell activation. Antibodies to activation antigens can also be used to measure in vitro activation after T cells have been incubated with mitogens or specific antigens.

In addition to IL 2 receptor antigens, there are other membrane antigens expressed on T cell membranes and released by T cells into the circulation that appear during different stages of T cell activation. For example, whereas the intensity of T cell membrane IL 2 receptors reaches a peak within one week of T cell activation and thereafter declines, another activation antigen, very late activation (VLA) antigen, reaches peak expression several weeks after activation and persists. T lymphocytes with late activation antigens are increased in some chronic inflammatory diseases, for example, rheumatoid arthritis. Activation antigens may be the receptors for lymphokines and other soluble mediators of lymphocyte activation.

In Vivo Evaluation of T Lymphocyte Function

A skin test for DTH is an effective method for evaluating T lymphocyte function in vivo. Most adults and older children will have been exposed to and will have mounted a primary cellular immune response to a number of antigens that are available for intradermal injection, for example, antigens derived from mycobacteria, candida, mumps virus, trichophyton, histoplasma, and tetanus toxoid. When one of these antigens is injected intradermally into an individual who has previously been exposed to it, a T cell-mediated anamnestic inflammatory response will take place at the site of injection. As was discussed earlier in this chapter, this results in an area of erythema and induration that reaches maximum size 24 to 48 hours after injection of the test antigen to which there is a response (Fig. 8–4 A). The *Mantoux test,* named after Charles Mantoux, is a DTH skin test that employs intradermal injection of a purified protein derivative (PPD) of *M tuberculosis.* The *tine test* is a modification that, instead of intradermal injection, uses multiple pinpoint punctures to introduce antigens into the skin. A positive DTH skin reaction indicates that cellular immunity and therefore T lymphocyte function is intact. A negative DTH skin reaction in response to antigens to which the individual has previously been exposed indicates a defect in cellular immunity and possibly in T lymphocyte function. Absence of DTH reactivity is called *anergy.*

DTH skin tests using common environmental antigens assess anamnestic or secondary cellular immune responsiveness. To test the ability to mount a new T cell-mediated immune response, an antigen to which an individual has never been exposed is applied to the skin. The most commonly used antigen is dinitrochlorobenzene (DNCB). Several weeks after the initial exposure to DNCB, DNCB is reapplied to the skin and the development of inflammation monitored. A negative DNCB–DTH skin test indicates defective cellular immunity.

In Vitro Tests for T Lymphocyte Function

When T cells are exposed in vitro to appropriate mitogens or antigens for which they have specificity, a number of events that can be measured in the laboratory should normally occur, including increased metabolism, DNA synthesis, blast transformation, generation of new membrane receptors, production of lymphokines, proliferation, and expression of functional activity, such as B cell help, B cell suppression, or cytotoxicity. The in vitro assays of T cell function that are used most extensively in clinical immunology laboratories are designed to measure (1) T cell blast transformation or proliferation stimulated by mitogen or specific antigen recognition; (2) T cell production of lymphokines, usually macrophage migration inhibition factor; or (3) T cell cytotoxicity toward a target cell.

In Vitro T Lymphocyte Stimulation

In vitro stimulation of T lymphocytes can be accomplished with mitogens or specific antigens for which the T cells have specificity.

Mitogens stimulate proliferation (mitosis) without specific recognition of antigens. T cells have membrane receptors for certain mitogens, and mitogen binding to these receptors stimulates proliferation. *Lectins* are substances that will agglutinate erythrocytes by binding to membrane glycosides. The plant lectins concanavilin A (Con A), extracted from jack beans, and phytohemagglutinin (PHA), extracted from red kidney beans, are mitogens for human T lymphocytes. Pokeweed mitogen (PWM), another plant lectin, stimulates predominantly B lymphocytes.

A convenient source of foreign antigens that should stimulate a patient's T cells in vitro is allogeneic lymphocytes, i.e., lymphocytes from another individual who has different MHC antigens. The cells that are used as the source of antigens are treated with mitomycin C to inhibit proliferation so that when the patient's cells and foreign cells are mixed together, any proliferation observed will be by the patient's cells. This type of assay for stimulation by allogeneic cells is called a *mixed lymphocyte culture (MLC)* or *mixed lymphocyte reaction (MLR)*. MLC can be used as a measure of compatibility between donor and recipient of a graft as well as a measure of T lymphocyte function. For the former, mitomycin C-treated donor lymphocytes are mixed with recipient lymphocytes.

Lymphocyte stimulation induced by mitogens or allogeneic cells can be measured by a variety of methods, including microscopically enumerating transformed blasts, measuring tritiated thymidine incorporation into DNA, measuring the production of lymphokines such as MIF, measuring de novo expression of T cell activation antigens, and measuring the ability of T cells to lyse target cells.

Methods for Measuring in Vitro T Lymphocyte Stimulation

Lymphocytes are incubated with mitogen or antigen source (e.g., allogeneic lymphocytes) at 37°C, physiologic pH, and 5% CO_2. The optimum incubation time varies depending upon the means of stimulation and the stimulation parameter to be measured, usually ranging from 2 to 7 days.

The simplest method of measuring stimulation is to microscopically count the percentage of blast cells (i.e., cells with large nuclei, pale chromatin, and prominent nucleoli) among the lymphocytes that were incubated with mitogen or antigen and to compare this to the percentage of blasts in control cells from the same individual that were incubated under identical conditions except for the absence of mitogen or antigen. This *stimulation index (SI)* for the patient should be compared with the stimulation index obtained with lymphocytes from one or more normal individuals. The *relative proliferation index (RPI)* is the ratio of patient SI to normal SI. Elevated RPI values indicate hyper-reactivity; reduced values indicate hyporeactivity.

One of the most widely used methods for assessing in vitro lymphocyte stimulation is the measurement of tritiated *thymidine incorporation* into DNA. After an initial incubation of isolated mononuclear cells with mitogen or antigen, for example, for 72 hours, tritiated thymidine is added and the culture is further incubated, for example, for 18 hours. The cells are harvested, washed, and the radioactivity counted. Radioactivity incorporated into DNA is directly proportional to lymphocyte stimulation. This can be expressed as the difference in radioactivity (counts per minute, cpm) between stimulated and unstimulated patient cells, as the ratio of stimulated cell cpm to unstimulated cell cpm (SI), or as the ratio of patient SI to normal control SI (RPI).

Stimulation can be measured by the de novo expression of *activation antigens,* such as IL 2 receptors and DR antigens, on stimulated T cells. This approach is gaining popularity in clinical immunology laboratories because of the availability of flow cytometers to analyze the results. After incubation with mitogen or antigen, mononuclear cells are immunostained with fluorochrome-conjugated monoclonal antibodies specific for activation antigens, usually IL 2 receptors (CD 25) or DR (MHC class II) antigens. Flow cytometry is used to quantitate the proportion of stimulated and unstimulated cells expressing the activation antigen. From these data a SI and RPI can be calculated.

Lymphokine production can be measured as an indicator of in vitro T cell stimulation. This approach is not widely used in clinical laboratories. Measurement of macrophage migration inhibitory factor (MIF) and leukocyte migration inhibitory factor (LIF) have been used most extensively. Assays for these lymphokines are based on the ability of MIF to inhibit macrophage migration and LIF to inhibit neutrophil migration. Direct MIF and LIF assays have the migrating cells admixed with lymphocytes during stimulation, whereas indirect assays test the ability of culture supernatants from stimulated lymphocytes to inhibit migration of normal macrophages or neutrophils. The indirect method using migrating cells that are known to be normal is better for testing the ability of a patient's T lymphocytes to respond to stimulation in vitro. Any reduction in migration inhibition can then be attributed to defective lymphokine production rather than defective macrophage or neutrophil mobility.

For the indirect MIF and LIF assays, culture supernatant is collected after isolated mononuclear cells have been incubated with mitogen or antigen, for example, for 48 hours. A commonly used procedure for LIF uses wells cut in agar. Dilutions of culture supernatant from stimulated and unstimulated patient lymphocytes and known normal lymphocytes are added to aliquots of neutrophils and the mixtures placed in agarose wells. After incubation, for example, for 18 hours, the diameter of the zone of migration around each well is measured. The percent migration inhibition is calculated by comparing diameter of neutrophil migration with supernatants from stimulated lymphocytes to that with supernatants from unstimulated lymphocytes. This LIF assay procedure can be modified to assay for MIF by substituting guinea pig peritoneal macrophages for neutrophils.

The cytotoxic function of T lymphocytes can be measured in vitro, but this is rarely done in clinical immunology laboratories. The most commonly used in vitro assay of T lymphocyte-mediated cytotoxicity measures cytoplasmic *radioactive chromium (^{51}Cr) release* from killed target cells. ^{51}Cr-release assays can also be used to evaluate cytotoxicity mediated by macrophages, NK cells, and K cells. Target cells are incubated with ^{51}Cr, which diffuses into the cells and is integrated into the cytoplasm and cannot diffuse out of the viable cells. The labeled target cells are then incubated with the cells that are to be tested for cytotoxicity. Target cells that are killed release ^{51}Cr into the supernatant. Therefore at the completion of the test the amount of radioactivity in the supernatant is directly proportional to the cytotoxic activity of the effector cells tested.

Discussion of the Illustrative Case

The individual in the illustrative case developed pulmonary tuberculosis. In this person, as in the typical case of tuberculosis, the initial infection with mycobacteria probably occurred many years earlier but was suppressed by a competent immune system. Reactivation of the tuberculosis was prompted by the debilitation associated with advancing age and alcoholism. Because the patient was already exposed to the mycobacterial antigens, this renewed proliferation of the pathogen in the lung resulted in a very destructive T lymphocyte-mediated inflammation, including granulomatous inflammation. This infiltration of inflammatory cells into the lung tissue produced the radiographic opacities. Tissue destruction by the mycobacteria and inflammation led to cavitation in the lung and hemoptysis. A facsimile of the pulmonary chronic inflammation was produced in the skin by the intradermal injection of mycobacterial antigens. This delayed hypersensitivity skin test indicated exposure to mycobacteria, whereas the identification of mycobacteria in sputa by staining and culture was strong evidence for active pulmonary infection.

QUESTIONS

1. What three stimuli are required for antigen-induced T lymphocyte proliferation to occur?

2. Discuss the cell distribution of class I and II HLA molecules and the receptors for these molecules. How does interaction between these molecules and receptors play a role in T lymphocyte–antigen recognition?

3. Describe, in chronological order, the events that take place at the tissue site of antigen-induced–T lymphocyte-mediated inflammation.

4. Why does T lymphocyte-mediated–delayed hypersensitivity take longer to develop than B lymphocyte-mediated–immediate hypersensitivity?

Chapter

9 B Lymphocyte Activation and Antibody Synthesis

OBJECTIVES

1. To discuss molecular properties of antigens.
2. To discuss factors that influence humoral immune responses.
3. To outline the events from introduction of antigen to antibody secretion.
4. To discuss the role of T lymphocytes in humoral immune responses.
5. To define and compare the molecular structure and properties of the classes of immunoglobulins.
6. To discuss isolation and purification of antibodies.
7. To discuss quantitative and functional evaluation of B lymphocytes.

Illustrative Case

A 30-year-old male developed severe abdominal pain 5 months after having a portion of his large intestine removed after an accidental gunshot wound. Physical examination revealed a distended abdomen, and radiographic studies indicated bowel obstruction caused by fibrous adhesions. Surgery was scheduled to relieve the obstruction, and three units of blood were ordered to be held on standby. Blood bank found 2 of 3 off-the-shelf units of blood to be compatible; however, the third unit was incompatible. Panel cell screening on patient serum plus a series of reagent red blood cells of known surface antigen composition found that the patient's serum agglutinated or reacted with the Le^a Lewis blood cell antigen. The red blood cells in the incompatible unit also were found to have

175

Le^a, but the cells in the compatible units did not. The patient's red blood cells were Le^a negative.

HISTORICAL PERSPECTIVE

The humoral immune response (antigen-induced antibody production) has been recognized and studied longer than the cellular immune response. Vaccination procedures for stimulating active immunity were developed late in 1700 and early in 1800 by Jenner for smallpox and by Pasteur for rabies. In the late 1800s the theoretical basis for clinical laboratory serology was discovered. Widal described the agglutination of typhoid bacilli with serum from individuals who had suffered from typhoid fever. This serologic method, the *Widal test,* was used to screen for antibodies in patients' sera in the diagnosis of typhoid fever. Pfeiffer found the clinically useful phenomenon of *Vibrio cholerae* lysis by sera from patients having the disease. Von Behring received the Nobel prize for his discovery of passive immune therapy against diphtheria and tetanus.

There are several types of immunity. *Active immunity* results from injection of antigens (vaccination) that stimulate the recipient to develop his or her own immune elements. *Passive immunity* results from the injection of antibodies that were synthesized in some other individual or animal that had been exposed to the antigen against which immunity is desired. *Adoptive immunity* results from the transfer of immune system tissue from an individual who is immune to some other individual who adopts the transferred tissue as his or her own and thereafter utilizes it to develop immunity. Because passive immunity is dependent upon the action of injected antibodies; it is effective immediately and remains effective for the lifetime of the administered antibodies. Active and adoptive immunity require time to become effective, but once active they remain effective for years to a lifetime. In the twentieth century there has been an explosion of knowledge concerning the production, structure, and function of antibodies. Landsteiner's immunochemical studies of blood group antigens and antibodies laid the foundation for modern immunohematology. Haurowitz's *template theory* (instructive theory) suggests that a portion of an antigen acts as a template around which lymphocytes synthesize specific antibodies. An alternative theory that is backed by substantial data is Burnet's *clonal selection theory* which suggests that each individual is innately endowed with genetic information required to produce antibodies of specificities for all antigens that he or she will ever encounter. When antigens are encountered they selectively stimulate only those lymphocytes that contain the genetic machinery to produce antibodies against them.

Porter and Edleman were the first to define the basic immunoglobulin structure of four protein chains (two heavy and two light). Subsequently there has been a detailed elucidation of the structure, biochemistry, and biosynthesis of antibody molecules and the antigens that they bind. A more recent development that has aided research in immunology and that has found application in the clinical laboratory is the ability to synthesize monoclonal antibodies with tissue-cultured hybridomas. *Hybrido-*

mas are clones of a cell, all of which produce *monoclonal antibodies* or antibodies with the same specificity for antigen.

ANTIGENS

The type and the extent of an immune response to antigen stimulation depends upon many factors, such as properties of the antigen, genetic and immune system constitution of the responding individual, and route by which the antigen is introduced into the body. Some of these factors only influence the immune response, whereas others are requirements for an immune response.

Molecular Requirements of Antigens

Antigens bind to antibodies, B lymphocyte receptors, and T lymphocyte receptors. That portion of an antigen that actually binds to antibody is called an *epitope* or an *antigenic determinant.* Most, but not all, antigens will stimulate an immune response. This capacity to stimulate an immune response is called *immunogenicity.* Antigens that stimulate immune responses are called *immunogens.*

Most important among the properties required for immunogenicity is that the antigen be *foreign* or "nonself." The greater the difference in molecular structure from self (the responder), or the greater the degree of foreignness, the better the immune response. For example, antigens from geese do not stimulate good humoral responses in ducks, whereas more foreign antigens from plants will stimulate good humoral responses in ducks.

A second property essential for an antigen to stimulate an immune response is that it be a *macromolecule* of a minimum size around 10,000 daltons. Smaller molecules are poor immunogens, possibly because they are not processed or phagocytized very well by macrophages.

A third essential property of immunogenic antigens is that they be of sufficient *molecular complexicity.* They should consist of as many different units as possible, that is, different amino acids in proteins and different sugars in carbohydrates. Large homopolymers, even though they are of sufficient molecular weight, are not good antigens due to lack of complexity. Nylon, Teflon, and polystyrene, for example, are nonantigenic. Because there are many different units or amino acids from which to build, proteins are the best antigens. Carbohydrates have fewer different units of sugars from which to build and are the next best antigens. There are even fewer different nucleosides from which to build nucleic acids, and there are only several fatty acids from which to build lipids. Data in the literature varies; however, our experience is that neither pure nucleic acids nor pure lipids are immunogenic by themselves. Either may, however, act as a hapten.

A *hapten* is a molecule that binds to specific antibodies but that cannot, by itself, initiate an immune response. Antibodies specific for haptens are produced by linking hapten with a carrier and then using the hapten-carrier complex as an immunogen. A *carrier* is a molecule that by itself is immunogenic and that when combined with hapten to form an immunogenic complex provides stimulation for production of antibodies specific to the hapten. Thus a hapten-carrier complex would stimulate production of a pool of antibodies, with some being specific for individual epitopes on the carrier, some being specific for the hapten, and some being specific for neoepitopes formed by hapten and juxtaposed parts of the carrier (Fig. 9–1).

For an immune response to occur, the individual receiving the immunogen must have appropriate *immune response genes* (IR or DR or Class II) MHC. These genes were discussed in Chapter 8. Individuals who develop immune responses to particular antigens are termed *responders*. Individuals who do not develop immune responses to particular antigens due to lack of the appropriate DR genes are termed *nonresponders*.

Other Factors That Influence Immune Responses

The *age* of the individual receiving the antigen influences the resultant immune response. In general, older individuals have decreased responses to immunogens. Cancer and other diseases that are thought to develop as a result of some defect in normal immune defenses are known to occur at a much higher rate in older individuals whose immune systems are waning. Neonates are another example of age influencing immune responses. Their immune systems are not yet totally developed, and therefore they do not demonstrate complete immune responses to antigenic stimuli. Neonates' humoral responses are essentially limited to IgM production.

Route of inoculation influences response to an antigen. Antigens can enter the body by way of inhalation, ingestion, intravenous injection, or subcutaneous injection. Persons suffering from allergies to ragweed pollen have developed an immune response to inhaled allergens. A somewhat successful therapy for these individuals is to intrader-

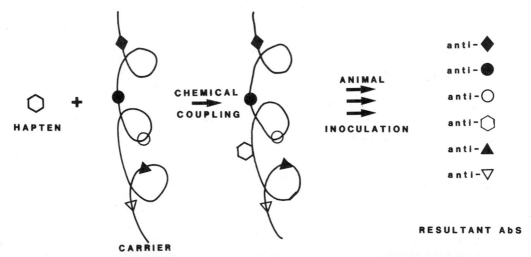

Figure 9–1. Hapten Carrier as Immunogen and Resultant Antibodies. When a hapten is covalently linked to a carrier and the complex is injected into an animal to stimulate an immune response, resulting antibodies will show specificity to the epitopes of the carrier plus to the hapten.

mally inject the same allergens to which they are allergic and thus stimulate a different type of immune response. The new route of inoculation causes IgG production, whereas the inhaled route stimulates mostly IgE production.

Another example of the route of inoculation affecting the immune response is the polio vaccine. This virus is initially ingested orally, establishes itself along the intestinal tract, enters the blood, and then invades the central nervous system. The original Salk vaccine consisted of intramuscular injections of formaldehyde-inactivated polio virus. This vaccine stimulated development of immunity that offered protection from paralytic and systemic poliomyelitis but did not protect an individual from infection by the polio virus. Intramuscular vaccination provided antibodies to neutralize blood-borne virus particles and thus prevented spread to the central nervous system. Although intramuscular vaccination prevented the recipient from suffering paralytic polio, it did not prevent that person from undergoing polio infection and passing that virus to other persons. In fact, individuals who had nonsymptomatic infections of the polio virus were found to be major contributors to epidemics of the disease. These individuals, or carriers of the polio virus, were unknowingly transmitting the disease. Sabin therefore developed an oral vaccine that consisted of live, attenuated polio virus. This vaccine stimulated immune responses to provide not only protection from the paralytic stage of polio but also protection from infection by the virus. The oral preparation stimulated production of secretory IgA in the intestinal tract to inhibit localized establishment of the polio virus. Thus carriers were eliminated. As far as benefit to the vaccinated individual, probably both Salk and Sabin vaccines were equally effective; however, the Sabin vaccine eliminated carriers and thus spread of the infection.

The *amount of antigen* used to stimulate the immune system influences the response. An example is the vaccination of mice with pneumococcal polysaccharide. Injections of small amounts of antigen (3 mg) stimulates immunity to subsequent challenge with the organism. However, injections of larger amounts of antigen (300 mg) induce a state of *tolerance* or paralysis of the immune system, and subsequent challenge results in infection and death to the animal.

Adjuvants are substances that are mixed with antigens to increase the resultant immune response. Aluminum salts form insoluble complexes with antigen. The complexing prevents rapid dissemination of soluble antigen from the injection site and thereby prolongs the existence of a reservoir of antigen for immune stimulation. Aluminum salt complexes also increase the size of antigenic particles and thus enhance processing by macrophages. Adjuvants commonly used to stimulate antibody production in animals are Freund's complete and Freund's incomplete. *Freund's complete adjuvant* is given with initial antigen injections of animals and consists of mineral oil, emulsifier, and killed mycobacterium. Antigen is mixed with the adjuvant to form an emulsion that is then injected. *Freund's incomplete adjuvant* lacks the mycobacteria and is mixed with subsequent injections of antigen into animals to boost their immune response. Freund's incomplete adjuvant is thought to increase the number of macrophages participating in antigen processing and to enhance processing by macrophages. Because Freund's adjuvants incite granulomatous inflammation, they are not used in humans. *Muramyl dipeptide* (MDP) is another adjuvant derived from mycobacteria, and it is sometimes used in human cancer therapy.

Modified Antigens

Antigens used to stimulate immunity against infectious diseases include toxoids and attenuated pathogens. *Toxoids* are bacterial exotoxins that have been treated (e.g., heated) to destroy their toxicity but not their immunogenicity. Diphtheria and tetanus toxoids are used to produce immune antisera to be used in passive immune therapy. Pathogenic effects of diphtheria and tetanus are caused by exotoxins, and antibodies that inactivate them prevent the disease.

Attenuated microorganisms are microorganisms that have been grown under special conditions to cause them to lose their virulence but not their immunogenicity. Passing microorganisms through different hosts (animals) or through growth media will sometimes change the microorganism's metabolism and/or structure so that it is no longer pathogenic to man. Rabies vaccine and Sabin vaccine are examples that use attenuated microorganisms as antigens. One possible complication of attenuated microorganisms in vaccines is that they may regain their virulence after several passes through normal hosts. Stringent quality control measures must be enforced to ensure patient safety in regard to attenuated preparations.

CELLULAR EVENTS IN THE HUMORAL IMMUNE RESPONSE

Antigens may be either T dependent (require T cell participation to elicit a humoral response) or T independent (do not require T cell participation to elicit a humoral response). Most antigens are T dependent. Large homopolymers are examples of T-independent antigens, and they stimulate only IgM type antibody production. Stimulation of the humoral immune response by T-dependent antigens begins with processing of antigen by the macrophage or other accessory cell, as described in Chapter 8. The macrophage or equivalent cell phagocytizes antigen and processes it for presentation to lymphocytes. This processing induces the macrophage to synthesize and secrete a series of *monokines* (Table 9–1). Other pertubations of the macrophage membrane, such as association with an uningestable fungus, can also stimulate monokine secretion.

Once processing of Ag has been accomplished, membrane immunoglobulin on the B cell will bind with its specific complementary epitope being offered by the macrophage or equivalent antigen-presenting cell (APC; Fig. 9–2). A T helper (T_H) simultaneously binds both to the APC and to the B cell via its receptors for Class II major

TABLE 9–1. MONOKINES: SOME OF THE SUBSTANCES SYNTHESIZED AND SECRETED BY MACROPHAGES AND MONOCYTES

Interferon
Interleukin 1
Complement factors
Coagulation factors

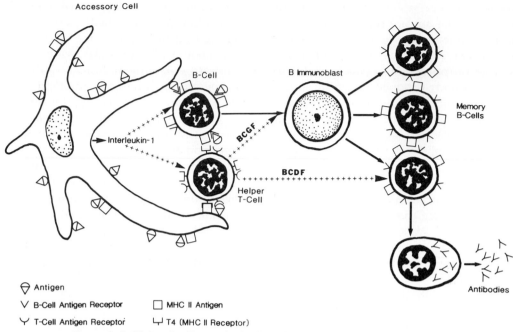

Figure 9–2. Molecular Events in Antigen Stimulation of B Lymphocytes.

histocompatibility complex (MHC) molecules on the surface of both of the other cells. This tricellular complex activates the resting B cell to transform into a blast and to generate receptors on its surface for the lymphokine *B cell growth factor* (BCGF).

Binding of BCGF secreted from activated T_H to the B cell receptors prompts the B cell to undergo cell division and to produce many daughter cells with identical Ag receptors on their surfaces. One feature that distinguishes these new daughter cells from the original adult B cell is their receptors for B cell differentiation factor.

At this point one of two things can happen. Daughter B cells can bind B cell differentiation factor (BCDF), which prompts them to undergo differentiation into terminal plasma cells and to synthesize and secrete many antibodies. Alternatively, daughter cells may not bind BCDF and instead may become memory cells. These memory cells have IgD and IgM receptors for that specific antigen that stimulated their production, and they also have receptors for BCDF.

Presence of memory cells explains the faster and heightened antibody response to antigen upon subsequent exposures. Memory cells and their ability to immediately differentiate to plasma cells upon binding of BCDF could also explain the nonspecific polyclonal antibody stimulation associated with some viral infections. *Polyclonal stimulation* is nonspecific stimulation of many different B cell clones with different Ab specificity from each clone. This stimulation has been related to production of BCDF as a result of the presence of the virus.

Humoral immune stimulation may be depressed by T suppressor cells (T_s). Exactly where the suppression occurs is still under investigation, although there are data to indicate several points of action. The secretion of essential BCGF and BCDF lympho-kines can be suppressed. There is evidence that different BCGF, BCDF, etc. are re-quired to stimulate IgM, IgG, etc. synthesis. Selected suppression of one type BCDF may occur while total BCDF is present in normal amounts. There is also evidence for selected suppression of B cells with specificity toward one antigen.

Antibody production can be suppressed by the production of anti-idiotypic anti-bodies. An idiotype is the portion of an antibody molecule that reacts with the antigen epitope. The idiotype is on secreted antibodies as well as immunoglobulins, such as IgM and IgD, that are functioning as B lymphocyte membrane receptors for antigen. An individual develops antibodies against idiotypes on antibodies and B lymphocytes that are increased during a humoral immune response. These *anti-idiotypic antibodies* suppress this specific immune response. This network of idiotypes and anti-idiotypic antibodies, along with suppressor T cells, serves to down-regulate humoral immune responses once the antigen that initiated the response has been eliminated.

STRUCTURE AND NOMENCLATURE OF IMMUNOGLOBULINS

Each basic antibody unit is composed of 2 light (L) chains and 2 heavy (H) chains (Fig. 9–3). These four polypeptide chains contain several *domains* of similar length formed into loops by intrachain disulphide bridges. L chains consist of two domains, a variable region domain and a constant region domain. The variable portion is the amino termi-nal half of the protein chain and has an amino acid sequence that varies among anti-body molecules having different antigen specificity. In tertiary structure this variable region of the L chain plus the variable region of the H chain form the binding site for antigen. The variable domain of the L chain is referred to as the V_L. The other domain of the L chain, the carboxyl end, is referred to as the C_L and contains the amino acid sequence that categorizes the L chain as κ or λ (Table 9–2). All normal individuals have both types of L chains. Each antibody molecule, however, has only one type of L chain. All the immunoglobulins produced by B cells arising from the same stimulated B cell have the same type of L chain. About 67% of human L chains are of the κ type. Within the λ chains, there are some *isotypes* or nonallelic markers (variation in amino acid sequences called Mcg, $Ke^-O_2^-$ and $Ke^-O_2^+$. There are no known allotypes of λ chains. Three *allotypes* (different genetic types in different individuals of the same spe-cies) are associated with κ chains and are called Km(1), Km(2), and Km(3). The older nomenclature for the κ chain allogeneic forms was Inv.

H chains consist of at least four, and sometimes five, domains V_H, C_H1, C_H2, C_H3, and, in the case of IgM, IgD and IgE, C_H4. The variable H chain domain together with the V_L form that area of the antibody molecule where antigen is bound. Variable areas of immunoglobulin molecules are of different amino acid sequence for each antigenic specificity. This unique amino acid sequence is the basis of antibody *idiotypes,* which will be explained later in this chapter. The constant domains of the H chains are the basis for classification of antibodies into major isotypes of IgM, IgG, IgA, IgE, and IgD. The corresponding H chains are μ, γ, α, ϵ, and δ. These H chain constant domains also are the basis for the subgroup isotypes of IgG1, IgG2, IgG3, IgG4, IgA1, IgA2, IgM1,

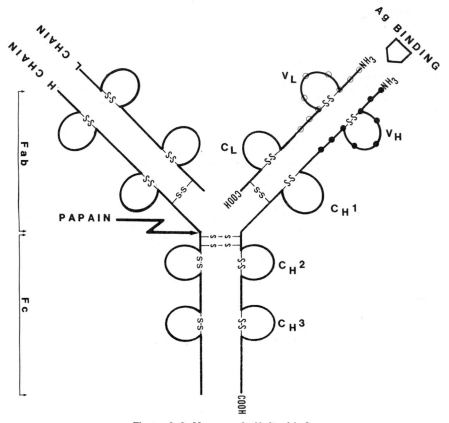

Figure 9-3. Monomeric Unit of IgG.

and IgM2. Allotypes based upon amino acid sequences in the constant region of the H chain are the basis for the 25 Gm types and the 2 Am types.

The 2 H and 2 L chains of the basic antibody unit are held together by interchain disulphide bonds (Fig. 9-3). In addition to the H and L chains of immunoglobulins, all antibodies consisting of 2 or more basic units (H_2L_2) have a J chain attached to hold the units together (Fig. 9-4). IgG, IgA, IgE, and IgD normally occur as the single unit form. Serum IgA occurs mostly as a monomer; however, small amounts of dimers with attached J chain are not uncommon. Serum IgM is a pentamer with attached J chain. Of the antibody classes, IgM is the most susceptible to disassociation by treatment with mild sulfhydral ($-SH$) reagents. IgG is stable to such treatment. This difference in susceptibility to $-SH$ is used in blood banks to distinguish between IgG and IgM type antibodies. Secretory IgA found in saliva and other body secretions consists of a dimer with attached J chain plus an additional polypeptide, the *secretory component* (SC).

The region between the C_H1 and C_H2 actually bends upon association of antibody with antigen and is therefore called the *hinge region*. When *papain* is used to digest the antibody molecule (Fig. 9-3), it cleaves at the point of the hinge region to give 2 Fab

TABLE 9–2. IMMUNOGLOBULINS

Class	IgG	IgA	IgM	IgD	IgE
Subclass	IgG (1–4)	IgA (1–2)	IgM (1–2)		
Allotype	Gm (1–25)	A2m (1–2)			
H chain	γ	α	μ	δ	ϵ
L chain	κ, λ	κ, λ	κ, λ	κ, λ	κ, λ
Molecular formula	H_2L_2	$(H_2L_2)_2J$	$(H_2L_2)_5J$	H_2L_2	H_2L_2
% CHO	4	10	15	12	12
Molecular weight	150,000	170,000	950,000	185,000	200,000
$S_{20,w}$	7	7,10	19	7	8
$t_{1/2}$	21	6	9	3	2
Crosses placenta	+	−	−	−	−
Classical complement activation	+	−	+	−	−
Serum concentration mg/dl	1200	250	125	3	0.01
C_H domains	3	3	4	4?	4?
Resistance to −SH	high	low	low	low	low
Stable at 56°C, 30 min	+	+	+	−	−
Secretory form + SC	−	+	+	−	−

Abbreviations: MW SC = 70,000; MW J chain = 15,000

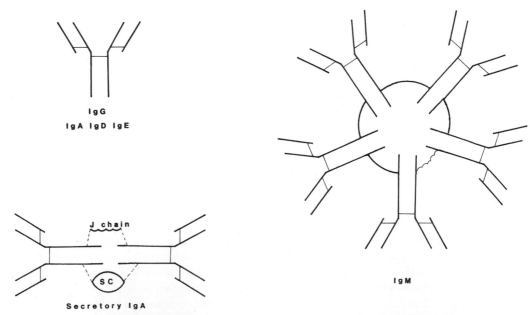

Figure 9–4. Molecular Configurations of Immunoglobulins. SC = secretory component.

(antibody fragment) pieces and one *Fc* (crystallizable fragment) piece. The cleavage point is before the inter-H-chain disulfide bonds so that the constant regions of the H chains remain bound together by the disulfide bonds. The Fab fragments have nothing to hold them to each other after cleavage and, therefore, fall apart into 2 separate V_HV_L pieces. *Pepsin* is another commonly used protease that will cleave the antibody unit further down below the inter-H-chain disulphide bonds to give one F(ab')$_2$ and several pieces of the Fc' region. The interchain bonds remain with the Fab' piece and hold the antigen-binding sites together. Therefore a Fab fragment has 1 antigen combining site, whereas a F(ab')$_2$ fragment has 2 combining sites. Fab fragments are useful in those assays that utilize labeled antibody to identify membrane antigen on cells that have membrane receptors for the Fc portion of antibody. These assays are based upon the labeled Ab reacting with Ag. If labeled Ab is bound to a cell via its Fc component, false labeling occurs. Think about the Fab and the F(ab')$_2$ fragments and their ability to mediate agglutination.

MOLECULAR EVENTS IN SYNTHESIS OF ANTIBODIES

Synthesis of the H, L, and J chains occurs in B cells to a limited extent and in plasma cells to a vast extent. Stimulation of the B cell to differentiate to a terminal plasma cell occurs as outlined earlier in this chapter. Antigen-specific receptors on the mature B cell membrane are mostly IgD and IgM. These receptors have been synthesized by the B cell and determine which Ag will stimulate the B cell. Processed Ag presented by the APC binds to one of the receptors to initiate the primary humoral immune response. The H, L, and J chains are synthesized according to the usual translational process for any protein. Messenger RNA for L chains is formed according to Figure 9–5. Each B cell has multiple V_L regions, several joining L chain regions, and either a λ or a κ C_L region. Selection of one of the variable segments and one of the joining segments with DNA rearrangement produces one intact gene segment from the previous two pieces. Another gene segment codes for C_L. Transcription and RNA splicing produce a single mRNA for the entire L chain. Similarly, 3 segments of DNA are rearranged to form the V_H, which is transcribed together with a DNA segment for the constant region. Splicing produces a single mRNA for the total H chain. These L and H chain templates then code for antibodies produced by that B cell.

The B cell sequentially incorporates different constant DNA regions on the H chain to explain the isotype switching of antibody classes during the life of a B cell. In a primary humoral response, IgM is always the first class of Ab to be produced by the terminal plasma cells. A terminal cell does not undergo further transformation during its life. After initiation of synthesis and secretion of IgM, the plasma cell can switch to other H chain isotypes further down the gene μ, δ, γ_3, γ_2, γ_1, α_1, γ_4, ϵ, and α_2. The V_H and the L chain V_LC_L mRNA remain constant to preserve antigen specificity throughout the life of the plasma cell. H, L, and, if applicable, J chains are translated as separate proteins. Their carbohydrate moieties are attached to the H chain constant region while it is still nascent. Later the free chains combine to form the complete antibody molecule, which is then secreted. The IgM pentamer seems to be assembled into its multiunit form concomitant with secretion from the cell.

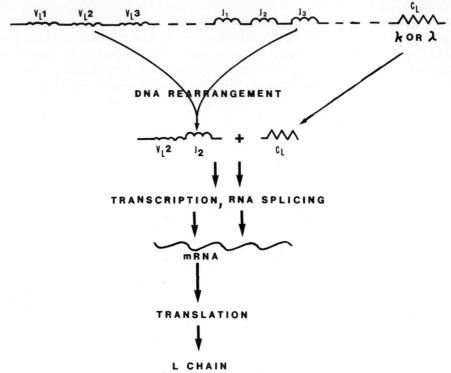

Figure 9-5. Rearrangement of Gene Portions and RNA Splicing to Form a Single mRNA for a Light Chain.

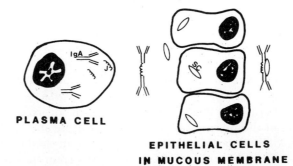

Figure 9-6. Formation of Secretory IgA.

Secretory IgA (Fig. 9–6) has an additional protein chain, the SC, incorporated into its structure. SC is not synthesized by the B cell but rather is synthesized by epithelial cells lining the mucosal areas of the body. After the dimeric form of IgA with attached J chain leaves the plasma cell, it migrates through the epithelial lining and, during this migration, picks up the SC. Therefore the IgA found in saliva, lacrimal fluid, colostrum, nasal fluid, and intestinal fluid has the SC and is called secretory IgA.

PHYSICAL, BIOLOGICAL, AND CHEMICAL PROPERTIES OF IMMUNOGLOBULINS

Properties of antibodies are summarized in Table 9–2. The L chain has a molecular weight of about 23,000 daltons, the H chain about 50,000 daltons plus carbohydrate moiety and fourth domain amino acids, the J chain 15,000 daltons, and the SC 70,000 daltons.

IgG

IgG is the antibody class of highest concentration in normal human serum. It is also the only antibody that can cross the placental barrier. The newborn's major antibody defense is maternal IgG because its immune system is incompletely developed and not yet capable of developing humoral immune responses other than IgM. IgG has the longest peripheral circulation half-life, 30 days, of any immunoglobulin class. The C_H2 domains of IgG3, IgG1, and IgG2 are capable of activating complement via the classical pathway in the decreasing order listed. IgG4 is incapable of activating complement via the classical pathway. Macrophages have specific receptors (Fc receptors) for the C_H3 portion of IgG1 and IgG3. In normal serum the IgG1 constitutes about 65% of total IgG, IgG2 about 25%, IgG3 about 7%, and IgG4 about 3%. IgG resists both treatment with mild $-SH$ and with heating at 37°C for 30 minutes.

IgA

IgA is the next most concentrated antibody type in normal human serum, and it occurs mostly in the monomer form. Secretory IgA is the most concentrated antibody type in body secretions. Of all classes of antibodies, IgA is the most effective in defense against viral infections, since viral pathogens most often enter the body at mucosal surfaces, for example, the respiratory and gastrointestinal tracts.

IgM

IgM is the third most concentrated antibody class in normal human serum and is the most efficient activator of the classical complement pathway. Because it is the first antibody class to be formed in humoral immune responses, its presence suggests current infection with those specific organisms to which it binds. IgM along with IgD are the antigen-specific membrane receptors on B cells. IgM is the most efficient Ab in agglutination of bacterial, blood, and other cells. IgM is denatured by exposure to mild $-SH$ and has an extra constant domain to give a total of 4 C_H domains.

IgD

IgD is highly susceptible to denaturation by heating. This class antibody is incorporated into the membrane of B cells where it functions as an antigen receptor. Because it occurs in such small concentrations, little is known about this antibody class.

IgE

IgE is best known for its role in immediate type I hypersensitivities or allergies. The pathophysiology of IgE will be discussed in Chapter 11. IgE is called a *cytotropic antibody* because it binds with high affinity to mast cells that have receptors for its Fc portion. IgE is sometimes called *reagin* in relation to its role in allergies. It is unfortunate that this term is the same applied to the unrelated nonspecific antibody formed in syphilis. Antigens that stimulate IgE production are termed *allergens*. Vollmer's in vivo patch tests are allergen assays that create wheal and flare reactions in sensitized patients. IgE is highly susceptible to heating at 37°C for 30 minutes and like IgM, contains an extra C_H4 domain.

MOLECULAR SPECIFICITIES OF ANTIBODIES

Antibodies have an incredible specificity toward the particular antigen that stimulated their production (Fig. 9–7). This specificity is capable of distinguishing different glycose units, ortho, meta, and para isomers, and different ionic radicals. Nonionic radicals are not, however, distinguishable. Figure 9–7 depicts the results of dialysis experiments with similar haptens to demonstrate the specificity of antibodies toward that

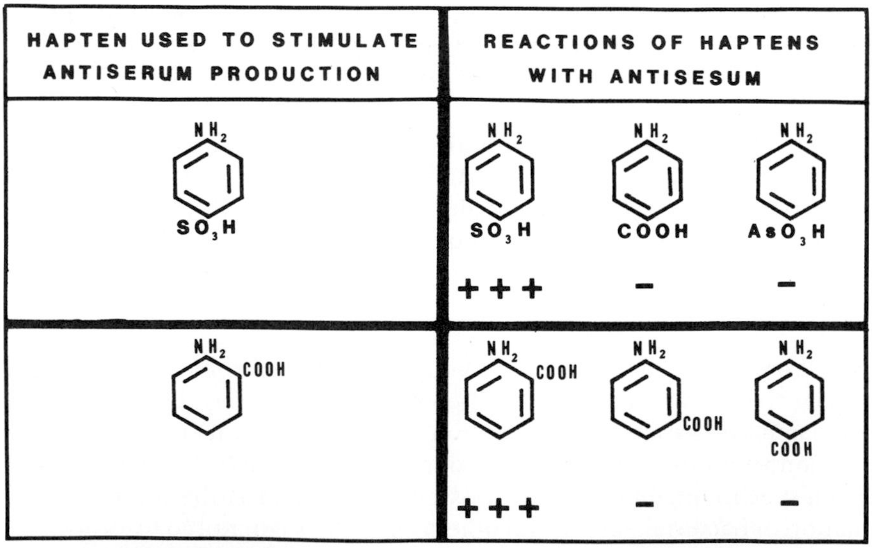

Figure 9-7. Antibody Specificity. The hapten on the left is used to produce antiserum that is tested for its binding to the original and to similar molecules.

specific hapten that participated in their stimulation. Antibodies will cross-react with antigens or haptens that are similar in structure to the antigen that initiated their production; however, binding affinities are strongest for the stimulating epitope. The Weil–Felix diagnostic laboratory test is one assay that makes use of the cross-reactivity of antibodies to rickettsial antigens with proteus antigens.

MONOCLONAL ANTIBODY PRODUCTION

A strategy for collecting large amounts of homogenous antibody is to culture clones of plasma cells, all of which produce identical antibody. The first large quantity of identical antibody that was used for amino acid sequencing was obtained from myeloma patients. *Myelomas* are neoplasms of plasma cells that secrete large amounts of identical antibody. Identifying high concentrations of this myeloma protein in serum is an important basis for diagnosis of the disease. Serum electrophoresis usually detects this abnormality. Hybridomas (Fig. 9–8) may be formed by fusion of spleen cells, which do not normally grow in any medium, with myeloma cells, which readily grow. A hybrid cell has the growth and antibody synthetic properties of a plasma cell and the antigen specificity of the spleen cell. Antigen is injected into a mouse to stimulate an immune response. A few days thereafter the spleen, containing stimulated B cells as well as T cells, is removed. These cells are mixed with myeloma cells in the presence of polyethylene glycol (PEG), which "melts" cytoplasmic membranes and allows adjacent cells to fuse. When the PEG is removed, the membranes become rigid again. Resulting fused cells are plated onto hypoxanthine, aminopterin, and thymidine (HAT) medium. Myeloma cells fail to grow on the HAT medium because they lack hypoxanthine transferase. Spleen cells fail to grow because they are incapable of growing for extended periods on any medium. The only cells that do grow are the hybridoma cells, which are myeloma cells that have acquired the transferase from spleen cells. These cells are then plated out and assayed for production of that antibody specific for the antigen, which was originally used to stimulate the spleen cells. Availability of monoclonal antibodies has revolutionized the clinical laboratory as well as the science of immunology. More and more clinical assays in all areas of the laboratory are being converted to methods involving monoclonal antibodies. A new technique for inducing clones of human antibody-producing B cells is to infect human B cells with Epstein–Barr virus.

SPECIAL TERMS FOR SOME CLINICALLY IMPORTANT ANTIBODIES

The pathophysiology of the antibodies mentioned in this section will be discussed in detail in Chapter 11. *Cryoglobulins or cold antibodies* are immunoglobulins, mostly of the IgM class, that precipitate in the cold (4°C) and that redissolve when warmed to 37°C. Detectable cryoglobulins are associated with a number of diseases, for example, lymphomas and myelomas, rheumatoid arthritis, and systemic lupus erythematosus (SLE). They are also found after a number of infections, for example, cytomegalovirus (CMV),

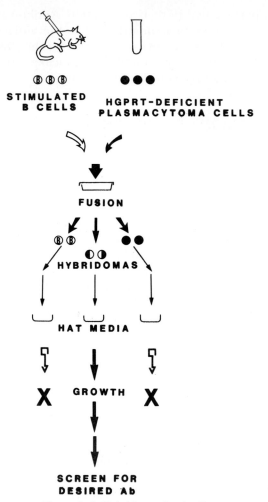

Figure 9-8. Hybridoma Production

infectious mononucleosis (IM), and mycoplasmal pneumonia. IgM cryoglobulins are often specific for blood group antigens, usually anti-I, but anti-i and anti-P have also been found. Individuals with cryoglobuins may demonstrate symptoms upon exposure to the cold, which precipitates the cryoglobulins. One symptom is Raynaud's phenomenon, which is a turning blue of the fingers, toes, and ear lobes. Other symptoms are vascular purpura, bleeding tendencies, and thrombosis with gangrene of distal extremities. Cryoglobulins may interfere with laboratory assays by precipitating and removing factors from serum during storage in the cold. Redissolving by heating will not replace these factors such as complement.

Donath–Landsteiner antibody is an IgG cold antibody that binds to (sensitizes) erythrocytes below 15°C. When warmed the cells will hemolyze and cause hemoglobinuria. *Paroxysmal cold hemoglobinuria* is the term applied to the symptoms of hemolysis and hemoglobinuria after exposure to cold. Associated symptoms may include pallor, fatigue, and pains in the arms and legs.

Warm antibodies are antibodies, mostly of IgG class, that sensitize and hemolyze erythrocytes at 37°C. Patients with these antibodies will have a positive direct Coombs' test and usually have anemia, splenomegaly, and fever. Warm antibody autoimmune hemolytic anemia may be idiopathic or may be associated with some other disease such as leukemia, lymphoma, or SLE.

Incomplete antibodies are antibodies that actively combine with antigens but that do not cause agglutination. Incomplete antibodies are commonly found in *hemolytic disease of the newborn* (HDN), which is a disease caused by maternal IgG Abs, usually of anti-Rh specificity, coating fetal blood cells and mediating hemolysis. During pregnancy of an Rh-negative mother, if there is a leakage of Rh-positive erythrocytes from the fetus into the mother's blood, the mother will be stimulated to anti-Rh Ab production. Since these Abs are IgG, they cross the placenta and attach to fetal erythrocytes. Rh-negative mothers who have never received blood transfusions have no problems with their first Rh-positive fetus. However, a B cell immune response against fetal Rh-positive cells may have occurred during the first gestation or parturition, so that subsequent pregnancies with Rh-positive fetuses may result in HDN. Anti-Rh serum, called RHOGAM, is given to Rh-negative mothers immediately after delivery of Rh-positive newborns to prevent possible generation of the anti-Rh antibodies that could harm subsequent Rh-positive fetuses. Rarely do ABO incompatibilities cause HDN.

The Coombs' test was devised to detect the presence of antibody-coated erythrocytes in HDN as well as in any other hemolytic disease. Many antierythrocyte antibodies are incomplete and cannot mediate agglutination. These antibodies are therefore not detected by the usual laboratory agglutination assays. *Coombs' serum* is anti-human gamma globulin that will bind to incomplete antibody coating the erythrocyte and will mediate agglutination by bridging antibody-coated erythrocytes. The *direct Coombs' assay* (Fig. 9–9) detects antibody-coated erythrocytes in a patient's blood.

There are instances when it is useful to know whether a patient has antibodies in his or her serum to particular erythrocytes. Such is the case in patients who have had multiple blood transfusions or in women who are or who have been pregnant. For the patient who has received multiple blood transfusions, it is important to avoid subsequent administration of blood with antigens to which the patient has antibodies to

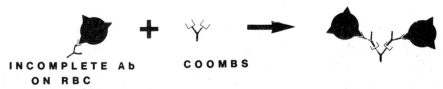

INCOMPLETE Ab   COOMBS
ON RBC

Figure 9-9. Direct Coombs' Test for Incomplete Antierythrocyte Antibodies.

prevent hemolytic or transfusion reactions. Pregnant women can be tested for the presence of antibodies to Rh factor to predict possible problems with Rh-positive fetuses. The *indirect Coombs' assay* (Fig. 9–10) is used to detect antierythrocyte antibodies in serum. This is a two-step procedure. During the first step patient serum is individually incubated with a panel of erythrocytes of known antigenic specificities. This provides opportunity for existing incomplete antibodies to coat the cells. In the second step Coombs serum is added, and if any antibody-coated cells are present, agglutination results.

   Bence Jones (BJ) proteins are abnormal L chains found in the urine of patients with multiple myeloma or other B cell neoplasms. When heated, BJ precipitate at 40 to 50°C and redissolve at 80 to 100°C. BJ proteins are monomers or dimers of L chains and may be of either isotype. BJ proteins are monoclonal proteins and can usually be identified by urine immunoelectrophoresis.

ANTIBODY ISOLATION AND PURIFICATION

Initial Precipitation From Protein Pool

Immunoglobulins are glycoprotein macromolecules and are isolated and purified as any glycoprotein would be according to methods based upon their physical–chemical properties. The usual first step in isolation of a protein from a pool of proteins is *precipitation*. This step can be accomplished by any one of several methods and yields a precipitate of high concentration of the desired protein plus small amounts of contaminating proteins. *Ammonium sulphate* is a salt commonly used in the initial precipitation step for IgG isolation. Salt concentration affects protein solubility. Low concentrations enhance antibody solubility by decreasing interaction of the solute molecules with one another. This phenomenon of adding small amounts of salt to bring protein

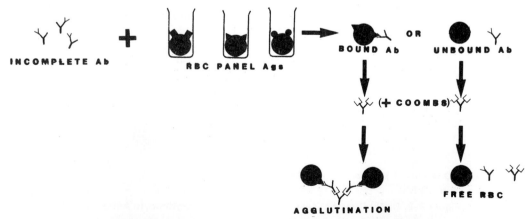

Figure 9-10. Indirect Coombs' Test for Antierythrocyte Antibodies.

into solution is sometimes called *salting in.* Small ions of salts interact with the ionic groups of protein molecules to diminish protein interactions and thus increase solubility. Globulins require a low-salt concentration for solubility, thus dialysis against water will precipitate globulins out of solution as the salt concentration is reduced. High-salt concentrations also precipitate or *salt out* proteins from solution. In this case the salt molecules dehydrate the protein by attracting around themselves the polarizable solvent molecules, which are then unavailable for interaction with the protein molecules. The salt precipitate may be collected by centrifugation and dialyzed to replace the solvent with an appropriate buffer. The pH also affects solubility of antibodies, because they are ampholytes and can be ionized as either anions or cations. Prior to initial salt precipitation the pH of the solvent is adjusted as close as possible to the pI of the antibody to be isolated. This is the pH at which the protein has a net zero charge and is least soluble.

Further Purification

Initial precipitation yields a protein solution with a high concentration of antibodies and substantial amounts of other proteins from the original pool. Further steps are required to obtain purified immunoglobulins. Possible methods include sucrose density gradient ultracentrifugation, preparative gel electrophoresis, ion exchange chromatography, molecular sieve chromatography, and affinity chromatography. All of these methods may be used in the purification of any glycoprotein. Although the clinical laboratory normally uses only the molecular sieve technique, the principles of these methods are helpful in understanding laboratory techniques utilizing purified antibodies.

Sucrose density gradient ultracentrifugation begins with preparation of a sucrose density gradient in a centrifuge tube to provide a gradually increasing concentration of sucrose from top to bottom. Automatic mixing devices are used to prepare the gradients. A sample of the previously precipitated gammaglobulins is carefully layered onto the top of the gradient. As this tube is centrifuged, solutes or proteins with different sedimentation characteristics will separate into discrete zones as they move through the gradient. Sedimentation rates are directly proportional to the size and density of the particle. When the density of the particle equals the density of the liquid, there is no sedimentation. Because the viscosity of the liquid causes frictional hindrance to particle migration through it, the greater the viscosity the less the rate of sedimentation. After centrifugation the separated zones of proteins may be collected either by allowing the gradient to drop out the bottom of the tube or by forcing the gradient upward through a collecting device with a much denser concentration of sucrose. A spectrophotometer scan during the collection of the gradient locates the protein zones. IgM is much heavier than other antibodies and is easily separated by this method. Antibodies with similar molecular weights are not separated with this technique.

Preparative gel electrophoresis is another method used to further purify antibodies from an initial salt precipitation of serum. The same theory, principles, and molecular influences apply to both preparative gel electrophoresis and analytic gel electrophoresis discussed in Chapter 4. Preparative gels allow application and electrophoresis of large amounts of sample and are designed to isolate or purify selected molecules, whereas analytic gels are designed to use small amounts of sample and to analyze individual protein constituents. A large block of starch gel may be used to further purify IgM or IgG from the initial salt precipitate. After electrophoresis the separated protein is easily eluted from the gel by homogenizing the gel and washing with buffered isotonic saline or other appropriate solvents. Large gels of polyacrylamide may also be used for preparative techniques; however, to collect separated proteins from the gel, a more extensive method such as electrophoresing off the gel into a solution is required. A major difference in starch and polyacrylamide is that the latter has a matrix that affects migration of molecules by retarding the larger ones. Thus molecular size plays a role in protein separation on polyacrylamide gels, whereas it has little importance in starch gels. Protein separation in starch gel is mainly due to the molecule's electrical charge in the electrophoresis buffer. Different pHs are used to isolate various proteins.

Ion exchange chromatography is a good method for further purifying IgG from an initial salt precipitate. The previously discussed ultracentrifugation and starch gel electrophoresis are best used in purifying IgM. In diethylaminoethyl (DEAE) cellulose chromatography, a solid phase is composed of polymers formed into beads with ionizable chemical groupings. DEAE cellulose is an *anion exchanger* (has positively charged groups on its surface). Usually the DEAE cellulose is used in the form of its chloride salt, in which negatively charged chloride anions are associated with the positive groups on the polymers. As ampholyte proteins are passed through a column filled with these beads, negatively charged solute molecules will exchange with the chloride ions and become electrostatically attached to the column. This process is an ion exchange, and this example is an *anion exchange*. As the column is run, anions are constantly associating, disassociating, and reassociating with the beads in the packed column. This process retards the migration of the charged molecules down the column. The greater the charge on the protein molecule, the slower it migrates down the column. A fraction collector can collect small fractions of column eluent, and spectrophotometric scanning can indicate which fractions contain the protein. By changing the ionic strength of the buffer passing through the column, different proteins can be eluted or released. The principle of *cation exchange chromatography* is the same, except that the beads used to pack the column have negative charges to which positively charged salt ions, usually sodium, are associated. Proteins displace or replace the positive sodium ions.

Molecular sieve chromatography (Fig. 9–11) is column chromatography based upon separation of molecules according to their size. Sephadex is one of several polymers that is available in beads with tunnels of fixed sizes. Tunnel size is determined by the degree of cross-linking during polymerization. As a protein migrates down a column filled with these beads with tunnels, those molecules larger than the tunnel size will be excluded from entering the tunnel and will progress rapidly down and out the column. Smaller molecules, however, will enter the tunnels, and their migration down the column will be hindered and slowed by passing through the tunnels. The smaller the molecules, the greater the hindrance, the slower the migration down the column. Fractions of molecules can be collected as they exit the column in decreasing molecu-

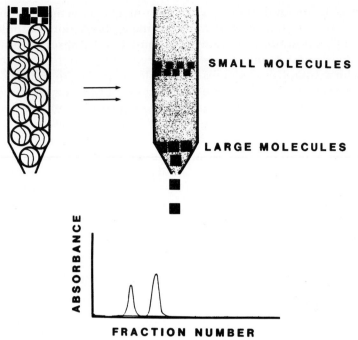

SMALL MOLECULES

LARGE MOLECULES

Figure 9-11. Molecular Sieve Chromatography.

lar size. The largest molecules will exit first and the smallest last. This method is some-times referred to as *molecular exclusion chromatography*. IgM is easily separated from other immunoglobulins by molecular sieve chromatography, as it is a much larger molecular weight than the other classes of antibodies.

Affinity chromatography differs from the above purification methods in that it iso-lates antibodies according to their specificity. The previous methods are nonspecific methods in that they are used to purify any antibody or protein having the required molecular properties. Specific methods isolate antibodies according to their specificity for particular antigen. *Solid phase chromatography* or *affinity chromatography* is column chromatography through a solid substrate to which antibodies or antigens have been covalently linked. For example, Sepharose that contains activated cyanogen bromide as the coupling agent to which proteins (antibody, antigen, or protein A) may be coupled is a frequently used affinity chromatography material. Antibody is covalently attached to the stationary phase used to pack the column. As a protein pool is passed through the column, the fixed antibodies will bind and take out of the pool those specific antigens that associate with their Fab regions. All other proteins will pass through and out the column. Later, altering the pH or the salt concentration of the buffer will cause disassociation of the desired protein from the solid phase antibodies, and a fraction collector with ultraviolet (UV) scanner can identify specific fractions containing the desired proteins. When Protein A from *Staphylococcus aureus* is attached to the solid phase, it binds the Fc portion of IgG and takes it out of the protein pool traveling down the column.

Absorption is the removal from a pool of immunoglobulins those antibodies having affinity for a particular antigen. When performing agglutination inhibition assays for identification of viral antibodies, many sera must first be absorbed by mixing with erythrocytes. This removes interfering, nonspecific inhibitors of agglutination. Absorption may be accomplished by mixing soluble antigens with the sera and then removing the antigen:antibody complexes. More commonly, absorption is accomplished by mixing antigen-coated particles (erythrocytes, Sepharose cyanogen bromide beads, latex beads) with the serum. The antigen-coated beads used here may be the same as those used in solid phase affinity chromatography. Antibodies in the serum attach to the specific antigens bound to the surface of the beads. The beads and attached antibody are then easily removed. Once the antibody:antigen:bead complex is removed from the serum, the attached antibodies may be released and recovered by changing the pH or salt concentration.

CHANGING SOLVENTS

After isolation procedures the desired immunoglobulin often is in an undesirable solvent or is too dilute. *Dialysis* against the desired buffer is one method to replace the solvent. Another method is to run the purified immunoglobulin through *molecular sieve chromatography* using the desired buffer. Both dialysis and molecular sieve chromatography usually yield diluted samples that must be concentrated before use.

CONCENTRATING SAMPLES

In the clinical laboratory urine samples must be concentrated before some assays are performed. One method for accomplishing this is to expose the specimen to hydrophilic materials that absorb out water. The hydrophilic material may be added directly to the sample, or it may be applied around a dialysis membrane sack that contains the specimen. Some commercially available hydrophilic materials are Sephadex, Carbowax, Aquacide, Ficoll, and Lymphogel.

Other concentration methods that are more commonly used in the research laboratory include *lyophilization* or freeze drying (sublimation of water from the frozen specimen under high vacuum), *pervaporation* (evaporation of water by passing a current of air around a dialysis sack containing the specimen), and *ultrafiltration* (removal of salt and water molecules by forcing the sample under nitrogen pressure through a semipermeable membrane that retains macromolecules).

EVALUATION OF HUMORAL IMMUNE SYSTEM

Quantitation of B Cells

B lymphocytes are identified by unique properties of their membranes (Table 9–3). About 15 to 20% of circulating lymphocytes are type B, and about 65 to 70% are type T. Properties unique to B lymphocytes include surface membrane proteins that can be detected by identifying their receptor activity, for example, C3b receptors, or by

TABLE 9-3. SURFACE ANTIGENS AND RECEPTORS OF B LYMPHOCYTES

PWM receptor				
EBV receptor				
C3b receptor				
Fc receptor				
Surface Ab				
pan-B	CD22	Leu-14		
pan-B	CD20	Leu-16	B1	
pre-B and pan-B	CD19	Leu-12	B4	
CALLA, pre-B	CD10	CALLA	J5	OKB-CALLA
B-CLL, pan-T	CD5	Leu-1	T1	OKT1

Abbreviations: CD = World Health Organization; Leu = Becton–Dickinson; B-J-T = Coulter; OK = Ortho Diagnostics; CLL = chronic lymphocytic leukemia; CALLA = common acute lymphoblastic leukemia antigen.

demonstrating reactivity with antibodies specific for the membrane proteins. Any one of the properties unique to B lymphocytes may be used to quantitate them. One assay for B cell quantitation utilizes the membrane receptors for the Fc portion of IgG. In humans B cell IgG Fc receptors associate with isogeneic or homogeneic Abs that have been either aggregated or bound to Ag. These Fc receptors will not bind the Fc of soluble or free native antibodies nor will they bind most heterogeneic antibodies. Rabbit antibodies will associate with human B cell Fc receptors; however, sheep, goat, and chicken antibodies do not. Due to the fact that blood from which lymphocytes are isolated may have circulating immune complexes, the B cells are first treated to release any attached antibodies by incubating at 37°C for 15 minutes. These cells are then washed to eliminate released antibody. The assay is continued by mixing the treated B cells with erythrocytes that have been coated with sheep antierythrocyte antibody (hemolysin). The Fc portion of the antibody coating the red blood cell will associate with Fc receptors on the B cell membrane, and microscopic examination reveals (erythrocyte: ½ antibody) EA rosettes around each B cell. Interpretation is similar to that of (erythrocyte) E rosettes, which were used to quantitate T cells in Chapter 8. Alternatively, heat aggregated, fluorochrome-conjugated IgG may be used to identify Fc receptor-carrying B cells. The aggregated IgG attaches to the Fc receptors on the B cells and can be detected under the fluorescence microscope.

Another assay for quantitation of B cells is based upon their membrane receptor for C3. Erythrocytes may be coated with antibody and then reacted with C5-deficient complement. This leads to binding of C3 to the erythrocytes, but the lack of C5 prevents hemolysis. This erythrocyte: antibody: C3 (EAC) reagent is mixed with the lymphocyte preparation and incubated. EAC rosettes identify the B cells.

B cells are also quantitated by identifying *membrane-integrated antibody* that is the antigen receptor for B cells. Immunoglobulins of more than one class can be present on a single B cell, but only one type of L chain will be present. IgD and IgM are the predominant antigen receptors with some IgG and IgA. Fluorochrome-labeled antibodies against immunoglobulin H and L chains may be used to identify the B cells. Rabbit antiserum should not be the fluorescent reagent because it binds via its Fc portion to B cells. To avoid this nonspecific attachment, either Fab or F(ab')₂ fragments or antisera prepared in some other animal, preferably sheep, are used. Some patients will have antilymphocyte antibodies attached to their lymphocytes, and these will bind the fluorescent-labeled anti-Ab. As above, before performing this assay the B cells need to be treated to remove any antibody attached via membrane Fc receptors. This assay should be evaluated as soon as possible if the preparation remains at room temperature in buffer; otherwise capping will complicate interpretation. Binding of 2 or more membrane-integrated B cell immunoglobulins leads to a phenomenon called *patching* or *capping*. Once surface antigens are cross-linked, they will migrate in the fluid bilipid membrane and form patches of immunofluorescing spots on the B cell. The migration proceeds to form a cap at one pole of the cell. The complexes are then internalized or shed. Cooling after mixing fluorochrome-labeled anti-immunoglobulin will slow patching and capping. If the stained cells are to be examined microscopically, capping can be prevented by drying the cells onto a slide after immunostaining and mounting them in glycerol for fluorescence microscopy.

With the advent of monoclonal antibodies, most clinical laboratories now quantitate B cells with assays for specific B cell antigens. An antibody for a selected B cell antigen is labeled with fluorochrome. Fluorescing cells may be manually counted or, as in most larger laboratories, evaluated by flow cytometry.

FUNCTIONAL EVALUATIONS

The functional status of an individual's B lymphocytes may be indicated by a well taken patient history. Repeated infections may indicate some abnormality. More specifically, the status of B lymphocytes may be determined by examining a patient's serum for total and individual antibody type concentration and by evaluating the ability of the patient's lymphocytes to respond to stimulation by mitogens or antigens.

The most general evaluation is to do a serum electrophoresis with total gamma globulin quantitation as described in Chapter 4. In diseases involving B cell deficiency, such as X-linked hypogammaglobulinemia, gamma-globulin levels will be low or undetectable. In multiple myeloma and some other B cell neoplasms, the levels will be increased. These clones of neoplastic cells produce large amounts of a single type of antibody molecule. This results in a *monoclonal gammopathy* in which the electrophoretic gamma-globulin peak is sharp and increased in concentration. This mass of identical antibodies is sometimes referred to as *paraproteins* or *monoclonal proteins*. Hyperplasia of many different clones of B cells produces a *polyclonal gammopathy* in which the gammaglobulin peak will be broader and increased in concentration.

Any abnormal gamma-globulin level found in serum electrophoresis is evaluated further by *immunoelectrophoresis* or *immunofixation electrophoresis* to identify which major type of chains are involved. Both of these electrophoresis assays were discussed in Chapter 4.

Automated nephelometry and radial immunodiffusion are used to quantitate concentration of *individual antibody classes*. This information together with the patient history and serum electrophoresis provide a good screening of the humoral immune system.

Isohemagglutin titers of a patient's natural blood group antibodies is performed on those patients who are likely to have B cell insufficiency. Normal values are 1 : 16 to 1 : 32 for anti-A and anti-B. Any titers lower than 1 : 4 are abnormal. Patients with transient hypogammaglobulinemias will demonstrate normal isohemagglutinin levels, whereas patients with hereditary hypogammaglobulinemias will have low or no levels.

Most individuals in the United States have had diphtheria, tetanus, pertussis (DTP) vaccination. Resultant humoral immunity would indicate functional B cells, whereas absence of humoral immunity would indicate nonfunctional B cells. The *Schick test* is a test for measuring immunity to diphtheria toxoid. Diphtheria toxin is injected intracutaneously, and 24 to 48 hours later the area of injection is observed for erythema and edema. A positive response indicates lack of neutralization of the toxin. A negative response indicates presence of antibodies to the toxin.

The above assays for evaluating B cell function have been directed toward evaluating B cell products. There are also assays to evaluate the B cell itself. Normal B cells are stimulated to blastogenesis by pokeweed mitogen and by staphylococcal protein A. Uptake of ^{3}H-thymidine is used to determine stimulation just as it was used in the T cell evaluations described in Chapter 8. Quantitative and qualitative evaluation of B cells and antibodies are also discussed in Chapters 6 and 7.

Discussion of the Illustrative Case

The patient described in the illustrative case had been transfused with 4 units of blood at the time of his gunshot wound and surgery. At that time the antibody screening test was negative for patient antibodies to the panel of red blood cell antigens. Five months later the patient's serum showed antibody to Le^a as described. A review of the phenotype of the transfused units revealed that one was Le^a positive.

This patient developed a humoral immune response against the blood group antigen Le^a as a result of blood transfusion therapy. Laboratory crossmatching followed by analysis of the patient's serum for antibodies to the allogeneic blood antigens found the antibody and prevented a possible transfusion of incompatible donor cells into the patient. If this patient had been transfused with the Le^a positive red blood cells, a transfusion reaction would most probably have occurred.

QUESTIONS

1. What are three important properties for immunogenicity?
2. Trace the stimulation of a humoral immune response and include diagrams. Include DNA rearrangement and isotype switching.
3. Describe the process for producing a monoclonal antibody.

4. Define and give the clinical significance of
    - C5 in the preparation of EAC reagent
    - cryoglobulins
    - cold Abs
    - warm Abs
    - incomplete Abs
    - direct and indirect Coombs' tests

5. List B cell membrane receptors and antigens used to evaluate B lymphocytes.

6. Use diagrams and explain how to purify antirabbit erythrocyte antibody from a pool of sheep antiserum made by injecting rabbit erythrocytes.

10 The Complement Systems and Other Humoral Mediators of Inflammation

OBJECTIVES

1. To describe in detail the classic and alternative pathways of complement activation.
2. To describe the activation of terminal complement components and the generation of the membrane attack complex.
3. To discuss the mediation of biological processes, including inflammation, by activated complement proteins and their fragments.
4. To discuss laboratory methods for evaluating the complement system.
5. To briefly discuss the interaction of complement, coagulation, plasmin, and kinin systems in amplifying the effects of antigen–antibody interactions.

Illustrative Case

A 10-year-old boy developed severe facial swelling after a visit to the dentist. The swelling was not associated with urticaria or itching and persisted for 2 days. During this time he was seen by a physician who obtained a history of recurrent, colicky abdominal pain and several episodes of swollen extremities over the preceding 3 years. No family history of similar symptoms could be elicited. On the basis of the presumptive diagnosis, a CH_{50} assay and nephelometric immunoassays for C3 and C4 were ordered. The CH_{50} and C3 levels were slightly reduced, and C4 was undetectable.

MOLECULAR MEDIATOR SYSTEMS ACTIVATED BY ANTIGEN–ANTIBODY INTERACTIONS

When an antigen binds to the antigen-binding site of an antibody, a number of physiologic processes can be initiated. The initiation of these processes often results from the generation of biologically active factors in the plasma, lymph, or interstitial fluid surrounding the site of antigen binding. These soluble or humoral factors directly or indirectly activate complex molecular and cellular systems that mediate many of the effects of the antigen–antibody union. This activation of mediator systems is responsible for much of the molecular, cellular, and tissue destruction produced by antibody recognition of antigen. Mediators of tissue injury also are released from cells, especially inflammatory cells that have been attracted to the site of antigen–antibody binding by activated humoral mediators.

Antibody–induced destruction can be beneficial to an individual, as in the case of immune elimination of a staphylococcal skin infection; or detrimental, as in the case of autoimmune attack on the skin in a patient with pemphigus (see Chap. 11). Thus mediators activated by antigen–antibody interaction can play a role in both physiologic defense and pathophysiologic disease induction. In either case the mechanisms of tissue injury are the same and involve the activation of humoral cellular mediator systems.

Four of the most important humoral mediator systems will be discussed in this chapter: the complement, plasmin, kinin, and coagulation systems. Cell-derived mediators, such as granule and lysosome contents, and lipid metabolites also will be discussed briefly.

THE COMPLEMENT SYSTEM

Complement is so named because it was first recognized as a factor in plasma that assisted (complemented) antibodies in the killing of bacteria. Complement is now known to be a group of approximately 20 plasma proteins that circulate in the blood in an inactive form. Certain stimuli can initiate activation of all or a portion of the complement components, resulting in mediation of a number of processes, such as immune clearance of circulating molecules and cells and induction of tissue inflammation. Figure 10–1 is a diagram of complement system activation. There are two pathways of complement activation, the *classic pathway* and the *alternative pathway*. Both pathways lead to the activation of the central complement component, C3, and the terminal complement components that comprise the *membrane attack complex*. As for all mediator systems, there are inhibitors of activated complement components that control the system by negative feedback.

The classic activation pathway was discovered before the alternative pathway. Classic pathway and terminal components are designated by the letter C followed by a number (Table 10–1). The exceptions to this are the three components of the C1 complex, which are designated C1q, C1r, and C1s. Fragments of complement components produced during activation and inactivation are designated by the name of the parent component followed by a lower case letter (e.g., C3a). Individual and com-

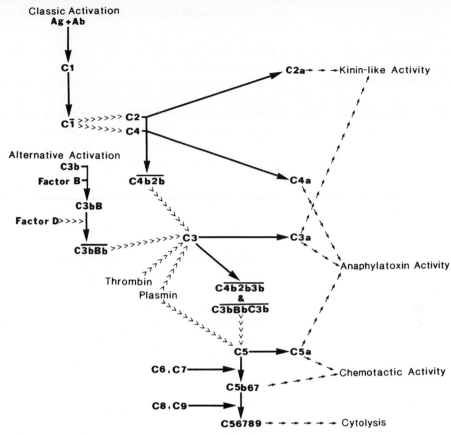

Figure 10-1. Complement Activation. Diagram of classic and alternative complement activation pathways. Note that prior to 1983 C2a was called C2b, and C2b was called C2a.

TABLE 10-1. COMPLEMENT COMPONENT DESIGNATIONS

Classic Pathway	Terminal Components
C1q	C5
C1r	C6
C1s	C7
C4	C8
C2	C9
C3	
Alternative Pathway	**Control Proteins**
C3	C1̄ inhibitor
Factor B (B)	C4 binding protein
Factor D (D)	Factor I (I)
Properdin (P)	Factor H (H)
	S protein (S)

plexed-activated complement components are denoted by a bar placed over the num-ber or letter designation for the components (e.g., $\overline{C4b2b}$).

Most complement proteins are proenzymes, that is, they are the inactive precur-sors of enzymes. When activated, usually by proteolytic cleavage, they become active proteolytic enzymes (proteases). Each active complement protease has specificity for the next complement component to be activated. Thus there is sequential activation of complement components by successive conversions of proenzymes to proteases that activate the next proenzyme of the complement system cascade.

CLASSIC ACTIVATION PATHWAY

The most important activators of the classic pathway are complexes of antigens with specific IgG or IgM antibodies. The antigen can be a determinant on a soluble mole-cule, the surface of a microorganism, or the membrane of a cell. The results of com-plement activation will depend upon the nature and location of antigen to which IgG or IgM is bound. For example, complement activation on the surface of a bacterium will produce opsonization and phagocytosis; complement fixation on the membrane of an erythrocyte will produce lysis via the membrane attack complex; and comple-ment activation by complexes of molecular antigens and antibodies lodged in vessel walls will produce acute inflammation.

The ability of IgG and IgM to activate the classic pathway is dependent upon the recognition of a portion of the Fc region of immune-complexed IgG and IgM by C1. In plasma C1 is a trimolecular complex of C1q, C1r, and C1s. C1q binds to the Fc region of IgG or IgM when these immunoglobulins are complexed with specific anti-gens. C1q does not bind to free IgG or IgM. C1q binds better to complexed IgG1 and IgG3 than to IgG2 but not at all to IgG4. The binding of C1q enables $\overline{C1r}$ to enzymati-cally activate C1s.

Activated C1s is a protease that enzymatically cleaves C4 and C2, producing the bimolecular complex $\overline{C4b2b}$, which is bound at the site of activation. Two smaller cleavage fragments, C4a and C2a, are released in this reaction. Until 1983 the desig-nations for the C2 fragments were opposite what has just been stated, and this must be taken into consideration when reading books published prior to that time. There-fore, for example, prior to 1983, the $\overline{C4b2b}$ complex was designated $\overline{C4b2a}$.

$\overline{C4b2b}$, also called C3 convertase, is a protease that cleaves C3 into C3a and C3b. C3b can localize near $\overline{C4b2b}$, producing the active enzyme complex $\overline{C4b2b3b}$. This protease activates C5, which initiates activation of the terminal complement compo-nents and generation of the membrane attack complex.

Classic activation of complement is counteracted by certain control proteins (Ta-ble 10–1). *$\overline{C1}$-inhibitor* inactivates active C1, as well as a number of other biologically active mediator molecules, such as kallekrein, plasmin, and Hageman factor. *Factor I* inactivates C3b and C4b by proteolytic cleavage. C3b inactivation by factor I is en-hanced by *factor H* and C3b receptors on cell membranes. *C4 binding protein* and C3b receptors assist factor I in the inactivation C4b.

ALTERNATIVE ACTIVATION PATHWAY

Classic pathway activation is the usual immune mechanism of complement activation, since the recognition of antigen by antibody is the most common initiating event. Alternative pathway activation is usually nonimmune, since no specific recognition of antigen is required. Probably the most important mechanism of alternative pathway activation is initiated by microbial constituents such as polysaccharides, lipopolysaccharides, and teichoic acid (Table 10–2). This leads to complement activation on the microorganism and elimination by lysis or opsonization-induced phagocytosis. Therefore alternative-pathway–complement activation is a rapid means of nonimmune defense against infectious microorganisms that does not require prior immunization.

C3b is an important component of the alternative pathway. There is a normal steady state of C3b production from C3, but this C3b is inactivated, primarily by the complement control proteins factor I and factor H. Activators of the alternative pathway provide a site where C3b is protected from inactivation and is allowed to interact with *factor B* to form $C\overline{3bB}$. Cleavage of factor B in the $C\overline{3bB}$ complex by *factor D* produces the active enzyme $C\overline{3bBb}$. This is the C3 convertase of the alternative pathway, being functionally analogous to $C\overline{4b2b}$, the C3 convertase of the classic pathway. *Properdin* stabilizes $C\overline{3bBb}$, thus enhancing C3 convertase activity. C3b generated by the classic and alternative pathways can participate in $C\overline{3bBb}$ formation, leading to amplification of complement activation. This is counteracted by the control proteins factors I and H.

TERMINAL COMPONENT ACTIVATION AND THE MEMBRANE ATTACK COMPLEX

The classic pathway C3 convertase, $C\overline{4b2b}$, and the alternative pathway C3 convertase, $C\overline{3bBb}$, both produce C3b from C3. C3b joins with these complexes to produce C5

TABLE 10–2. ACTIVATORS OF CLASSIC AND ALTERNATIVE COMPLEMENT PATHWAYS

Classic Pathway Activators
  IgG and IgM antibody–antigen complexes
  Aggregated immunoglobulins
  Trypsin-like enzymes
  C-reactive protein complexed to phospholipids
  Staphylococcal protein A complexed to IgG

Alternative Pathway Activators
  Polysaccharides
  Lipopolysaccharides (including those in gram-negative bacteria)
  Teichoic acid (including that in gram-positive bacteria)
  Some viruses, fungi, and parasites
  Aggregated immunoglobulins IgG and IgA
  Trypsin-like enzymes

convertases, that is, $\overline{\text{C4b2b3b}}$ and $\overline{\text{C3bBb3b}}$, that cleave C5, resulting in C5a and C5b. C5b forms a trimolecular complex with C6 and C7, that is, C5b67, that can bind to membranes. This is inhibited by the binding of *S protein* to the C5b67 complex. Lysis of membranes begins when C8 joins the complex on the membrane, but optimum cell lysis requires that multiple molecules of C9 (poly C9) also join the complex to complete the *membrane attack complex (MAC)*, C5b6789. The MAC forms channels through the membrane resulting in osmotic cell lysis.

MEDIATION OF BIOLOGICAL EVENTS BY COMPLEMENT

Activation of complement mediates a variety of biological events, such as cytolysis, opsonization, alterations in vascular permeability and perfusion, smooth muscle contraction, attraction and activation of inflammatory cells, and modulation of immune responses (Table 10–3). These processes are involved in defense and response to injury.

Complement-mediated cytolysis by the MAC was discussed above. Mac-mediated lysis can destroy erythrocytes, some leukocytes, platelets, bacteria, and some viruses. Complement also can mediate cell lysis by opsonization, leading to destruction within phagocytes.

Complement components, especially C3b and C4b, are important *opsonins*. This facilitates the phagocytosis by polymorphonuclear leukocytes and macrophages of molecules or cells bearing complement components. Neutrophils, monocytes, and macrophages have surface receptors for C3b and C4b, allowing them to bind to and engulf molecules, particles, and cells coated with C3b and C4b. For example, invading bacteria can become coated with C3b, either by specific binding of antibodies to bacterial antigens followed by classic pathway activation or by alternative pathway activation initiated by bacterial polysaccharides. These opsonized bacteria would then be phagocytosed and destroyed by neutrophils and macrophages.

Activated complement components and complement fragments are important mediators of acute inflammation. They can produce vascular changes and recruit inflammatory cells. Complement fragments released during complement activation can have *kinin-like* and *anaphylatoxin* activity. C2a and C3a have kinin-like activity, such as the ability to increase vascular permeability, which results in edema at the site of com-

TABLE 10-3. BIOLOGICAL ACTIVITIES OF COMPLEMENT

Component	Activity
C3b, C4b	Opsonization
C2a, C3a	Kinin-like
C3a, C4a, C5a	Anaphylatoxin
C3e	Induces leukocytosis
C5a, C5b67	Leukocyte chemotaxis
C5b678, C5b6789	Cytolysis

plement activation. C3a, C4a, and C5a are anaphylatoxins, which means that they mediate inflammatory events similar to those occurring during anaphylactic responses (see Chap. 11). For example, they can cause increased vascular permeability, contraction of smooth muscle, and degranulation of certain leukocytes and mast cells, causing release of vasoactive mediators such as histamine. C5a is particularly important in the mediation of inflammation because of its effects on granulocytes. These effects include granulocyte chemoattraction, degranulation, toxic oxygen radical production, and increased arachidonic acid metabolism. This last effect leads to the production of prostaglandins and leukotrienes, including leukotriene B4, which is a potent neutrophil chemotactic factor. C5a also stimulates the release of interleukin 1 (IL1) from macrophages. As discussed in Chapter 8, IL1 enhances immune responses and mediates some systemic effects of inflammation, for example, fever. Anaphylatoxins are inactivated by the control protein *carboxypeptidase N*.

C5a and C5b67 are *chemotactic* for leukocytes, especially neutrophilic polymorphonuclear leukocytes. Therefore at sites in tissue where complement is activated, neutrophils accumulate, resulting in acute inflammation. C5a promotes the release of lytic enzymes, toxic oxygen radicals, and lipid metabolites such as leukotrienes from granulocytes, further augmenting tissue destruction. The recruitment of leukocytes is enhanced by C3e, which causes increased release of leukocytes from the bone marrow and blood leukocytosis.

Thus complement activation by either the classic or alternative pathway will mediate acute inflammation in tissues. There will be increased vascular permeability, causing edema; chemoattraction of leukocytes, causing the influx of numerous neutrophils; and release of lytic enzymes and other destructive products from neutrophils, causing necrosis. This inflammatory response can be beneficial by destroying noxious foreign material, such as bacteria; but tissue injury is also occurring and must be taken into consideration in the final cost : benefit ratio for the individual.

COMPLEMENT DEFICIENCY SYNDROMES

It is clear from congenital complement-deficiency states that an intact complement system is important for controlling infections and reducing the incidence of immune complex-mediated diseases. The kinds of diseases that are most common in individuals with different complement-protein deficiencies suggest that early classic pathway components are most important in clearing immune complexes from the blood or in mobilizing them from tissues, while alternative and terminal pathway components are most important in defense against certain bacteria, especially *Neisseria*.

Individuals with congenital deficiencies of C1q, C1r, C1s, C4, and C2 are susceptible to the development of immune complex-mediated inflammatory diseases, especially systemic lupus erythematosus and immune complex-mediated glomerulonephritis (see Chap. 11). It is postulated that the absence of early classic pathway components results in inadequate opsonization of immune complexes, leaving them available to localize in tissues and induce inflammation. Complement may also play a role in the mobilization of immune complexes in tissues, a function that would be defective in classic pathway deficiencies.

C3, C5, and factor B deficiencies result in marked susceptibility to infections with pyogenic bacteria. Deficiencies of C6, C7, and C8 are associated with severe recurrent infections with *Neisseria gonococcus* and *N meningococcus*.

Individuals with C9 deficiency have no clinically apparent associated diseases.

Congenital deficiencies of complement control proteins can also cause diseases. The most common is *hereditary angioedema*, caused by a deficiency of $\overline{C1}$-inhibitor. These individuals develop uncontrolled activation of early, classic, pathway-complement components with production of kinin-like factors and anaphylatoxins. $\overline{C1}$-inhibitor is also a control protein for the kinin system, thus its absence allows uncontrolled kinin generation. Abnormal activation of complement and kinin generation cause increased vascular permeability, resulting in edema, especially in the larynx, gastrointestinal tract, genitourinary tract, and skin. These individuals have episodes of severe abdominal and pelvic pain caused by gastrointestinal and genitourinary edema. They can die from strangulation resulting from laryngeal edema. The most consistent and readily determined laboratory abnormality in individuals with $\overline{C1}$-inhibitor deficiency is a markedly reduced serum C4 level.

Immunoassays or functional assays can be used to assay $\overline{C1}$-inhibitor. Most individuals with hereditary angioedema will lack $\overline{C1}$-inhibitor molecules and be identified by either a functional or immunochemical assay. A minority, however, will have a nonfunctional molecule that will give abnormal results in a functional assay but not in an immunochemical assay.

Factor H and factor I deficiencies cause a marked consumption of C3 by the uncontrolled activation of C3 by $\overline{\overline{C3bBb}}$. These individuals are susceptible to pyogenic infections.

Acquired reductions in complement components also occur. These are usually induced by the consumption of complement during inflammatory diseases, especially immune complex-mediated diseases such as systemic lupus erythematosus and certain forms of immune complex-mediated glomerulonephritis. Laboratory analysis of these reductions in complement components are useful in diagnosing and assessing the activity of the underlying disease.

LABORATORY EVALUATION OF THE COMPLEMENT SYSTEM

The most widely used laboratory test of complement function is the total hemolytic complement (CH_{50}) assay. Individual complement components and activation fragments can be assessed by specific immunochemical and functional assays. Both the functional and antigenic characteristics of complement proteins are very heat liable and undergo rapid in vitro degradation. Therefore if laboratory evaluation of complement is to be accurate, great care must be taken to quickly remove serum from clotted blood and to store it at $-70°C$. Blood should be clotted at room temperature, however.

The CH_{50} assay measures the ability of serum to lyse 50% of a suspension of sheep erythrocytes (E) coated with an optimum amount of rabbit anti-E antibody (A). Antibody-coated erythrocytes (EA) are incubated with different dilutions of test serum, followed by centrifugation to pellet intact EA. The supernatant is then analyzed spectrophotometrically for the amount of hemoglobin released by EA lysis. The percent lysis is calculated by comparison with 100% lysis of EA by water-induced hypotonic lysis. The volume of serum required to lyse 50% of EA is determined from a graph on which percent lysis is plotted against amount of serum. This volume of serum is then considered to contain 1 CH_{50} unit and is used to calculate the CH_{50} units per milliter of test serum. The reference range of CH_{50} must be determined empirically in each laboratory because values will vary depending upon the sources and amounts of reagents used.

The CH_{50} assay measures the function of the classic pathway and terminal complement components. This functional assay can be modified to measure the activity of individual complement proteins. To do this EA are incubated with test serum as well as a source for all the complement components except the one being tested.

Individual complement proteins can be quantitated using a number of immunochemical methods, most commonly radial immunodiffusion and nephelometry. C3 and C4 are the complement proteins that are measured most often.

A variety of disease processes can cause abnormal complement levels. Because complement proteins are acute phase reactants, the CH_{50}, C3, and C4 levels can be elevated in individuals with inflammatory diseases. Low levels result from complement consumption in individuals with immune complex-mediated diseases. A consistent finding in hereditary angioedema is markedly reduced C4. Reduced synthesis of complement proteins in patients with severe liver disease causes depressed complement levels. Most congenital complement deficiencies cause profound depression of CH_{50} values.

INTERRELATIONSHIP OF COMPLEMENT, COAGULATION, PLASMIN, AND KININ SYSTEMS IN IMMUNE-MEDIATED INJURY

The coagulation, plasmin, and kinin systems are humoral mediator systems that interact with the complement system in the pathogenesis of immune-mediated tissue injury. All four systems are characterized by the sequential activition of precursor proteins, leading to the production of biologically active molecules that mediate specific events such as leukocyte chemotaxis, altered vascular permeability, thrombus formation, and thrombus lysis. These mediator systems have interconnected activation, because some active intermediates in one system can activate components of one or more other systems (Fig. 10–2).

The major function of the *coagulation system* is *hemostasis* (stopping blood flow by occluding vessels). This is accomplished by forming a hemostatic plug, *thrombus*, composed predominantly of the cross-linked protein fibrin and platelets. Coagulation can be initiated by vascular injury via activation of *factor XII* (*Hageman factor*) by collagen exposed by endothelial injury (*intrinsic coagulation pathway*) or by contact of coagulation factors with thrombogenic tissue factors (*extrinsic coagulation pathway*). Both pathways lead to the generation of the protease *thrombin* from *prothrombin* (Fig. 10–2). Thrombin cleaves *fibrinogen* to produce *fibrin*, the major coagulation protein constituent of a

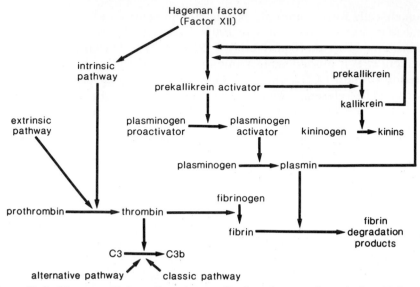

Figure 10-2. Diagram of Interactions Among the Complement, Coagulation, Kinin, and Plasmin Systems.

thrombus. Factor XII (Hageman factor) also activates the kinin and plasmin systems, and thrombin also activates C3 and the plasmin system.

The *plasmin system* counteracts the coagulation system by generating the proteolytic enzyme plasmin, which degrades fibrin and lyses thrombi (Fig. 10-2). The plasmin system is initiated by the activation of *plasminogen proactivator* to *plasminogen activator*. This is catalyzed by *prekallikrein activator* that is derived from factor XII (Hageman factor). Plasminogen activator then converts *plasminogen* to *plasmin*. Thrombin also can convert plasminogen to plasmin.

Kinins (bradykinin, lysyl-bradykinin, methionylilysyl-bradykinin) mediate a number of inflammatory processes such as leukocyte chemotaxis, increased vascular permeability, vasodilation, and smooth muscle contraction. Kinins are generated from *kininogen* by *kallikrein*; and kallikrein from *prekallikrein* by *prekallikrein activator* (Fig. 10-2). Activated factor XII (Hageman factor) is converted to prekallikrein activator by plasmin and kallikrein. Because plasmin and kallikrein are products as well as activators of kinin generation, they form a positive feedback loop that amplifies inflammatory events. C1-inhibitor is the major antagonist of the kinin system. Therefore the edema and other abnormalities in patients with hereditary angioedema are induced by uncontrolled kinin generation as well as complement activation.

When antibodies bind to antigens, activation of the complement, coagulation, kinin, and plasmin systems can occur, leading to mediation of inflammation. These humoral mediator systems amplify the biological consequences, both beneficial and detrimental, or antigen–antibody interactions. In Chapter 11 different mechanisms of antibody-mediated tissue injury will be discussed, all involving these humoral amplification systems.

Discussion of the Illustrative Case

The boy described in the illustrative case had hereditary angioedema caused by a congenital deficiency of the complement-control protein $\overline{\text{C1}}$-inhibitor. The clinical features are quite typical, except for the absence of a family history. This is, however, not that uncommon and indicates that this individual probably developed the deficiency as a result of genetic mutation. Sometimes the cutaneous swelling is incited by trauma, in this case dental work. The recurrent episodes of abdominal pain were caused by edema of the gastrointestinal tract. The absence of $\overline{\text{C1}}$-inhibitor allowed abnormal complement activation and kinin generation. Increased amounts of activated C1 caused the consumption of C3 and C4 identified in the laboratory. In this disease C4 reductions are most severe and persistent than changes in C3 and CH_{50}.

QUESTIONS

1. Diagram the activation sequence of the classic complement pathway.

2. List several activators of the classic complement activation pathway and the alternative complement activation pathway.

3. Does the activation of the alternative complement pathway by bacterial lipopolysaccharide involve immune recognition? Explain.

4. How do the terminal complement components mediate cell lysis?

5. List four biological processes mediated by complement activation.

6. What general categories of disease are caused by congenital deficiencies of early, classic, complement-pathway proteins and alternative pathway proteins?

7. State the basic steps in the CH_{50} assay of hemolytic complement activity in serum.

8. What are the four major humoral systems involved in the mediation of inflammation?

Chapter

11 Antibody-Mediated Injury

OBJECTIVES

1. To summarize the categorization of antibody-mediated injury.
2. To discuss IgE-mediated immediate hypersensitivity and allergic diseases.
3. To discuss antibody-mediated cytotoxicity and direct attack of tissues.
4. To discuss immune complex-mediated tissue injury.
5. To discuss autoimmune diseases.
6. To describe laboratory tests that are useful in the evaluation of antibody-mediated diseases, including autoimmune diseases.

Illustrative Case

A 10-year-old girl was playing in the woods behind her home when she fell and was bitten on the arm by a large copperhead snake. She was quickly transported to a hospital emergency department. The girl was complaining of severe burning pain at the bite site. Physical examination revealed two deeply penetrating fang marks just above the antecubital fossa of the right arm. The right arm was already markedly edematous, and there was a large ecchymosis around the wounds. The patient also had fever, nausea, vomiting, and increasing disorientation. A decision was made to treat with antivenin (horse antipit viper venom antiserum). After intradermal injection of normal horse serum did not elicit a positive immediate-type skin test reaction, antivenin was given intravenously. The patient's symptoms quickly improved, and she was discharged from the hospital after several days. She did well until 10 days after the snake bite, when she developed fever, pruritus, arthralgias, and lymphadenopathy. Laboratory tests ordered by the physician to whom she was taken revealed a mild neutrophilia with increased bands, slight CH_{50} reduction, negative antinuclear antibody test, 2+ proteinuria, and 10 to 15 red blood cells per high-powered field in the urine. The serum creatinine and blood urea nitrogen were normal. The patient was treated with aspirin, and her symptoms resolved over several days. Repeat laboratory tests 3 weeks later revealed no abnormalities.

CATEGORIZATION OF ANTIBODY-MEDIATED INJURY

Antibody-mediated attack on molecules, cells, and tissues is usually beneficial to the individual in whom the immune attack is taking place. For example, antibody-mediated attack is an important means of defense against the injurious effects of molecular toxins, such as bacterial endotoxins and exotoxins, and cellular pathogens, such as bacteria and fungi. Even when participating in such appropriate immune defense, however, antibody-mediated immune reactions can contribute to the pathogenesis of diseases. For example, antibody-mediated immune response to a bacterial infection in the lungs, by activating the mediator systems discussed in Chapter 10, incites an acute inflammation with extensive infiltration of lung tissue by polymorphonuclear leukocytes. This inflammatory disease of the lungs, bacterial pneumonia, is caused in part by the antibody-mediated immune response against the bacteria. Even though the antibody-mediated inflammatory process destroys some lung tissue, the overall effect is beneficial if the infection can be eradicated and the inflammation resolved without extensive permanent impairment of lung function. The antibody-mediated inflammation, however, can be so severe that it causes respiratory failure and death.

Every antibody-mediated inflammatory reaction is a double-edged sword. On the one hand such reactions are required for defense against injurious agents such as microbial pathogens, but on the other hand they can cause tissue injury and even death. Most of the time the cost:benefit ratio is in favor of the individual in whom the immune response is occurring. From the discussion of immune deficiency diseases in Chapter 6, it is clear that the risk of immune injury is worth taking, because lack of immune defense is even more dangerous.

Thus both an appropriate antibody-mediated immune response and too little antibody-mediated immune response can contribute to disease induction. Too much immune response can also cause disease. Too much immune response can be defined as a greater degree of immune activation of mediators than is warranted given the injurious potential of the antigen-bearing substance that the immune response is directed against. For example, the inhalation of pollen does not pose a major threat to an individual. In most people it is handled by immune and nonimmune defense mechanisms without the production of disease symptoms. In people who mount too much immune response against the pollen, however, rhinitis, conjunctivitis, and asthma are produced by antibody-mediated mechanisms. Diseases caused by too much immune response are called *allergies*.

In addition to too much, too little, and appropriate antibody response, misdirected immune response can produce disease. Because the appropriate aim of im-

TABLE 11-1. CATEGORIES OF DISEASE CAUSED BY THE IMMUNE SYSTEM

Nature of the Pathogenic Immune Response	Type of Disease	Example
Too little	Immunodeficiency	Agammaglobulinemia
Appropriate	Inflammatory	Bacterial pneumonia
Too much	Allergic	Allergic asthma
Misdirected	Autoimmune	Autoimmune hemolysis
Neoplastic	Lymphoma/leukemia	Multiple myeloma

mune responses is against nonself, inappropriate aim is against self. Immune attack against one's own constituents is called *autoimmunity*. For example, antibody-mediated attack against one's own red blood cells produces autoimmune hemolytic anemia.

Another category of diseases in which B lymphocytes can participate in disease production is neoplasms of B lymphocytes and plasma cells. Such neoplasms were discussed in Chapter 7.

Diseases that are caused by the immune system can be divided into the categories shown in Table 11-1. Another commonly used system of categorizing immune-mediated injury was devised by Gell and Coombs and is shown in Table 11-2. Types I, II, and III are antibody-mediated forms of immune injury, while type IV is cell-mediated immune injury. Type IV injury, which is mediated by T lymphocytes, was discussed in detail in Chapter 8.

TYPE I IMMUNE INJURY

Systemic and local *anaphylaxis* (type I injury of Gell and Coombs) are forms of immune injury produced by the release of mediators from mast cells and basophils. The stimulus for mediator release is the union of antigens with IgE antibodies that are bound to mast cell or basophil surface membranes via IgE–Fc receptors (Fig. 11–1). The stimulus for immune-mediated mast cell and basophil mediator release is bridging between the membrane-bound IgE molecules by antigens for which the IgE has specificity. In the cell this activates adenylate cyclase and methyl transferases. The former leads to cyclic adenosine monophosphate (cAMP) production from adenosine triphosphate

TABLE 11-2. GELL AND COOMBS' CATEGORIZATION OF IMMUNE-MEDIATED INJURY

Type	Mechanism	Example
I	Anaphylaxis	Allergic asthma
II	Cytotoxicity	Hemolytic anemia
III	Immune complex	Serum sickness
IV	Cell mediated	Contact dermatitis

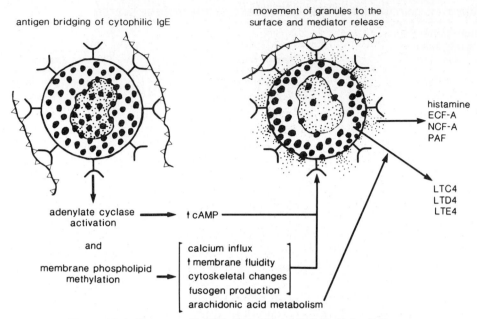

Figure 11-1. Diagram of IgE-Mediated Mast Cell Mediator Release.

(ATP), and the latter causes methylation of membrane phospholipids. These events peak within approximately 15 seconds. Thereafter there is a fall in cAMP. These changes in cAMP concentration and phospholipid methylation lead to intracellular influx of calcium, increased membrane fluidity, reorganization of the cytoskeleton that moves granules to the cell surface, production of a factor (fusogen) that promotes fusion of granule membranes with surface membranes, and ultimately the release of mediators from granules into the extracellular fluid. These mediators include *histamine, eosinophil chemotactic factor of anaphylaxis (ECF-A), neutrophil chemotactic factor of anaphylaxis (NCF-A)*, and *platelet activating factor (PAF)*. Phospholipid methylation and calcium influx along with phospholipase A2 stimulate arachidonic acid metabolism. Many of the resultant lipid metabolites are mediators of inflammation. The most important are the *leukotrienes LTC4, LTD4, and LTE4,* which mediate vasodilation and smooth muscle contraction. Before their biochemical characterization, these leukotrienes were known as *slow reacting substance of anaphylaxis (SRS-A)*.

Factors other than antigen binding to cytophilic IgE can stimulate mast cell and basophil degranulation and contribute to allergic symptoms. Complement anaphylatoxins stimulate degranulation. The autonomic nervous system also influences mast cells and basophils. Stimulation of cholinergic and α-adrenergic receptors stimulates mediator release, whereas stimulation of β-adrenergic receptors inhibits mediator release. This inhibition is caused by an increase in intracellular cAMP. Although intracellular production of cAMP is an early event in the antigen-IgE–mediated stimulation of mast cells and basophils, if there is a rise in intracellular cAMP prior to IgE bridging by antigen, there is suppression of the phospholipid methylation and calcium influx required for degranulation. Agents that influence adrenergic receptors and intracellular cAMP will have effects on mediator release. For example, beta adrenergic stimulation by epinephrine and isoproterenol suppress mediator release by stimulating adenylate cyclase to increase intracellular cAMP. Methylxanthines, such as theophylline, cause suppression by inhibiting the phosphodiesterase that converts cAMP, to AMP, thus resulting in increased cAMP and inhibition of degranulation.

The tissue reactions caused by mast cell mediator release occur so rapidly that this form of immune injury is also called *immediate hypersensitivity*. The symptoms and signs of systemic and local anaphylaxis are dependent upon the tissue in which the immediate hypersensitivity has been elicited (Table 11–3).

Pathogenic Mechanisms of Type I Immune Injury

The plasma concentration of IgE varies with age, sex, and antigen exposure but is normally very low (approximately 0.02 mg/dl). It is elevated in certain allergic diseases and infectious diseases in which it is involved in the pathophysiologic events that are taking place. IgE plays a role in the defense against some pathogens, especially helminths. In developed countries, however, most individuals with elevated IgE levels are not fending off helminth infections but are suffering from IgE-mediated allergic diseases. Susceptibility to developing allergic diseases is called *atopy*.

Allergens are antigens that induce allergic diseases. The IgE antibodies that react with allergens are sometimes referred to as *reagins* or *reaginic antibodies*. Because of its propensity to bind to mast cells and basophils, IgE is also called *cytotropic antibody*. IgE has a half-life of only a few days in the plasma but remains bound to mast cells in tissue for many months. Once IgE is bound to mast cells and basophils, these cells are able to specifically react with the allergens for which the bound IgE antibodies have specificity.

Mast cells and basophils are activated when IgE molecules fixed to membrane Fc receptors are cross-linked by binding to antigens (allergens). This stimulates the cells to release the contents of their cytoplasmic granules and to secrete other molecules such as lipid metabolites. The molecules released by activated mast cells and basophils are mediators of inflammation and include histamine, kallikrein, platelet activating factor, chemotactic factors for eosinophils and neutrophils, leukotrienes, and prostaglandins. At the site of mast cell activation these mediators cause vasodilation, in-

TABLE 11-3. RELATIONSHIP BETWEEN THE SITE OF TYPE I IMMUNE RESPONSE AND THE RESULTANT DISEASE

Disease	Site of Type I Response
Hay fever	Upper respiratory tract and eyes
Rhinitis	Nasopharynx
Conjunctivitis	Eyes
Atopic asthma	Lower respiratory tract
Urticaria and angioedema	Skin
System anaphylaxis	Throughout the body

creased vascular permeability, smooth muscle contraction, increased gland secretion, and influx of leukocytes, especially eosinophils.

Clinical Manifestations of Local and Systemic Anaphylaxis

The clinical manifestations of type I immune injury are determined by the site in the body where mast cells and basophils are activated by allergens (Table 11–3).

Hay fever is caused by type I immune injury occurring in the upper respiratory tract (*allergic rhinitis*) and conjunctiva (*allergic conjunctivitis*). Vasodilation causes reddening of the eyes and upper respiratory mucosa. Increased vascular permeability causes swelling (edema) of the conjunctiva and nasopharyngeal mucosa. Increased gland secretion causes runny nose (rhinorrhea) and watery eyes.

Allergic (atopic) asthma is caused by type I immune injury in the lower respiratory tract. Contraction of smooth muscle in bronchi and bronchioles (bronchospasm) along with mucosal edema narrows the airways. Increased mucous gland secretion causes mucus plugs in the airway lumens. The end result is difficulty breathing.

Type I injury in the skin causes *urticaria* and *angioedema*. Urticaria (hives) are well-circumscribed, raised areas on the skin caused by increased permeability in superficial vessels of the skin resulting in focal areas of edema. Angioedema is a more generalized swelling caused by increased permeability of vessels deeper in the skin and in subcutaneous tissues.

Activation of mast cells and basophils throughout the body causes *systemic anaphylaxis*, a potentially life-threatening form of type I immune injury. Injection of a drug to which a patient is allergic, such as penicillin or novacaine, is a common means of inducing anaphylaxis. Insect stings are another source of allergens that can induce systemic anaphylaxis. During systemic anaphylaxis there is increased permeability of vessels throughout the body, causing edema in many organs. In the skin this can manifest as urticaria. Edema also occurs in the respiratory tract, narrowing the airways. Severe laryngeal edema can cause acute strangulation. Bronchoconstriction further compromises respiratory function. The extensive loss of fluid from vessels reduces the blood volume, causing hypotension. Poor oxygenation of blood caused by narrowed airways and poor tissue perfusion caused by hypotension can lead to shock and death if not reversed by pharmacologic antagonists of type I injury such as epinephrine.

Laboratory Evaluation of IgE-Mediated Diseases

Skin tests for immediate hypersensitivity and laboratory determinations of total serum IgE levels as well as amounts of allergen-specific IgE are useful in the evaluation and management of individuals with type I immune-mediated diseases. Blood eosinophilia is also observed in some atopic patients.

Immediate hypersensitivity skin tests entail pricking or scratching the skin surface and applying a drop of antigen-containing fluid over the skin lesion. Often a battery of antigens will be tested simultaneously, for example, on the skin of the back or forearm. If one or more of the antigens is an allergen in the tested individual, edema (a wheal) and/or erythema will develop at the test site for that antigen.

Blood concentrations of IgE are usually expressed in international units (IU) per milliter. One IU equals approximately 2.4 ng IgE. Normal adults have serum IgE levels of approximately 50 to 100 IU/ml. Normally newborn children have no detectable serum IgE. At 6 months old serum IgE is approximately 10 IU/ml and usually remains less than 50 IU/ml until adulthood. Individuals with type I allergic diseases and helminth infections have elevated levels. Because of the small amounts in many individuals, serum IgE is usually quantitated by radioimmunoassay (RIA) or enzyme-linked immunoassay. Serum levels of IgE can be measured by a competitive (indirect) or noncompetitive (direct) *radioimmunosorbent test (RIST)* (Fig. 11–2). Both assays use anti-IgE insolubilized on particles or discs. In the direct (noncompetitive) RIST, the insolubilized anti-IgE is incubated with the serum sample, allowing IgE in the sample to bind to the anti-IgE. After washing, radiolabeled anti-IgE is added. This binds to IgE from the serum that attached to the insolubilized anti-IgE. After washing, the radioactivity of the insolubilized anti-IgE is directly proportional to IgE in the serum sample. In the indirect (competitive) RIST, the insolubilized anti-IgE is incubated with sample serum and radiolabeled IgE. IgE in the serum competes with the radiolabeled IgE for binding

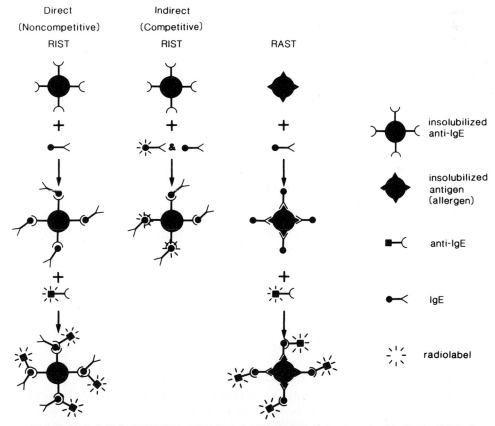

Figure 11–2. IgE Quantitation. Diagrams of the sequential events in the direct and indirect radioimmunosorbent test (RIST) for quantitating total serum IgE and the radioallergosorbent test (RAST) for quantitating IgE with specificity for a particular allergen.

to the anti-IgE. After washing, the radioactivity of the insolubilized anti-IgE is indirectly proportional to the amount of IgE in the serum. The quantity of IgE in an unknown serum sample is determined by comparing the unknown sample results with a standard curve derived from values obtained with samples containing known amounts of IgE.

IgE antibodies with specificity for specific allergens can also be measured. The most commonly employed assay for this purpose is the *radioallergosorbent test (RAST)* (Fig. 11–2). In this test allergen is bound to an insoluble substrate, such as cellulose beads. The substrate with bound allergen is incubated with serum. If IgE specific for the allergen is present in the serum, it binds to the immobilized allergen. The substrate is then incubated with radiolabeled anti-IgE. The radioactivity of the substrate, after washing, is a measure of the amount of allergen-specific IgE in the serum sample.

TYPE II IMMUNE INJURY

Direct antibody attack against cells and tissues, especially by complement-fixing IgG and IgM antibodies, causes injury categorized as type II by Gell and Coombs. Direct complement-fixing antibody attack against cells causes cytotoxcity, whereas attack against tissues causes acute inflammation. Direct antibody binding to antigens on cells can also cause events other than lysis, such as stimulation or blockade of hormone receptors. Type II immune injury is directed against either foreign antigens or self-antigens. The latter causes autoimmune diseases and is discussed in detail later in this chapter.

Cytotoxicity

When complement-fixing antibodies, IgG and IgM, bind to antigens on cells, they cause lysis by two mechanisms, complement-mediated membrane disruption and opsonization-induced phagocytosis.

IgG and IgM bound to cell membrane antigens activate the classic complement pathway, leading to generation of the membrane attack complex, C5b6789. Membrane attack complexes form cylindrical channels through cell membranes, leading to osmotic lysis.

IgG and complement, especially C3b and C4b, bound to antigens on cell surfaces act as opsonins. They are recognized by Fc and complement receptors on phagocytes, primarily macrophages and polymorphonuclear leukocytes, and initiate phagocytosis. The cells are phagocytosed into membrane-linked cytoplasmic vacuoles (*phagosomes*) that fuse with lytic enzyme-containing vacuoles (*lysosomes*), resulting in lysis of the cells.

Acute Inflammation Induced by Direct Antibody Attack

In addition to cytotoxicity, direct antibody attack can cause tissue inflammation if the antigen that the immune response is directed against is a constituent of tissue or has become tightly bound to tissue. If the antigen is a constituent of one's own tissue, the immune response against it is an autoimmune response.

The most often cited example of tissue injury induced by direct antibody attack is *Goodpasture's syndrome*. Individuals with this disease have autoantibodies against antigens in the basement membranes of renal glomerular capillaries and pulmonary alveolar septal capillaries. Binding of the antibasement membrane autoantibodies to the glomerular and alveolar capillaries initiates acute inflammation by activating mediator systems, such as complement. This causes glomerulonephritis and lung hemorrhage. Individuals with this disease develop hemoptysis and respiratory insufficiency. The laboratory manifestations of the glomerulonephritis include hematuria, proteinuria, and, if it is severe enough, elevated serum creatinine and blood urea nitrogen. Histologic examination of biopsied lung tissue reveals intra-alveolar hemorrhage, and renal tissue reveals glomerular inflammation. Direct immunofluorescence microscopy of glomeruli using fluorochrome-labeled anti-IgG antibodies demonstrates linear localization of IgG along the glomerular basement membranes (Fig. 11–3 A). The use of

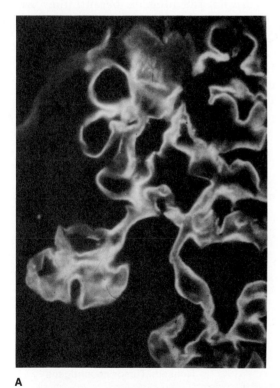 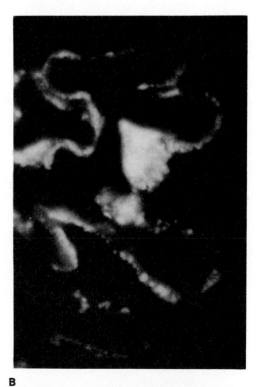

A   B

Figure 11-3. Immunofluorescence Microscopy of Glomerulonephritis. Direct immunofluorescence microscopy for IgG showing **(A)** linear staining of glomerular basement membranes indicative of antiglomerular basement membrane antibody-mediated glomerulonephritis, and **(B)** granular staining of glomerular capillaries indicative of immune complex-mediated glomerulonephritis.

direct and indirect immunofluorescence microscopy to detect autoantibodies and autoantibody-mediated tissue injury are discussed in more detail later in this chapter.

IMMUNE COMPLEX-MEDIATED INJURY

Immune complexes are formed by the union of antigens with specific antibodies. This term is almost always used to refer to complexes formed between antibodies and antigens that are not attached to cells or tissues, that is, antigens that are free floating in the plasma, lymph, interstitial fluid, or other fluids of the body. The antigen, however, could be shed from cells or tissues prior to or after complexing with antibody.

Antigens in immune complexes are of endogenous (produced by the body) or exogenous (produced by something other than the body) origin (Table 11–4). Endogenous antigens are usually self-antigens; therefore the antibodies complexed with them are autoantibodies. An exception to this would be neoantigens derived from neoplasms. These antigens are endogenous but are not self-antigens, because they are expressed by the aberrant cancer cells but not by normal body cells. The most common exogenous source for antigens in pathogenic immune complexes is infectious pathogens, especially bacteria and viruses.

The site of an infection that is releasing antigens that will form pathogenic immune complexes is often different from the site of immune complex-mediated injury. For example, in *poststreptococcal glomerulonephritis*, a group A β-hemolytic streptococcal infection of the oropharynx (strep throat) or skin (impetigo) releases streptococcal

TABLE 11-4. SOURCES OF ANTIGENS IN PATHOGENIC IMMUNE COMPLEXES

Exogenous	Endogenous

Drugs: Penicillin
    Sulfonamides
	Fungi: Candida
	    Coccidioides

Foreign Proteins: Antitoxins
    Antilymphocyte antibodies
    Therapeutic insulin
    Therapeutic procoagulants
    Bee and snake venoms
	Protozoa: Plasmodium
	    Toxoplasma
	Helminths: Schistosoma
	Self: DNA
	    Other nuclear antigens
	    Renal epithelium
	    Immunoglobulins
	    Thyroglobulin

Bacteria: Streptococci
    Staphylococci
    Neisseria
    Treponema
    Salmonella
	Nonself: Tumor neoantigens

Viruses: Hepatitis B
    Cytomegalovirus
    Epstein–Barr
    Varicella	

antigens into the blood. Subsequent production of antistreptococcal antibodies results in the localization of immune complexes in glomerular capillaries, where they mediate acute inflammatory injury.

Pathogenesis of Immune Complex-Mediated Injury

Immune complexes can form in the circulation and deposit in vessel walls or cross vessel walls to be deposited in tissues. Alternatively, immune complexes can form in situ in vessel walls or tissues, that is, uncomplexed antigens and antibodies come into contact in the vessel walls or tissues and form immune complexes in those sites. When immune complexes localize in vessel walls or tissues, by either *deposition* from the circulation or *in situ formation*, they induce injury (type III immune injury), primarily through mediating acute inflammation.

Figure 11–4 illustrates three mechanisms by which complement-fixing antibodies can induce acute inflammatory injury in vessel walls. Direct antibody attack is an example of type II injury, whereas in situ immune complex formation and immune complex deposition are examples of type III injury. In direct antibody attack the antigen to which

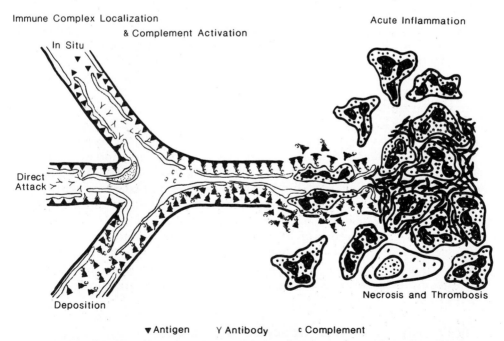

Figure 11–4. Immune Complex Localization in Vessels. Diagram depicting three mechanisms by which antibodies bound to antigens can occur in vessel walls and mediate inflammation: direct attack, deposition from the circulation, and in situ formation.

antibody binds is a fixed constituent of the vessel wall. In in situ formation the antigen and antibody reach the site of immune complex localization independently and then form immune complexes. In deposition immune complexes form in the circulation and then deposit at the site of localization. Once complement-fixing antibodies bound to antigens localize in vessel walls or tissues by any of these three mechanisms, they incite acute inflammation and tissue injury.

Immune complexes in tissues induce injury primarily by activating humoral mediator systems, such as the complement, kinin, coagulation, and plasmin systems. This causes increased vascular permeability resulting in edema and greater spread of inflammatory mediators through the tissues. Chemotactic factors generated by the mediator systems, such as C5a, C5b67, and kallikrein, attract polymorphonuclear leukocytes and macrophages. These inflammatory cells release lytic enzymes, toxic oxygen species, and lipid metabolites that further enhance the inflammation and cause tissue destruction.

Many factors determine the pathogenic potential of immune complexes. From the discussion above it is clear that the ability of the constituent antibody to activate complement and other mediator systems is important. Factors that allow immune complexes to deposit in tissues or to form in situ in tissues also are important.

The size of immune complexes affects their ability to deposit from the circulation. Immune complex size is related to antigen : antibody ratio. Immune complexes formed in the circulation at a ratio near equivalence are large, are poor at entering and crossing vessel walls, and are rapidly cleared from the circulation by phagocytes. Immune complexes formed in antibody excess are maximally opsonized and thus rapidly cleared from the circulation by phagocytes. Immune complexes formed in *antigen excess* are the most pathogenic, because they are least effectively cleared from the circulation by phagocytosis and are most able to penetrate vessel walls.

The charge of immune complexes and the constituent antigens and antibodies affects the ability to localize in tissues and the site of localization. Because vessel walls have anionic charges, cationic immune complexes are better able to penetrate them than are anionic immune complexes. Cationic antigens can bind to vessel walls and other anionic tissue sites, where they are then available to participate in in situ immune-complex formation. Such binding fixes antigens to tissues so tightly that the distinction between in situ immune-complex formation and direct antibody attack of a tissue-bound antigen becomes arbitrary.

The strength of the binding (avidity or affinity) between antibodies and antigens in immune complexes can also affect pathogenicity. For example, low avidity antibodies may allow immune complexes in the circulation to disassociate, penetrate vessel walls as uncomplexed antibody and antigen, and then reassociate to form immune complexes in situ.

The Clinical and Pathologic Spectrum of Immune Complex-Mediated Diseases

The clinical, pathologic, and laboratory manifestations of immune complex-mediated diseases are dependent upon the tissues in which the immune complexes have localized and are producing injury (Table 11-5).

TABLE 11–5. RELATIONSHIP BETWEEN SITE OF IMMUNE COMPLEX LOCALIZATION AND DISEASE INDUCTION

Localization Site	Disease Induced
Vessels	Vasculitis
Arteries	Arteritis
Venules	Venulitis
Skin	Dermatitis
Joints	Arthritis
Glomeruli	Glomerulonephritis
Muscles	Myositis
Lungs	Pneumonitis

The most common site for immune complex localization is within vessel walls, where they can cause acute inflammation, *vasculitis*. This process can affect vessels of different types, such as arteries (causing *arteritis*) or venules (causing *venulitis*). Figure 11–5 A is a photomicrograph of an artery from a patient with immune complex-mediated arteritis. At the bottom of the photomicrograph the wall of the artery is relatively normal, but at the top it is necrotic, and there is a marked infiltration of the wall and adjacent tissue by polymorphonuclear leukocytes, some of which are fragmenting. Figure 11–5 B is an immunofluorescence photomicrograph showing IgG granular staining of an artery, indicating the localization of IgG-containing immune complexes in the wall.

In most tissues that are injured by immune complex-mediated inflammation, at least part of the immune complex localization is in the microvasculature. Immune complex-mediated *glomerulonephritis* and *pneumonitis* are in fact vasculitis of glomerular capillaries and alveolar capillaries respectively. Figure 11–3 B shows granular immunostaining for IgG in glomerular capillaries of a patient with immune complex mediated glomerulonephritis.

The symptoms and signs of immune complex-mediated vascular inflammation depend on the location of the involved vessels and the type of injury produced. Patients with glomerulonephritis have hematuria, proteinuria, and renal failure. Patients with pneumonitis have cough and difficulty breathing (dyspnea). If small vessels in the skin are severely injured and rupture, the resulting hemorrhage produces irregular areas of cutaneous discoloration caused by blood in the dermis, *purpura* (Fig. 11–6). If the vascular injury affects arteries, blood flow can be interrupted by thrombosis or rupture of the artery, leading to necrosis of the tissue supplied by that artery, *infarction*. If this occurs in an abdominal organ, the patient experiences abdominal pain as a symptom of the immune complex-mediated arteritis. If the immune complex-mediated injury is in the muscle vasculature and surrounding tissue causing *myositis*, the patient complains of muscle pain and weakness. Immune complexes localizing in joint synovial tissue and fluid mediate inflammation that manifests as *arthralgia* and *arthritis*.

Many patients with immune complex-mediated disease will have combinations of the processes described in the preceding paragraph. This occurs when the components

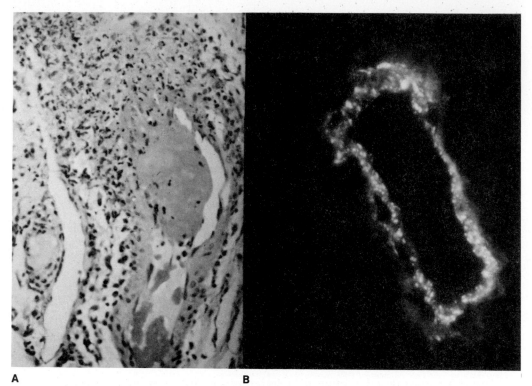

A   **B**

Figure 11-5. Immune-Mediated Arteritis. Photomicrographs of arteries from patients with immune complex-mediated arteritis. **(A)** Light microscopy showing acute inflammation with marked influx of neutrophils. **(B)** Immunofluorescence microscopy for IgG showing granular staining of the artery wall.

of the immune complexes are in the circulation and localize in more than one tissue. An example of this would be a patient with *serum sickness*. Serum sickness is caused by the administration to a patient of foreign proteins, for example horse antiserum (antitoxin) against tetanus or diphtheria toxins. After a latent period of approximately 1 to 2 weeks, during which time the patient is producing antibodies to the circulating horse proteins, the patient begins to develop signs and symptoms of systemic, immune complex-mediated injury. Fever, leukocytosis, and hypocomplementemia are manifestations of the systemic immune-complex formation and activation of mediator systems. Lymphadenopathy and splenomegaly result from the immune response to foreign antigen and the phagocytosis of immune complexes. Immune complex localization in multiple tissues produces concurrent arthritis with arthralgias, myositis and myalgias, and glomerulonephritis and hematuria and proteinuria.

Laboratory Evaluation of Immune Complex-Mediated Diseases

Table 11-6 lists a number of laboratory procedures that are useful in evaluating immune complex-mediated diseases. Nonspecific indicators of possible immune

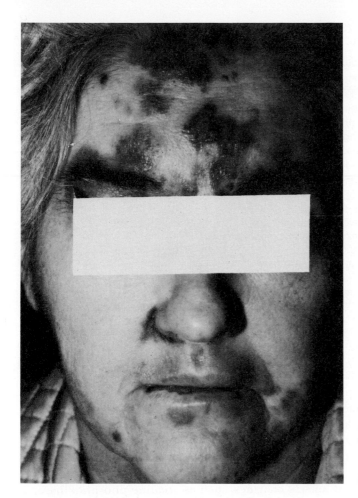

Figure 11-6. Immune-Mediated Vasculitis. A patient with immune complex-mediated vasculitis in the skin causing focal intradermal hemorrhages (purpura), most marked on the forehead.

complex-mediated injury are polyclonal hypergammaglobulinemia, leukocytosis with increased segmented and immature neutrophils, elevated sedimentation rate, and elevated acute-phase reactants such as C-reactive protein. These findings are indicative of inflammation but are not specific for the pathogenic mechanism that has elicited the inflammation. Hypocomplementemia can accompany immune complex-mediated diseases as a result of complement protein consumption during complement activation by immune complexes.

There are laboratory tests that can detect circulating immune complexes in blood. Some immune complexes will precipitate from serum when it is cooled to 4°C. Immunoglobulins that precipitate from serum in the cold are called *cryoglobulins*. Not all cryoglobulins are immune complexes, for example, monoclonal IgM produced by B cell lymphomas can form cryoprecipitates. Immune complexed, but not free, IgG and IgM can bind to C1q. Therefore there are a variety of *C1q-binding assays* that measure the ability of IgG and IgM in serum to bind to C1q. Immune complexes that have fixed

TABLE 11–6. LABORATORY TESTS USEFUL FOR EVALUATING IMMUNE COMPLEX-MEDIATED DISEASES

Immunoglobulin quantification
Blood leukocyte differential count
Complement quantification
Identification of circulating immune complexes:
    Cryoglobulin assay
    C1q-binding assays
    Raji cell assay
Acute-phase reactant and sedimentation rate evaluation
Organ-specific laboratory test:
    Urine analysis
    Joint fluid analysis
    Rheumatoid factor assay
    Muscle enzyme and myoglobin analysis
    Electromyography
Tissue biopsy evaluation:
    Light microscopy
    Immunofluorescence microscopy

complement will bind to B lymphocytes via Fc and complement receptors. The *Raji cell test* for immune complexes measures the binding of serum IgG to a tissue-cultured B lymphoblastic cell line derived from a patient with Burkitt's lymphoma (Raji cells). Another type of immune complex assay uses rheumatoid factors (anti-IgG autoantibodies) that preferentially bind immune complexes.

There are organ-specific laboratory tests that can be used to support the presence of immune complex-mediated injury in a particular tissue. For example, if immune complex-mediated glomerulonephritis is suspected, urine analysis for proteinuria and hematuria is useful for confirming the presence of glomerular injury. Myositis can be confirmed by detecting elevated muscle enzymes, such as creatine phosphokinase, in the blood and increased myoglobin in blood or in urine. Synovial fluid analysis helps differentiate between mechanisms of joint injury. Degenerative osteoarthritis is characterized by fluid with much less evidence for active inflammation than that from patients with immune complex-mediated arthritis. The latter is characterized by an elevated leukocyte count, increased protein concentration, reduced viscosity, and reduced complement level.

Light and immunofluorescence microscopic evaluation of biopsies from involved tissues can indicate an immune complex pathogenesis. Acute vascular inflammation (Fig. 11–5 A) and granular immunostaining for immunoglobulins and complement (Fig. 11–3 B and 11–5 B) are consistent with immune complex-mediated injury.

PATHOGENESIS OF AUTOIMMUNITY

Autoimmunity is immune response against one's own molecules. An *autoimmune disease* is a disease caused, in large measure, by an immune attack against one's own molecules, cells, or tissues. There are many theories that attempt to explain autoimmunity and autoimmune diseases (Table 11–7). Some are supported by a reasonable amount of data, but others are not. It is likely that different mechanisms and combinations of mechanisms are responsible for inducing different types of autoimmune phenomena.

Normally the immune system appears to show *tolerance* toward self-molecules and to mount immune attack only against nonself molecules. In the past it was theorized that lymphocytes with receptors for self-antigens were eliminated during embryonic or fetal development, thus preventing immune responses against self. On the basis of this theory, autoimmunity would result from the appearance of a so-called *"forbidden" clone* of self-reactive lymphocytes normally not present in an individual. This theory has been discredited by the demonstration that all individuals have lymphocytes with receptors capable of recognizing self-molecules. Therefore current theories propose that tolerance is the result of active regulatory suppression of potential immune responses to self-molecules. The converse to this theory is that autoimmunity is caused by defects in this homeostatic suppression of self-immune reactivity.

Another theory suggests that immune tolerance is due to the large amounts of self-molecules in effect overwhelming self-reactive lymphocytes. This implies that molecules sequestered inside tissues where lymphocytes normally do not contact them would cause an autoimmune response if released into the circulation by tissue injury. Some data supports this postulate. For example, injury to the eye can lead to the development of detectable autoantibodies directed against lens antigens, and injury to the testis can result in detectable levels of autoantibodies reactive with spermatozoa. However, there is also evidence that not only are such sequestered antigens released by injury, but they may also be somewhat altered, and this may be the important event in the induction of the autoimmune response. Because most clinically important autoimmune responses are not directed against antigens that would be considered sequestered, the sequestered antigen theory is not an adequate pathogenetic explanation of autoimmunity.

The pathogenetic theories receiving the greatest support at the present time suggest that clinically significant autoimmunity results from disturbed immune regulation. Many factors may play a role in the induction of this disturbance, for example, viral infections that perturb normal lymphocyte function or alterations in self-antigens such as linkage to drugs. Some individuals may be predisposed by genetic and hormonal factors to the development of particular autoimmune diseases. Genetic predisposition

TABLE 11-7. PATHOGENETIC THEORIES OF AUTOIMMUNITY

Developing "forbidden" clones of self-reactive lymphocytes
Release of sequestered self-antigens
Genetic and hormonal predisposition
Reduction in suppressor T lymphocytes
Increase in helper T lymphocytes
Disordered idiotype-anti-idiotype networks
Polyclonal B lymphocyte activation
Altered self-antigens

may be linked to immune response genes in the major histocompatibility complex. HLA-D typing identifies individuals at higher risk of developing certain types of autoimmune disease. For example, in white populations HLA alleles DR2, DR3, DR4, and DR5 are associated with a higher risk for a variety of autoimmune diseases.

A review of the complex regulatory mechanisms of the immune system discussed in earlier chapters will indicate the many potential regulatory defects that could act alone or synergistically to produce autoimmunity. There is evidence that although B lymphocytes are available to respond to self-antigens, tolerance is maintained by T lymphocyte suppression or lack of T lymphocyte help, with the latter being more likely. Immunoregulation by B and T lymphocyte idiotype–anti-idiotype interactions may be involved in tolerance, and dysfunction of this network could lead to autoimmunity.

Autoimmunity would arise when regulatory mechanisms are defective or bypassed. Alteration of antigens, for example, by linkage with drugs or viral antigens, could lead to T lymphocyte recognition and generation of helper activity to break B lymphocyte tolerance. The lack of T lymphocyte help could also be overcome by *polyclonal B lymphocyte activators*. These are substances that stimulate B lymphocyte proliferation and antibody production. Many bacteria, viruses, and parasites produce polyclonal B lymphocyte activators. It is possible that infections cause the development of some autoimmune diseases by producing polyclonal B lymphocyte activators that help stimulate autoreactive B lymphocytes even in the absence of T lymphocyte help.

CATEGORIZATION OF AUTOIMMUNE DISEASES

Autoimmune diseases can be classified on the basis of the specificity of the autoimmune response or on the basis of the type of autoimmune injury.

Autoimmune diseases can be divided into those that are *organ specific* and those that are *systemic* (Table 11–8). This approach, however, is imperfect, because some individuals have multiple organ-specific and/or systemic autoimmune diseases. Organ-specific autoimmune diseases have injury confined to one specific organ. In individuals with these diseases an autoimmune response to certain constituents of the injured organ can be demonstrated by laboratory tests. Systemic autoimmune diseases affect many different organs simultaneously. These individuals have autoantibodies specific for structures found at many sites in the body.

Autoimmune diseases can also be categorized on the basis of the mechanism by which the autoimmunity produces the disease (Table 11–9). An autoimmune response can lead to the destruction or altered function of macromolecules, cells, tissues, and organs by a variety of antibody-mediated and cell-mediated mechanisms. The pathophysiology of autoimmune responses is the same as that for appropriate immune responses, except that in the former the response is against self and in the latter the response is against nonself. For example, immune attack on red blood cells in the circulation employs the same immunopathologic mechanisms, whether it is appropriate destruction of mismatched red blood cells producing a transfusion reaction or autoimmune destruction of one's own red blood cells producing autoimmune hemolytic anemia.

TABLE 11–8. ORGAN-SPECIFIC AND SYSTEMIC AUTOIMMUNE DISEASES

Organ-Specific Autoimmune Diseases	
Disease	*Autoimmune Specificity*
Autoimmune thyroiditis	Thyroglobulin, microsomal thyroid antigens
Thyrotoxicosis	Thyroid-stimulating hormone receptors
Autoimmune hypoparathyroidism	Parathyroid cells
Insulin-dependent diabetes	Pancreatic islet cells
Insulin-resistant diabetes	Insulin receptors
Autoimmune hemophilia	Coagulation factors
Autoimmune adrenal failure	Adrenal cortical cells
Autoimmune atrophic gastritis	Gastric parietal cells
Myasthenia gravis	Acetylcholine receptors
Pemphigus	Epidermal cells
Pemphigoid	Skin basement membrane
Vitiligo	skin melanocytes
Autoimmune hemolytic anemia	Red blood cells
Autoimmune neutropenia	Neutrophilic granulocytes
Autoimmune thrombocytopenia	Platelets
Autoimmune male sterility	Sperm
Premature ovarian failure	Ovarian corpus luteum and interstitial cells
Systemic Autoimmune Diseases	
Disease	*Autoimmune Specificity*
Goodpasture's syndrome	Kidney and lung basement membrane
Systemic lupus erythematosus	Multiple nuclear antigens and many others
Other connective tissue diseases	Varied nuclear antigens and others
Rheumatoid arthritis	Immunoglobulins and others

LABORATORY EVALUATION OF AUTOIMMUNITY

To support a diagnosis of an autoimmune disease, laboratory data must be obtained documenting the presence of abnormal levels of autoantibodies or autoreactive lymphocytes. Most current laboratory tests for autoimmunity identify autoantibodies. Many different tests are used, including indirect immunofluorescence microscopy, RIAs, enzyme-linked immunoassays, agglutination reactions, immunoprecipitation, complement fixation, and bioassays. In all of these tests some self-antigens are being tested for reactivity with antibodies in a patient's blood.

Indirect immunofluorescence microscopy as well as *direct immunofluorescence microscopy* are often used to detect autoantibodies. As described in Chapter 4, immunofluorescence microscopy detects the binding of antibodies to cells or tissues by labeling the antibodies with a fluorescent compound (fluorochrome), usually fluorescein. Direct immunofluorescence microscopy is used to detect autoantibodies present in an indivi-

TABLE 11–9. AUTOIMMUNE DISEASES CLASSIFIED BY MECHANISM OF DISEASE PRODUCTION

Blood Cell Cytolysis	Tissue Inflammation and Injury
Autoimmune hemolytic anemia	Autoimmune thyroiditis
Autoimmune leukopenia	Autoimmune hypoparathyroidism
Autoimmune thrombocytopenia	Autoimmune adrenal failure
Inactivation of Biologically Active Macromolecules	Autoimmune atrophic gastritis
	Pemphigus
Autoimmune hemophilia	Pemphigoid
Blockade of Cell-Surface Receptors	Autoimmune male sterility
Insulin-resistant diabetes	Premature ovarian failure
Myasthenia gravis	Goodpasture's syndrome
	Systemic lupus erythematosus
Stimulation of Cell-Surface Receptors	Rheumatoid arthritis
Thyrotoxicosis	Insulin-dependent diabetes
	Vitiligo

dual's tissues, whereas indirect immunofluorescence is used to detect autoantibodies in blood. The tissue substrate for indirect immunofluorescence microscopy is chosen on the basis of the suspected specificity of the autoantibody being sought. For example, if an autoimmune skin disease is suspected, skin would be used as the substrate; if autoimmune kidney disease is suspected, kidney tissue would be used. For detecting some autoantibodies, human tissue must be used; for others, animal tissue is adequate.

RIAs, enzyme-linked immunoassays, agglutination assays, immunoprecipitation assays, and complement fixation assays for autoantibodies are technically identical to analogous serologic assays for antimicrobial antibodies, the only difference being that the antigen used in the assays for autoantibodies is one normally found in an individual's tissues rather than a microbial antigen. For example, patients with autoimmune thyroiditis have circulating antithyroglobulin antibodies that can be detected by hemagglutination of tanned red blood cells coated with thyroglobulin.

AUTOIMMUNE BLOOD CELL CYTOPENIAS

Any cellular component of the blood can be attacked and eliminated by an autoimmune response, producing a reduced number of that cell type in the blood, a *cytopenia*, such as anemia, neutropenia, lymphopenia, and thrombocytopenia. Cytopenias can also be produced by nonimmunologic mechanisms, such as suppression of hematopoiesis by drug toxicity.

Autoimmune destruction of blood cells occurs within the lumens of blood vessels, *intravascularly*, or within phagocytes, *extravascularly*. Intravascular lysis is mediated by complement activation and extravascular lysis by opsonization. When complement-fixing autoantibodies fix to the surfaces of blood cells, the complement cascade is activated, leading to the deposition of activated complement components on the cell surface membrane. As discussed in Chapter 10, the membrane-attack complex punches holes in cell membranes, resulting in intravascular lysis.

When blood cells are opsonized by autoantibodies and complement, they bind to phagocytes via Fc and complement receptors, are engulfed by phagocytosis, and are lysed within the phagocyte by lytic lysosomal enzymes.

Autoimmune Hemolytic Anemia

Autoimmune hemolytic anemias occur for no apparent reason (i.e., are idiopathic) or are induced by viral infection or drug administration. In a patient with an anemia, autoimmunity is incriminated as the mechanism of lysis by laboratory demonstration of autoantibodies bound to the surface of patient erythrocytes or of free autoantibodies in the serum. This is done by direct or indirect antiglobulin hemagglutination (Coombs') tests, respectively. In the *direct Coombs' test* patient red cells are incubated with antibodies specific for human immunoglobulin. If the patient's red cells are coated with autoantibodies, they will agglutinate. In the *indirect Coombs' test* patient serum is incubated with reagent red blood cells having known red cell antigens. Thereafter the reagent cells are incubated with the anti-immunoglobulin antibodies and are examined for agglutination. Agglutination indicates that the patient has circulating antibodies reactive with antigens on the surface of the reagent cells. By reacting the patient's serum with a variety of reagent cells having different red cell antigens, the specificity of the patient's autoantibody is determined.

In addition to detecting and identifying the specificity of red cell autoantibodies, Coombs' tests are used to assess certain functional characteristics of the pathogenic autoantibodies. Instead of using an anti-immunoglobulin antibody reactive with all immunoglobulins, antibodies specific for particular immunoglobulin classes and subclasses can be used. The direct Coombs' test can also be performed using an anticomplement antibody rather than an anti-immunoglobulin antibody. Agglutination with this antibody documents complement activation on the patient's red cells. Indirect Coombs' tests can be run in the presence of complement to test for lysis by examining the supernatant after sedimentation for released hemoglobin.

Indirect Coombs' tests are performed at different temperatures, usually 37°C and 4°C, to assess the optimum temperature at which the autoantibodies bind to the red cells. On this basis autoimmune hemolytic anemias are divided into *warm antibody induced* and *cold antibody induced*. Warm antibody hemolytic anemia is common. Warm antibody anemia is usually caused by IgG antibodies and cold antibody anemia by IgM.

Autoimmune Leukopenias

Autoimmune neutropenia and lymphopenia occur alone and in association with systemic autoimmune diseases, such as systemic lupus erythematosus and rheumatoid arthritis. Affected individuals may be asymptomatic or suffer from recurrent infections. Autoimmune neutropenia is more common than lymphopenia. Autoimmune leukopenias are usually caused by autoantibodies and complement by mechanisms analogous to those for autoimmune hemolytic anemias, but in some patients immune destruction of leukocytes involves K cells and antibody-dependent-cell-mediated cyto-toxicity (ADCC). Leukocyte autoantibodies are detected in the laboratory by direct and indirect leukoagglutination and leukocyte immunofluorescence assays.

Autoimmune Thrombocytopenia

Idiopathic thrombocytopenic purpura (ITP) is caused by destruction of platelets (thrombo-cytes) by autoantibodies. The blood platelet count is usually below 100,000/mcL and may be below 30,000/mcL. Individuals with ITP are prone to develop hemorrhages in many tissues, including multifocal skin hemorrhages called purpura.

Antiplatelet antibodies, especially autoimmune antiplatelet antibodies, are more difficult to detect than antileukocyte and antierythrocyte antibodies. One of the more widely used tests is an indirect immunofluorescence assay using paraformaldehyde-fixed normal platelets as the substrate. Radiolabeled or enzyme-labeled anti-immuno-globulins or staphylococcal protein A are also used to detect antiplatelet antibodies bound to platelets.

AUTOIMMUNE INACTIVATION OF BIOLOGICALLY ACTIVE MACROMOLECULES

Autoantibody-mediated inactivation or elimination by opsonization of macromole-cules required for normal homeostasis can cause diseases. The best known example is autoimmune inactivation of coagulation factors, sometimes causing acquired hemo-philia. Autoantibodies against many different coagulation factors have been identi-fied, including fibrinogen, prothrombin, and factors V, VIII : C, VIII : vWF, IX, and XI.

The best known anticoagulation factor autoantibody is *antifactor VIII*. Antifactor VIII antibodies occur in some patients with hemophilia A, presumably induced by the therapeutic administration of replacement coagulation factors from donor blood. These antifactor VIII antibodies more likely are alloantibodies rather than autoanti-bodies. Some individuals with no coagulation abnormalities develop antifactor VIII autoantibodies that may result in a severe bleeding disorder or be asymptomatic. Anti-factor VIII autoantibodies are seen most often in postpartum women, in older individ-uals, and in patients with autoimmune diseases, especially systemic lupus erythema-tosus.

Patients with lupus also can develop an antibody that reacts with phospholipid in some coagulation tests thus inhibiting the conversion of prothrombin to thrombin and resulting in an abnormal test value. This antibody is called the *lupus anticoagulant*. It occasionally is seen in patients who do not have lupus. This antibody is not known to cause abnormal bleeding in vivo, so its major significance is as a cause for abnormal coagulation test results in the laboratory.

Coagulation factor antibodies are usually identified in the laboratory by their inhibition of coagulation tests rather than by specific immunologic assays, although immunologic assays can be used to confirm the antibody nature of the inhibitor. Not all inhibitors are autoantibodies. When a coagulation test is prolonged, it could be the result of either a deficiency of coagulation factors or an inhibitor. The first step in identifying an inhibitor is to repeat the test after mixing normal plasma with the patient's plasma. If the prolongation of the initial test was due to a deficiency, the mix test will give a normal time, because normal coagulation factors have been added. If the prolongation was due to an inhibitor, the mix test will remain prolonged, because the inhibitor inhibits the coagulation factors in the normal plasma. An inhibitor is shown to be an antibody by neutralization of the inhibitor with antihuman immunoglobulin antiserum.

AUTOIMMUNE BLOCKADE OF CELL SURFACE RECEPTORS

One form of *insulin-resistant diabetes mellitus* results from the binding of autoantibodies to insulin receptors on cell surfaces so that insulin in the extracellular fluid is blocked from binding to the receptors. Therefore the cells are unable to respond to endogenous or exogenous insulin, resulting in abnormal carbohydrate metabolism that is more difficult to correct with insulin injection than that in the more common insulin-dependent diabetes mellitus.

Myasthenia gravis is a neuromuscular disease caused by an autoantibody that blocks the transmission of signals between motor nerves and muscles. Normally the neurotransmitter acetylcholine is released by the motor nerve endings, crosses the synapse between nerve and muscle, and binds to receptors on the muscle cell, initiating muscle contraction once enough acetylcholine has reacted with the receptors. In myasthenia gravis, autoantibodies bind to, block, and destroy acetylcholine receptors on muscle cells, preventing normal contraction in response to neural signals. The resultant symptoms are marked, voluntary muscle weakness and easy fatiguability.

Antiacetylocholine receptor antibodies are detected in serum by RIAs, enzyme-linked immunoassays, hemagglutination assays, and complement-fixing assays.

AUTOIMMUNE STIMULATION OF CELL SURFACE RECEPTORS

Graves' disease, a type of hyperthyroidism or thyrotoxicosis, is caused by an autoantibody that stimulates thryroid cells. Normally thyroid follicular cells are stimulated by thryoid stimulating hormone (TSH) that reacts with TSH receptors on cell membranes, resulting in increased thyroid hormone production. Individuals with Graves' disease have anti-TSH receptor autoantibodies that bind to TSH receptors, causing stimulation of thyroid cells and overproduction of thyroid hormones. This antibody is also called *long-acting thyroid stimulator (LATS)*. Laboratory evaluation of patients with Graves' disease reveals elevated blood levels of thyroxine and triiodothyronine. This hormonal excess causes hyperactivity, restlessness, hand tremors, weight loss, heat intolerance, and heart palpitations.

Anti-TSH receptor autoantibodies are detected using a bioassay that measures stimulation of test animal thyroids or isolated thyroid cells by patient immunoglobulin. Another approach for identifying anti-TSH receptors is to use a RIA that measures competition between patient immunoglobulin and TSH for TSH receptors.

AUTOIMMUNE-INDUCED TISSUE INJURY AND INFLAMMATION

Autoimmune injury to tissues can be mediated by autoantibodies and autoreactive T lymphocytes. Most autoimmune tissue injury is currently thought to be primarily mediated via autoantibodies. Autoantibodies often cause tissue injury by the induction of acute inflammation.

Autoimmune Injury to Endocrine Tissues

Many endocrine tissues are injured by autoimmune attack, resulting in hormonal deficiencies. The most commonly injured endocrine organs are the thyroid gland, parathyroid gland, adrenal gland, and pancreas. Individuals with predominant injury to one of these glands often have demonstrable autoantibodies specific for that organ and may also have autoantibodies against other endocrine glands, gastric parietal cells, ovarian follicle cells, or testicular interstitial cells.

As discussed previously, in Graves' disease autoantibodies cause increased thyroid function, hyperthyroidism, by stimulating TSH receptors. Autoimmunity of different specificity causes persistent destructive thyroid inflammation, that is, chronic thyroiditis. Individuals with this disease, called *Hashimoto's thyroiditis*, have multiple autoantibodies and autoreactive T lymphocytes with specificities for a variety of thyroid antigens. Laboratory tests, such as indirect immunofluorescence microscopy and hemagglutination, detect in these individuals autoantibodies specific for thyroglobulin, microsomal antigen in thyroid follicular cells, and colloid antigens of the extracellular material inside thyroid follicles. In addition to Hashimoto's thyroiditis, these autoantibodies are found associated with a number of other thyroid diseases.

In patients with *hypoparathyroidism* and parathyroid inflammation, autoantibodies specific for parathyroid cells can be detected in serum. This suggests an autoimmune pathogenesis.

Individuals with chronic adrenal failure, *Addison's disease*, have sustained injury to the cortex of the adrenal gland, resulting in adrenocortical hormone insufficiency. Because of this hormonal insufficiency, individuals with Addison's disease have weakness, anorexia, weight loss, hypotension, and hyperpigmented skin. Many different pathogenetic mechanisms, such as infection, neoplasia, and infarction, can injure the adrenal gland; however, in the United States autoimmune injury of the adrenal gland appears to be most common. Histologically the adrenal cortex in individuals with autoimmune adrenal failure has a reduction in the number of adrenal cells, a disorganization of the normal architecture, and infiltration of inflammatory cells, predominantly lymphocytes and monocytes. About 50% of patients with Addison's disease that is not caused by nonimmune mechanisms will have autoantibodies in their sera detectable by indirect immunofluorescence microscopy or other immunoassay techniques.

Insulin-dependent or type I diabetes mellitus results from a reduction in insulin production caused by destruction of the pancreatic islet cells that normally produce insulin. During the first year of recognized disease, approximately 75% of type I diabetic individuals have in their serum detectable autoantibodies against pancreatic islet cells. These antibodies are less commonly detectable later in the disease. *Anti-islet cell antibodies* are usually detected by indirect immunofluorescence microscopy using either normal human or nonhuman pancreas as substrate. Histologic examination of pancreatic tissue at different times during the course of type I diabetes demonstrates islet inflammation early and, later, marked reduction in islet cells, especially those islet cells that produce insulin.

Autoimmune Injury to the Stomach

Autoimmune attack against gastric cells produces a *chronic atrophic gastritis*, characterized histologically by marked influx of lymphocytes and macrophages and reduced numbers of mucosal epithelial cells (atrophy), especially parietal cells. Parietal cells produce intrinsic factor, which is required for vitamin B12 absorption from the gut. Individuals with chronic atrophic gastritis have autoantibodies against parietal cells, the intrinsic factor-B12 binding site and the intrinsic factor-B12 complex. This autoimmunity against cells and molecules required for vitamin B12 absorption causes a B12 deficiency that in turn produces a severe form of anemia called *pernicious anemia. Antiparietal cell autoantibodies* are usually detected by indirect immunofluorescence microscopy (Fig. 11–7) and anti-intrinsic factor autoantibodies by RIA or enzyme-linked immunoassay.

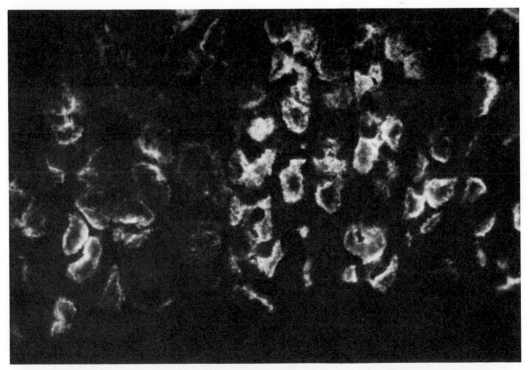

Figure 11–7. Antiparietal Cell Autoantibodies. Indirect immunofluorescence microscopy using serum from a patient with chronic atrophic gastritis demonstrating antiparietal cell autoantibodies staining parietal cells in the gastric mucosa.

Autoimmune Injury to Reproductive Organs

Both male and female infertility can be associated with autoantibodies specific for testicular or ovarian cells.

Individuals with autoimmune ovarian failure often also have some form of autoimmune endocrine disease such as thyroiditis, hypoparathyroidism, Addison's disease, or type I diabetes mellitus. By indirect immunofluorescence microscopy, autoantibodies reactive with the cytoplasm of theca interna cells of the ovarian follicles can be detected. These antibodies also react with adrenal cortical cells, and individuals with Addison's disease often have antibodies that react with ovarian theca interna cells. Autoantibodies that immunostain ovarian corpus luteum and interstitial cells are also found in individuals with autoimmune ovarian failure. The symptoms of this disease include reduced fertility and amenorrhea or premature menopause.

Both males and females can produce antibodies against sperm that can be associated with reduced fertility. These antibodies are detected in serum and semen, usually by agglutination, immobilization, cytotoxicity, or indirect immunofluorescence microscopy of spermatozoa. Rather than causing inflammatory injury to the testes, *antisperm autoantibodies* probably reduce fertility by inhibiting sperm motility. There is an increased frequency of sperm autoantibodies in homosexual men and in men who have undergone vasectomy.

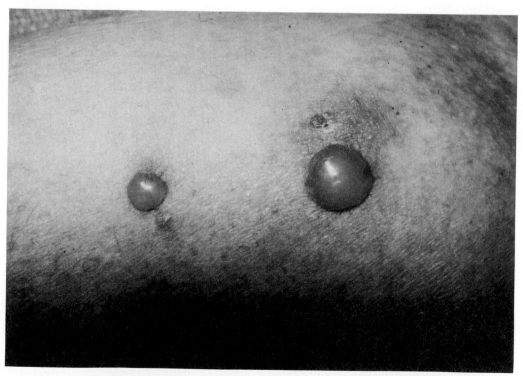

Figure 11–8. Immune-Mediated Bullae. Antiepidermal basement-membrane–zone-induced blisters (bullae) on the arm of an individual with pemphigoid.

Autoimmune Injury to Skin

Many different autoimmune mechanisms can injure the skin. As examples, pemphigus, pemphigoid, vitiligo, and lupus dermatitis will be discussed.

Pemphigus and *pemphigoid* are blistering (bullous) skin diseases (Fig. 11–8). Autoimmune attack on the skin produces clefts that fill up with fluid (blisters or bullae) and, especially in pemphigus, rupture to form shallow ulcers. In pemphigus, autoantibodies are directed against the surfaces of epidermal cells and cause the epidermal cells to detach from one another, thus producing bullae. In pemphigoid, autoantibodies are directed against the dermal–epidermal junction–basement-membrane zone and cause the epidermis to detach from the dermis, thus producing bullae. Direct immunofluorescence microscopy of skin biopsy tissue can differentiate between these clinically similar diseases by the site of localization of immunoglobulin within the skin, staining of epidermal intercellular substance in pemphigus (Fig. 11–9), and linear staining of the basement membrane zone in pemphigoid (Fig. 11–10). Serum samples can also be analyzed by indirect immunofluorescence microscopy using normal human or primate skin or esophagus as substrate. As in the direct procedure, the two diseases can be differentiated by the pattern of immunofluorescence.

Vitiligo is a disease characterized by skin depigmentation. It results from the de-

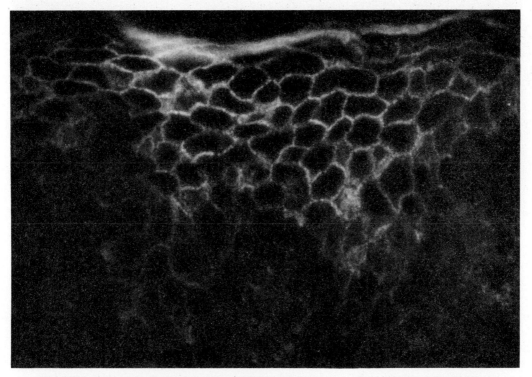

Figure 11-9. Immunohistology of Pemphigus. Direct immunofluorescence microscopy of a skin biopsy from a patient with pemphigus showing epidermal cell surface staining.

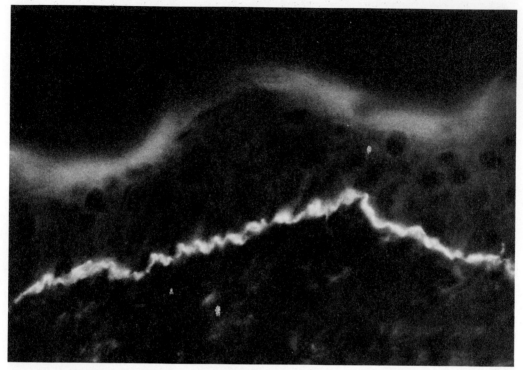

Figure 11–10. Immunohistology of Pemphigoid. Direct immunofluorescence microscopy of a skin biopsy from a patient with pemphigoid showing linear dermal–epidermal-basement-membrane zone staining.

struction of the pigment-producing cells in the skin, called melanocytes. These individuals have *antimelanocyte autoantibodies*, and it is likely that these autoantibodies mediate the melanocyte destruction. Vitiligo is sometimes associated with other autoimmune diseases, especially Addison's disease, thyroiditis, and chronic atrophic gastritis. Antimelanocyte autoantibodies are usually detected by indirect immunofluorescence microscopy.

Lupus dermatitis is caused by the localization of autoantibody-containing immune complexes at the dermal–epidermal junction and the resultant induction of inflammation (Fig. 11–11). As will be discussed later in this chapter, individuals with *lupus erythematosus* have many different types of autoantibodies, especially against nuclear antigens. The immune complexes causing lupus dermatitis are probably composed primarily of DNA and anti-DNA autoantibodies. The anti-DNA antibodies do not attack viable cells but complex with DNA released from dead cells. When these immune complexes accumulate at a particular site, they induce inflammation. Direct immunofluorescence microscopy of a biopsy of skin involved with lupus dermatitis demonstrates granular staining for immunoglobulin at the dermal–epidermal junction (Fig. 11–12), corresponding to the site of immune complex accumulation. This differs from the linear staining at the dermal–epidermal junction in pemphigoid.

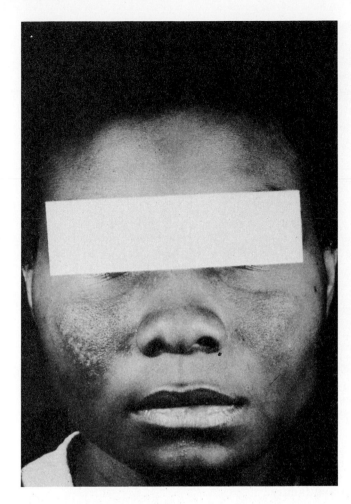

Figure 11-11. Lupus Dermatitis. Facial rash on the cheeks of a patient with systemic lupus erythematosus.

Lupus dermatitis occurs as one component of *systemic lupus erythematosus* or as an isolated process, called *discoid lupus erythematosus,* that may or may not develop into the systemic disease. Individuals with discoid lupus have immune deposits demonstrable only at the sites of dermatitis, whereas systemic lupus individuals usually have deposits in both inflamed and noninflamed skin.

Goodpasture's Syndrome

As mentioned earlier in this chapter, *Goodpasture's syndrome* is an autoimmune disease that affects the lungs and kidneys. It is caused by autoantibodies against the basement membranes of capillaries in lung alveolar and kidney glomeruli. Autoimmune-mediated destruction of pulmonary capillaries produces hemorrhage into the alveolar air spaces and impairment of the gas exchange surfaces of the lung that are required for oxygenation of blood. Autoimmune destruction of renal glomeruli produces hemorrhage and loss of protein in the urine and impairment of the filtration surfaces of

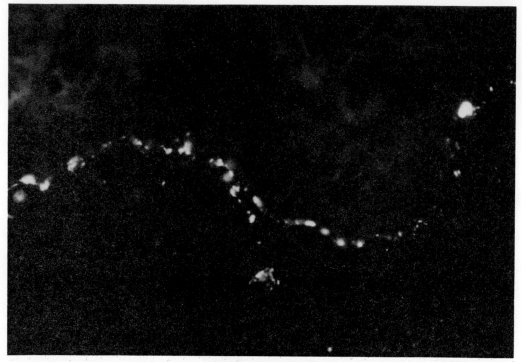

Figure 11-12. Immunohistology of Lupus Dermatitis. Direct immunofluorescence microscopy of a skin biopsy from a patient with systemic lupus erythematosus showing granular dermal–epidermal–basement-membrane zone staining.

the glomeruli that are required for elimination of nitrogenous wastes from the blood. Therefore individuals with this disease have hemoptysis, hematuria, and proteinuria and can die of respiratory and renal failure.

Antibasement membrane autoantibodies can be detected by direct immunofluorescence microscopy of kidney or lung biopsy tissue and by indirect immunofluorescence microscopy of serum using normal human lung or kidney as substrate. The characteristic finding is linear localization of IgG along the glomerular or alveolar basement membranes. RIA and enzyme-linked immunoassay for antibasement membrane autoantibodies are more sensitive than indirect immunofluorescence microscopy.

SYSTEMIC LUPUS ERYTHEMATOSUS

Systemic lupus erythematosus (SLE) is a systemic autoimmune disease that involves many different tissues of the body. It usually begins in late childhood or early adulthood and is more frequent in females than males and in blacks than whites. Individuals with this disease are prone to develop many different autoantibodies, including most of the autoantibodies discussed so far in this chapter. But the sine qua non of SLE is the development of autoantibodies against nuclear antigens, especially DNA.

Antinuclear autoantibodies do not produce tissue injury by cytotoxicity, because they cannot penetrate viable cells to interact with nuclear antigens. Instead, antinuclear antibodies form immne complexes with nuclear antigens released by the degradation of dead cells. These dead cells are primarily derived from the continual turnover of cells that occurs physiologically. The localization, by deposition from the circulation or in situ formation, of these antinuclear antibody-containing immune complexes in tissues induces acute inflammation.

The sites of immune complex localization determine the clinical manifestations of SLE in a given individual. As was discussed earlier, localization in the skin produces dermatitis, and when this is the only site of injury it is called discoid lupus erythematosus. In SLE many other tissues of the body can be injured by immune complex-mediated inflammation, especially the renal glomeruli, producing glomerulonephritis, and the joints, producing arthritis. Therefore frequent clinical manifestations of SLE are a facial rash caused by dermititis, joint pain and swelling caused by arthritis, and hematuria and proteinuria caused by glomerulonephritis.

The most life-threatening of these lesions is the glomerulonephritis, which can progress to complete renal failure. All individuals with lupus glomerulonephritis have immune complexes in their glomeruli. There are a number of pathologically distinct forms of lupus glomerulonephritis, determined by the site of immune complex localization within glomeruli. Direct immunofluorescence microscopy on renal biopsy tissue is used to assess glomerular immune deposits in SLE patients.

The screening test for antinuclear antibodies in the blood is indirect immunofluorescence microscopy using tissue sections or cultured cells as substrate. When present in serum, antinuclear antibodies will bind to nuclei in the substrate. Antinuclear antibodies with specificities for different nuclear antigens will produce different patterns of staining, usually designated homogeneous (diffuse) (Fig. 11–13), speckled (Fig. 11–14), nucleolar, or rim (peripheral). To a degree the pattern of staining indicates the predominant specificity of the antinuclear antibody producing it. A homogeneous pattern indicates a predominance of anti-DNA and anti-deoxyribonucleoprotein antibodies; speckled indicates a predominance of antibodies against a variety of saline-extractable, non-DNA nuclear antigens, including nonhistone proteins; nucleolar indicates a predominance of antinucleolar, including anti-RNA and anti-ribonucleoprotein antibodies; and rim indicates a predominance of anti-double-stranded DNA antibodies. Another pattern caused by anticentromere antibodies produces a uniform speckled pattern on tissue cell substrates. This antibody is accurately identified only using tissue culture cell with numerous mitotic figures in which localization of the immunostaining to the centromeres of chromosomes can be discerned.

Modern clinical immunology laboratory evaluation of antinuclear antibodies requires characterization by specific immunoassays in addition to indirect immunofluorescence microscopy screening. Assays used to determine specificity include RIA, enzyme-linked immunoassay, counterimmunoelectrophoresis, and double immunodiffusion. Identification of the specificity of antinuclear antibodies can be useful in differentiating between SLE and various SLE-related diseases (Table 11–10).

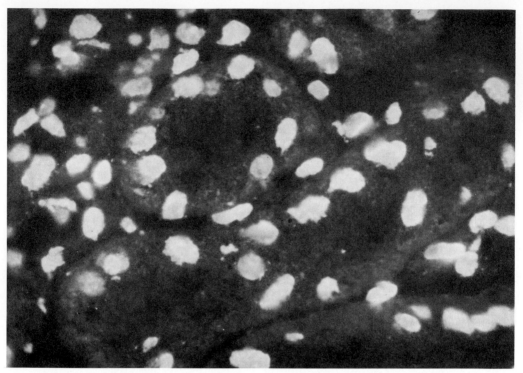

Figure 11–13. Homogeneous Antinuclear Antibody Reaction. Indirect immunofluorescence microscopy using lupus serum showing a homogeneous antinuclear antibody reaction.

A commonly used laboratory test for native, double-stranded DNA employs the hemoflagellate organism *Crithidia lucilia* as the substrate for serum indirect-immunofluorescence microscopy. This organism has a large modified mitochondrion called a kinetoplast that contains a large amount of double-stranded DNA. Indirect immunofluorescent staining of this kinetoplast using an individual's serum indicates the presence of antidouble-stranded DNA autoantibodies. As shown in Table 11–10, demonstration of anti-DNA antibodies is more specific for SLE than is the standard indirect immunofluorescence antinuclear antibody test, although the latter is more sensitive. The presence of autoantibodies against Smith (Sm) antigen is also relatively specific for SLE but not very sensitive, because it is identified in only about 30% of SLE patients.

Individuals with SLE can have a variety of autoimmune processes simultaneously, such as autoimmune cytopenias (especially hemolytic anemia), autoimmune anticoagulants, autoimmune endocrinopathies, and the SLE-related diseases discussed in the following section. This relationship is probably due to a genetic predisposition determined by genes in the major histocompatibility complex that regulates immune responses.

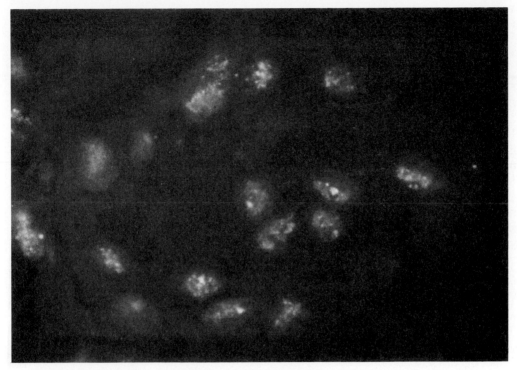

Figure 11-14. Speckled Antinuclear Antibody Reaction. Indirect immunofluorescence microscopy using mixed connective-tissue disease serum showing a speckled antinuclear antibody reaction.

DISEASES RELATED TO SLE

SLE and a group of related diseases are often grouped under the designations *connective tissue diseases* or *collagen vascular diseases*. These diseases are clinically and pathologically diverse but share the laboratory finding of antinuclear autoantibodies. As shown in Table 11-10, however, the specificity of antinuclear antibodies varies among these diseases, as do the clinical and pathologic characteristics.

The most distinctive feature of *progressive systemic sclerosis* is increased collagen deposition (scarring or sclerosis) in tissues, including the skin (*scleroderma*). This causes increased skin thickness and impaired flexibility, especially in the hands (*sclerodactyly*). The most life-threatening injury is to lungs, kidneys, and gastrointestinal tract. A common symptom of progressive systemic sclerosis is *Raynaud's phenomenon*, which is the occurrence in the fingers and toes of sudden episodes of pallor or cyanosis, coolness, numbness, and pain initiated by cold or emotional upset. Laboratory evaluation of individuals with progressive systemic sclerosis reveals about a 75% incidence of antinuclear antibodies that produce a speckled or nucleolar pattern, and 50% incidence

TABLE 11–10. FREQUENCY OF DIFFERENT TYPES OF ANTINUCLEAR AUTOANTIBODIES (ANA) IN SLE AND SLE-RELATED DISEASES

ANA Specificity	Frequency[a]						
	SLE	**DLE**	**MCTD**	**PSS**	**CREST**	**SS**	**PDM**
Fluorescent ANA[b]	+ + + +	+ + + +	+ + + +	+ + +	+ + +	+ + +	+ +
Double-stranded DNA	+ + +	+	+	+	+	+	+
Nuclear histones	+ + +	+ + + +	+	+	+	+	+
Ribonucleoprotein	+ +	+	+ + + +	+ +	+ +	+	+
Smith (Sm)	+ +	+	+	+	+	+	+
Scl-70	+	+	+	+ +	+	+	+
Centromere	+	+	+	+ +	+ + +	+	+
SS-A (Ro)	+ +	+	+ +	+	+	+ + +	+
SS-B (La)	+ +	+	+	+	+	+ + +	+
Jo-1	+	+	+	+	+	+	+ +

Abbreviations: SLE = systemic lupus erythematosus; DLE = discoid lupus erythematosus; MCTD = mixed connective tissue disease; PSS = progressive systemic sclerosis; CREST = calcinosis, Raynaud's phenomenon, esophageal dysmotility, sclerodactyly, telangiectasia syndrome; SS = Sjörgren's syndrome; PDM = polymyositis-dermatomyositis.
[a] + = <10%, + + = 10% to 50%, + + + = 51% to 90%, + + + + = >90%.
[b] Positive standard indirect immunofluorescence assay.

of a relatively specific autoantibody designated Scl-70, which is usually detected by immunodiffusion.

The *CREST syndrome* is a variant of progressive systemic sclerosis characterized by calcinosis (subcutaneous calcification), Raynaud's phenomenon, esophageal dysmotility, sclerodactylyl, and telangiectasia. Using indirect immunofluorescence microscopy on tissue culture cell preparation containing mitotic figures, approximately 80% of individuals with CREST syndrome are found to have anticentromere autoantibodies that are specific for kinetochore proteins.

Polymyositis–dermatomyositis is an inflammatory disease of muscle and skin. Approximately half of the individuals with this disease have demonstrable autoantibodies against a variety of nuclear, nucleolar, and cytoplasmic antigens, including a number of transfer RNA synthetases. For example, Jo-1, an autoantibody associated with this disease, is specific for a histidyl-tRNA synthetase.

Individuals with *mixed connective tissue disease* have combined features of SLE, progressive systemic sclerosis, polymyositis–dermatomyositis, and rheumatoid arthritis. One of the most characteristic features of this disease is the presence in the serum of high titers of antinuclear autoantibodies that produce a speckled pattern. These autoantibodies are specific for nuclear ribonucleoprotein.

Sjögren's syndrome is an inflammatory disease that primarily affects the salivary and lacrimal glands, causing dry mouth (xerostomia) and dry eyes (keratoconjunctivitis sicca). In about half of the individuals with this syndrome there will be concomitant rheumatoid arthritis, SLE, or another SLE-related disease. Over 75% of these individuals have rheumatoid factor and antinuclear antibodies, usually giving a speckled pattern. Some of these autoantibodies are specific for acid-extractable nuclear antigens called SS-A (Ro) and SS-B (La) that are somewhat specific for Sjögren's syndrome (see Table 11–10).

RHEUMATOID ARTHRITIS

Rheumatoid arthritis is a destructive, chronic inflammatory joint disease of poorly understood pathogenesis, but autoimmunity is thought to play an important role. The characteristic laboratory abnormality found in individuals with rheumatoid arthritis is the presence of *rheumatoid factors* in serum and joint fluid. Rheumatoid factors are autoantibodies specific for antigens on the Fc region of IgG; therefore they are anti-antibodies. Most rheumatoid factors that are detected are IgM, but IgG and IgA rheumatoid factors also occur.

Laboratory detection of rheumatoid factors often entails agglutination or flocculation of IgG-coated particles, such as latex, bentonite, charcoal, and erythrocytes. These tests are most sensitive for IgM rheumatoid antibodies, because they are most efficient at producing agglutination. Additional tests that can detect and distinguish between different rheumatoid factor isotypes employ RIAs, enzyme-linked assays, or nephelometry.

Rheumatoid factors are found in over 75% of individuals with rheumatoid arthritis. They are not completely specific for this disease, however, because they are present at lower frequency in a number of other diseases, such as SLE and SLE-related disease (especially Sjögren's syndrome).

Another serologic marker of rheumatoid arthritis (RA) is the presence of antibodies to RA-associated nuclear antigen (RANA). These antibodies react with extracts of Epstein–Barr virus (EBV)-infected human B lymphocytes. Anti-RANA are detected in approximately 80% of patients with rheumatoid arthritis.

Discussion of the Illustrative Case
The patient described in the illustrative case had serum sickness. She developed antibodies against the horse proteins in the antivenom that she was given, leading to the formation of pathogenic immune complexes. Systemic and local activation of inflammatory mediators produced the signs and symptoms that appeared 10 days after the administration of the horse protein. The arthralgias were caused by immune complexes localizing in joints and the proteinuria and hematuria by immune complex-mediated glomerulonephritis. Serum sickness induced by a single exposure to antigen is usually a self-limited disease that responds well to anti-inflammatory medications such as aspirin. Once the immune complexes have been cleared from the circulation and degraded by phagocytes and the local inflammatory responses, the disease resolves. A repeat exposure to the same antigen may elicit a life-threatening anaphylactic response. This is why the patient was given a skin test with horse serum prior to the intravenous injection of the antivenom.

QUESTIONS

1. Discuss the Gell and Coombs' categorization system for immune-mediated injury.

2. If hay fever and allergic asthma both are mediated by the same mechanism of immune injury, why are their symptoms so different?

3. What are the two mechanisms by which antibodies can cause red blood cell lysis?

4. What is the difference between deposition of immune complexes and in situ formation of immune complexes in tissues?

5. How does localization of immune complexes in tissues cause acute inflammatory injury?

6. Define immune tolerance and autoimmunity in terms of immune regulation.

7. Give the most important clinical, pathologic, and serologic features of one autoimmune cytopenia.

8. Give the most important clinical, pathologic, and serologic features of one systemic autoimmune disease.

9. Suggest why there is a genetic predisposition for many autoimmune diseases.

Section V

Immunology and Serology of Infectious Diseases

Chapter 12

Immunology and Serology of Bacterial and Fungal Diseases

OBJECTIVES

1. To discuss the immune response in bacterial and fungal diseases.
2. To discuss serologic assays for bacterial and fungal infections.

Illustrative Case

A 48-year-old woman came into the hospital complaining of repeated febrile episodes during the last 3 years. Fever was accompanied with chills, headache, and weakness, but no other complaints were noticed by the patient. She lived on a farm where the entire family drank fresh cow's milk. None of the other members of the family had the same chronic symptoms. The patient had never been more than 100 miles from home. Stool examination for ova and parasites was negative. Blood count and urinalysis were normal. The slide agglutination assay of *Brucella abortus* antigens mixed with patient serum was positive (or the patient serum contained antibodies to the *B abortus* antigen and agglutinated the antigens). Antibodies for *Francisella* were not detectable.

THE IMMUNE RESPONSE IN BACTERIAL DISEASES

The humoral immune system is, in general, more important than the cellular immune system in preventing bacterial diseases. Bacterial infections stimulate antibody production toward the infecting organism and/or toward products released by the infecting

251

organism. Antibodies to the organism itself may protect against infection. Antibodies toward products secreted by the bacteria, for example, exotoxins, may not protect against infection but may protect against the pathologic consequences of the infection, for example, the myocardial and neural complications of diphtheria. The logic of administering antisera in passive immune therapy to patients already showing symptoms of a bacterial disease is based upon this latter premise.

The most effective defenses against bacterial infections involve phagocytosis. Although phagocytes do ingest bacteria without opsonins, the coating of bacteria with antibodies and complement greatly enhances both internalization into the phagocyte and destruction of the bacteria thereafter. IgG or IgM antibodies bind to the bacterial cell via the antigen-binding sites in their Fab regions. Complement may be activated to mediate bacterial lysis via the membrane attack complex. More often, opsonized bacteria are bound via the Fc regions of the coating antibodies to specific membrane Fc receptors on neutrophils and macrophages. Likewise, complement-coated bacteria are bound by complement receptors on phagocytes. Immobilized bacteria are then ingested and destroyed.

Antibodies also protect against infection by binding to and covering that part of the bacterial cell that attaches to specific receptors on an epithelial cell. Essentially all bacteria require attachment to membrane receptors on living cells as the initial step in their infective process. When the attachment is prevented by antibodies covering up the specific sites on the bacteria, infection is prevented. Antibodies to group A streptococci are an example of this protective process. Secretory IgA prevents attachment of bacteria to epithelial cells of the mucosal linings. *Mycoplasma pneumonia, Vibrio cholerae, Shigella, and Salmonella* are examples of bacteria whose invasion may be prevented by secretory IgA.

Some bacteria resist phagocytosis or intracellular destruction after phagocytosis. *Streptococcus pyogenes,* for example, synthesize M protein that inhibits phagocytosis. Mycobacteria have a cell wall that provides resistance to intracellular destruction after their ingestion. The mycobacteria actually live within the phagocyte and are isolated from the humoral immune system. In this type of intracellular bacterial infection, the cellular immune system is most important in defense. Other examples of intracellular survival of bacteria include *Rickettsia, Brucella,* and *Francisella.*

Bacterial antigens may be classified into 5 types. (1) K antigens, or envelope antigens, surround the bacteria and are mostly heat labile. In *Salmonella,* the K antigens are referred to as Vi antigens; in *Escherichia,* they are the L, A, and B group antigens. (2) O antigens, or somatic antigens, are located on the cell surface and are mostly heat stable. When K antigens are present they may cover the O antigens. (3) H antigens are on the flagella and are also heat labile. (4) F antigens are on the fimbriae and are not species specific. (5) External secretions of exotoxins and enzymes when uniquely synthesized and secreted by a pathogen may provide the basis for serologic diagnosis.

PRINCIPLES OF SEROLOGIC ASSAYS FOR BACTERIAL INFECTIONS

Bacterial antigens are present in the patient upon initial infection long before the immune response has had time to develop. Many infections do not exhibit clinical

symptoms until the bacteria have had time to multiply and produce masses of pathologic agents. By this time antibodies are usually present. To date most clinical assays
for bacterial infections are designed to detect specific antibody; however, the trend in
technology is toward developing methods that detect antigen. DNA probe techniques
which test for the presence of specific bacterial DNA, by annealing to a known radioisotope labeled complementary DNA strand, are rapidly developing. However, latex
agglutination is now the most popular method for assaying for bacterial antigens.

Bacteria stimulate predominantly a humoral immune response. IgM antibodies
are the first to appear, and thereafter IgG and other classes of antibodies appear. IgM
antibodies usually disappear rapidly whereas IgG antibodies remain for lengthy periods. Many bacterial diseases do not have clinical symptoms until the infection has
progressed to the IgG antibody producing stage. Some adverse effects of bacterial diseases appear long after the infection has been resolved, for example, rheumatic fever
and glomerulonephritis induced by streptococcal infection. At this time the IgM antibodies have usually disappeared, whereas the IgG antibodies are still present.

The goals in serologic diagnosis of bacterial diseases are demonstration of (1)
antibodies to secretory products or to antigens unique for a particular bacterial species
to establish a past infection, for example, DNAse B of streptococci; (2) a rising titer of
antibodies to secretory products or antigens for a particular bacterial species to establish an ongoing infection; (3) a single high antibody titer as presumptive evidence for
ongoing infection when the patient is at the peak of antibody stimulation and will not
have an increasing titer; (4) unique bacterial antigens to establish ongoing infection.
DNA probes are not serological techniques and will not be discussed.

SEROLOGIC ASSAYS FOR SPECIFIC BACTERIAL INFECTIONS

Salmonella

Salmonella causes diseases with persistent fever as a symptom. *Salmonella typhi* causes
typhoid fever, a systemic disease, with the gastrointestinal tract being the route of introduction. Contaminated food and water are the usual sources of the organism. From
the gastrointestinal tract organisms enter the intestinal mucosa and spread into the
lymphatics and peripheral blood. Salmonellae multiply within phagocytes. The gall
bladder sometimes harbors residual Salmonellae after recovery and periodically sheds
them via the feces and urine. If this situation occurs, food handlers can pass the disease
on to many persons. Salmonellae also cause *paratyphoid fever,* which is symptomatically
similar to typhoid fever. The causative agent is *Salmonella enteritidis* with paratyphi serotypes. Paratyphoid fever is usually less severe and does not develop carriers.

Originally a French physician, Widal, introduced an agglutination assay for detecting serum antibodies to *Salmonella.* This assay was called the *Widal's test* and assayed
for agglutination of H and O *Salmonella* antigens, by patient serum. A positive agglutination for antibodies to Salmonella O and H antigens, however, is not diagnostic and
must be followed by cultures to isolate the organism. Today the agglutination assay for
Salmonella is not utilized due to its inability to define the strain of *Salmonella* and
due to its cross-reactivity with other bacterial antigens, for example, *Brucella.* Because

of the poor specificity and sensitivity of serologic tests, a diagnosis of typhoid or para-typhoid should be confirmed by culture.

Brucellosis

Brucellosis, or *undulant fever* is an infection that causes fever. *Brucella* is transmitted via animals, especially cattle, and grows well in phagocytes. Animal tissue or unpasteurized milk is the usual means by which humans are infected. Cases are rare, often go undetected, and develop into chronic and recurrent episodes of the disease. Culture isolation is difficult so that diagnosis is usually based upon laboratory serology. *Brucella* antibodies cross-react with *Vibrio cholerae* and *Francisella tularensis.* Direct agglutination assay is a commonly used serologic test for *Brucella* infection.

Tularemia

Tularensis causes *tularemia,* another febrile disease. It can be carried by rabbits who can infect hunters that have contact with them during skinning. Ticks may also transmit the organism. Organisms enter the blood via lymphatics and multiply with phagocytes to eventually form granulomas with necrosis in the infected tissues. *Francisella* is dangerous to isolate. The most commonly used serologic test for tularemia is a direct agglutination assay for antibodies using formalin-treated bacteria. ELISA is more sensitive for *Francisella* infection, but is less widely available.

Syphilis

Treponema pallidum is the etiologic agent of *syphilis.* The disease process begins with a *primary stage* during which a chancre appears. Later the chancre enlarges and develops necrosis. Pus, which usually accompanies bacterial lesions, is absent. Dark-field examination of a wet mount of the chancre fluid may reveal many treponemes. In the early syphilis the only diagnostic assay is the darkfield examination of chancre material because the humoral response has not yet had time to develop. Later in primary syphilis a humoral, immunologic response occurs (Fig. 12–1). One response results in antibodies to a nontreponeme antigen, Venereal Disease Research Laboratory (VDRL) antigen or *reagin.* The other response results in antibodies specific to the infecting treponemes. The primary chancres will heal spontaneously.

In untreated patients about 2 months later a *secondary phase* of the disease begins with a generalized rash. Secondary chancres appear and contain treponemes that are detectable with darkfield microscopy. Primary and secondary stages are those in which spirochetes may be found. These secondary chancres also heal spontaneously. During the secondary stage the humoral, immune response is stimulated, producing increased titers of antibodies.

The untreated patient will next enter a *latent phase,* with no clinical symptoms or signs except a positive serology. Sometimes later, even as long as years later, a *tertiary stage* of syphilis appears. In this stage the lesions do not contain treponemes. A delayed-type hypersensitivity to the treponemes is demonstrable in this stage whereas it is not during the primary and secondary stages.

Syphilis may be transmitted maternally to fetuses. Due to normal transplacental transfer of maternal IgG, serologic tests for neonatal syphilis infection should be spe-

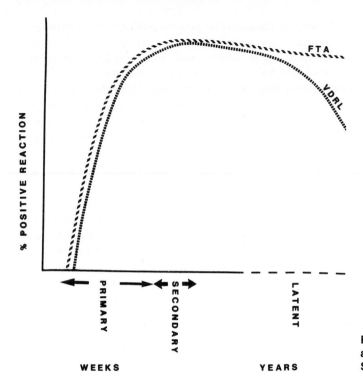

Figure 12-1. Reactivity of VDRL and FTA in Various Phases of Syphilis.

cifically for IgM antibodies. Alternatively, demonstration of treponemes from lesions on the newborn may be used in diagnosis.

There are two main types of serologic assays used to detect patient antibodies in the diagnosis of syphilis: (1) nontreponemal antigen tests, and (2) treponemal antigen tests. *Nontreponemal tests* utilize extracts of beef heart (cardiolipin) that react with the syphilis-induced, nontreponemal antibody *reagin*. Unfortunately this is the same term that is used for IgE antibodies that are involved in allergies. Because of the nonspecificity of reagin, nontreponemal assays are screening assays and only indicate possible syphilis. Therefore any positive result must be confirmed by a treponemal assay that uses antigen of the etiologic agent.

Nontreponemal assays that are used to screen for syphilis today are the VDRL and the rapid plasm reagin (RPR) tests. Historically Wasserman designed a complement fixation assay to test for antibodies to cardiolipin antigen that is still sometimes called *Wasserman antigen*. Both VDRL and RPR tests use the nontreponemal antigen or Wasserman antigen.

The VDRL test has microscopic flocculation detected with a microscope as the end point, while the RPR test uses macroscopic agglutination easily detected with the eye as the end point. In both assays the antigen is made part of a larger particle to provide a more sensitive assay than liquid precipitation. In the VDRL flocculation assay, beef cardiolipin antigen is combined with cholesterol to provide the larger antigen particles. Lecithin is added to the antigen complex to increase reproducibility.

Reconstitution of the lyophilized antigen reagent just before performing the assay is essential for correct results. Old antigen may give false-positive results. Heat inactivation of patient serum immediately before the assay is also essential for ridding the serum of interfering factors. If the serum has been heat inactivated the day before, it should be inactivated again immediately before the assay is performed.

The *RPR macroscopic agglutination assay* uses less equipment (no water bath and no microscope) and does not require heat inactivation. Heparinized blood from a finger stick can be directly assayed on a paper card, making the RPR test most useful for field conditions. The RPR test is more sensitive than the VDRL test because it uses charcoal particles to provide a large antigen particle. The charcoal particles allow agglutination by positive sera to be seen with the naked eye. Although the RPR test is more sensitive than the VDRL test, there are more false positives that must be confirmed.

False-positive results with nontreponemal assays are seen in infectious mononucleosis, vaccinia, viral pneumonia, malaria, leprosy, infectious hepatitis, autoimmune diseases, heroin addiction, and in patients undergoing antihypertensive drug therapy. Cross-reactions may occur in other treponemal conditions such as yaws. In either the VDRL or the RPR tests, prozone phenomena may cause suspicious but not definitely positive reactions. In these cases the assay should be redone on dilutions of patient serum. Any positive result obtained with either of the nontreponemal screening methods, VDRL or RPR, must be confirmed with a treponemal assay.

The *treponemal assays* for syphilis utilize antigens from the treponemes to detect specific antibodies. The *treponemal pallidum immobilization* assay is one of the earlier treponemal tests. *Nichols strain* of treponema (the pathogenic strain) is isolated from rabbit testes, incubated with patient serum and complement, and observed by dark-field microscopy for immobilization of the organisms. If antibodies are present in the patient serum, they combine with the organisms and immobilize them. Few laboratories are able to maintain cultures for the TPI assay, and there is potential danger involved with maintaining the cultures. Therefore today this assay is rarely used.

The most commonly used assay for confirming a positive screening test for syphilis is the fluorescent assay. These assays originally resulted in many false positives due to nonspecific antibodies reacting with the animal tissue that surrounded treponemal antigen on the slides. This problem was solved by using the nonpathogenic *Reiter treponemal strain* to first absorb out of patient serum any nonspecific antibodies to animal tissue. Then the absorbed serum was used to perform the fluorescent assay for antibodies to the Nichols pathogenic strain. This absorption assay is termed the *fluorescent treponemal antibody-absorption assay* (FTA-ABS assay). It is a very sensitive assay and is positive about 2 weeks into the primary stage of the disease.

Poststreptococcal Diseases

Rheumatic fever is a systemic inflammatory disease that appears after a pharyngeal infection with group A *streptococci*. Antibodies against the group A streptococcal antigens are stimulated by infection. These antibodies then may cross-react with cardiac tissue antigens and cause carditis, polyarthritis, and fever. Rheumatic fever can resemble systemic lupus erythematosus (SLE) and juvenile rheumatoid arthritis. Rheumatic fever does not induce antinuclear antibodies, LE cells, or erosive joint disease.

Acute glomerulonephritis may follow pharyngeal or skin infections with streptococci with specific M types. It usually occurs about 2 weeks after the primary infection and is mediated via immune complex deposition in the kidney. Disease manifestations include proteinuria, hematuria, hypertension, impairment of renal function, and edema. There is hypocomplementemia in the first several weeks of the acute phase. The disease is usually self-limited, especially in children.

Serologic assays are important in the differential diagnosis of poststreptococcal diseases. The most common assays test for patient antibodies to enzymes secreted by the streptococci. Extracellular enzymes secreted by streptococci include streptolysin O; DNAse types A, B, C, and D; hyaluronidase; streptokinase, and nicotinamide adenine dinucleotidase. Of these, assays for antibodies to streptolysin O and to DNAse B are used most often. Anti-DNAse type B correlates best with group A streptococcal infections because the other groups of streptococci produce insignificant or no amounts of DNAse B. A rise in titer of DNAse B antibodies is much more definitive than is a single higher titer.

The antistreptolysin O assay (ASO) is based upon the ability of patient antistreptolysin O antibodies to inhibit the hemolytic activity of streptolysin O. Varying dilutions of patient serum are incubated with constant amounts of streptolysin O. Erythrocytes are then added, and the highest dilution of patient serum that completely neutralizes the streptolysin is noted. Assays are reported in Todd units, which are the reciprocal of the noted dilution. ASO titers peak about 3 weeks after onset of infection and fall to preinfection levels within 6 weeks. An alternative method for detecting ASO antibodies is the use of streptolysin O-coated latex particles in an agglutination assay. An elevated ASO level indicates recent streptococcal infection. This is a precondition for developing both rheumatic fever and poststreptococcal glomerulonephritis. ASO reference ranges are difficult to define, because the titer varies with age and environment. The ASO titer is not greatly affected by skin streptococcal infections. Spuriously high ASO titers may be due to hypergammaglobulinemia or liver disease.

Another assay for streptococcal infections tests for antibodies to DNAse B, another enzyme secreted by streptococci. The *anti-DNAse B* (ADN-B) assay is based upon the ability of patient antibodies to inhibit the depolymerizing ability of DNAse-B. Patient serum is incubated with DNAse-B, after which time DNA reagent is added. Polymerized DNA reagent retains methyl green dye, whereas depolymerized DNA reagent will not. The final reaction mixture is spectrophotometrically analyzed for extent of remaining color in polymerized DNA. Alternatively, alcohol may be added to precipitate any polymerized DNA. Depolymerized DNA will not precipitate. ADN-B antibodies appear later than ASO antibodies and persist for a longer time. ADN-B titers increase with skin streptococcal infections, whereas the ASO titer does not. False positives are not seen in liver disease. False negatives may occur in the presence of endogenous DNAse, such as in hemorrhagic pancreatitis. ADN-B assays are not affected by oxidation of the reagents, whereas the ASO titer is affected by oxidation of the streptolysin O. Again, reference normal titers vary with age, with the highest levels in school-age children.

Other tests for streptococcal infections are available. Antibodies against other enzymes secreted by streptococci, such as hyaluronidase and streptokinase, can be measured. There is a commercial assay called the *streptozyme* assay that uses latex particles coated with a combination of streptococcal antigens. There is also a commercial kit that uses antibody-coated latex beads to establish presence of group A streptococci in throat or other swabs.

Meningitis

Diagnosis of meningitis with characterization of the etiologic agent is important for the survival of the patient, who is often a child under the age of 5. Fever and irritability may be the only signs of the potentially lethal central nervous system infection. Many different agents may cause meningitis. Latex agglutination has now replaced counter immunoelectrophoresis as an assay for antigens of the most common causes of meningitis—group B streptococci, *Hemophilus influenzae, Neisseria meningitidis, and Streptococcus pneumoniae* (Table 12–1).

Actinomyces Hypersensitivity or Farmer's Lung

Actinomycetes are filamentous bacteria that are difficult to culture. Infections are most frequent in the oropharyngeal soft tissues. Actinomycetes can also cause hypersensitivity pneumonitis, or Farmer's lung. Chills, fever, cough, and dyspnea occur 4 to 6 hours after inhalation of the antigen. A positive immunodiffusion for antibodies is diagnostic.

FUNGAL INFECTIONS

Immunology

There is not a great deal of knowledge about the role of the immune system in fungal infections; however, the prevailing evidence is that both cellular and humoral immunity are important, with the former being more important. Phagocytes cannot ingest the large mycelia, but they do attach to them, and this causes a pertubation of the cell membrane to initiate release of lysosomal enzymes that damage the organism. Respiratory mycoses caused by histoplasmosis and coccidioidomycosis suggest a need for cellular immune system involvement in protection from infection, because these diseases are usually limited to patients with impaired cellular immune functions. Infections by ubiquitous *Candida albicans* occurs in patients with decreased T cell function, such as in patients with Swiss immunodeficiency, DiGeorge's syndrome, and AIDS.

TABLE 12–1. PERCENT OF CASES OF PROMINENT MENINGITIS-CAUSING ORGANISMS IN DIFFERENT AGE GROUPS

Age Group	Streptococcus pneumoniae	Hemophilus influenzae	Neisseria meningitidis	Group B Streptococci
Adult	50	3	25	———
Child	20	45	40	———
Infant	5	———	———	95

Laboratory Diagnosis of Fungal Diseases

Culture and histologic examination are usually used to diagnose fungal diseases, but application of these methods is not always possible. Therefore immunologic assays are used to assist in diagnosis.

Candidiasis

Candidiasis, also called candidosis, occurs most often in patients with depressed cellular immunity. *Albicans* is ubiquitous and is a common inhabitant of the mucosal surfaces and gastrointestinal tract. Fetuses are normally exposed to the organism during passage through the birth canal. Because all normal individuals have been exposed to candida and have developed cellular immune responses to it, the DTH skin test to candida antigen is a common method of assessing cellular immune function. Diagnosis of candidiasis may be made with assays for systemic antigen by latex agglutination, immunodiffusion, or counterimmunoelectrophoresis. Neither a positive DTH skin test nor presence of specific antibody is diagnostic of active infection because healthy individuals have both. Absence of specific antibody in the absence of immunosuppressive conditions rules out the infection.

Coccidioidomycosis

This pulmonary infection by *Coccidioides* is sometimes referred to as valley fever because of its frequency in the San Joaquin Valley of California. The DTH skin test against *Coccidioides* antigens is diagnostic and is positive in about 85% of patients. Immunodiffusion can be used to identify specific fungal antigens. Anticoccidioidin antibodies indicative of coccidioidomycosis can be identified in serum and CSF by complement fixation, immunodiffusion and latex particle agglutination assays.

Histoplasmosis

Histoplasma capsulatum infection may be acquired through inhalation of spores that live in the soil, deposited there by avian droppings. The disease is usually found in the very young and very old and in immunosuppressed patients. DTH skin test and serologic assays for antibodies against histoplasmin antigen are used for diagnosis. The most commonly used serologic tests are immunodiffusion, complement fixation, and latex particle agglutination.

Blastomycosis

This disease is a chronic granulomatous disease usually following pulmonary infection with *Blastomyces dermatitidis*. Inhalation of spores from the soil may lead to spreading to the lymphatics and blood. There is a low-grade fever, cough, and malaise. Ulcerative skin lesions, if present, demonstrate pus and yeast cells. Diagnosis may be by histology and direct examination followed by culture. Immunodiffusion and complement fixation assays are used for serologic diagnosis. More sensitive methods of radioimmunoassay (RIA) and enzyme-linked immunoassay (EIA) are available. Because of cross-reactivity, some patients who have been exposed to *Histoplasma* or *Coccidioides* will have a false-positive serologic test for blastomycosis.

Cryptococcosis

This disease is a subacute fungal disease that may show pulmonary, systemic, or meningitic forms. It is seen most often in immune deficient patients and is common in patients with acquired immune deficiency syndrome (AIDS). Cryptococci may be demonstrated in cerebrospinal fluid from meningitic patients by mixing with India ink and observing a halo produced by the polysaccharide capsule around the organism. Most laboratories now prefer to use agglutination of latex beads covered with antibody to detect the cryptococcal antigen in cerebrospinal fluid. In severe infections cryptococcal antigens can be identified in serum by latex particle agglutination. False-positive results can be caused by rheumatoid factor.

Aspergillosis

Aspergillus infection results in three major clinical syndromes. Growth of a mass of fungi in a pulmonary cavity caused by some other disease, such as tuberculosis or emphysema, produces a fungus ball or aspergilloma. A hypersensitivity response to inhaled *Aspergillus* causes allergic bronchopulmonary aspergillosis. The most injurious form of infection is invasive aspergiollsis. This is most common in immunocompromised individuals. The most frequently used diagnostic serologic test is an immunodiffusion assay, but complement fixation and ELISA assays can also be used. Serologic tests are positive in most patients with aspergilloma and allergic bronchopulmonary aspergillosis but are usually negative in patients with invasive aspergillosis. Because *Aspergillus* antigens have C-substance that forms a precipitate with C-reactive protein (CRP) common to inflammatory diseases, the assays using precipitation as an end point may be falsely positive in the absence of antibody.

> ### Discussion of the Illustrative Case
>
> The patient had typical undulant fever or brucellosis. Serology is very important in the diagnosis of this disease, since culture of the organism is difficult. Currently the disease is of low incidence in the United States; however, it is prevalent in those areas of the United States and third world countries where pasteurization of milk is not practiced. Antibody titers arise with each recurrent episode.

QUESTIONS

1. Discuss the streptococcal antigens and their clinical importance.

2. Outline the general immune defenses toward bacterial and toward fungal infections.

3. Discuss the assays for syphilis, and relate them to the immune response during the stages of the disease.

4. Relate the clinical importance of the DTH skin test to *Candida albicans*.

Chapter

13 Viral, Parasitic, Rickettsial, and Chlamydial Infections

OBJECTIVES

1. To discuss events from viral inoculation to clinically apparent infection, including the related appearance of nonspecific and specific body defenses.
2. To relate characteristics of viruses and viral-infected cells to specific body defenses.
3. To discuss tactics viruses use to evade body defenses.
4. To discuss immunologic diagnosis of viral infections.
5. To briefly describe the clinical features and laboratory findings in some common viral diseases.
6. To discuss the immunologic diagnosis of parasitic, rickettsial, and chlamydial infections.

Illustrative Case

A 21-year-old woman who had no prenatal care was admitted to the hospital through the emergency department; she delivered a term infant. The neonate had recurrent seizures beginning shortly after birth. Physical examination of the infant revealed hydrocephalus, jaundice, hepatosplenomegaly, and retinochoroiditis. The mother had noticed no illness during the pregnancy. The leading clinical diagnosis was congenital toxoplasmosis. Sera samples for serologic testing were obtained over the next 3 months. During this period there was a greater than fourfold rise in antitoxoplasma antibody titer by complement fixation assay. The

Sabin–Feldman dye test was persistently positive. An immunofluorescence microscopy assay (IFA) for toxoplasma-specific IgM was positive.

THE INFECTIVE PROCESS IN VIRAL DISEASES

Viruses are obligate intracellular parasites consisting of a core of nucleic acid enclosed by a protein capsid. There may be an additional enclosure or envelope of lipoprotein around the nucleocapsid (Fig. 13–1). Extracellular forms of viruses, with or without an envelope, are called virions and are infective. Viruses usually lack some enzymes required for their own proliferation. After invading host cells viruses use the host enzymes for their own reproduction. Viral infections may result in asymptomatic infections, acute diseases, chronic diseases, alterations in immune defenses, and induction of tumors. Viruses are generally not sensitive to conventional antibiotics, and many have evaded control by standard vaccination techniques and by passive immune therapy.

The process of viral infection (Fig. 13–2) may be divided into attachment; penetration of virus into cell; uncoating; and, when it occurs, integration into host genomes, replication, maturation, and release and spread of virions to other host cells. Attachment is the binding of specific capsid or envelope viral proteins with their matching receptor sites on the host cell. This anchors the virion to the host cell membrane to enable the next step in viral infection. This requirement of a complementary and specific host cell membrane receptor for each individual virus explains why human cells are resistant to most animal cell viruses, since animal and human cells have different receptors. Viral envelopes are lipoprotein and, after attachment occurs, will fuse with host cell membrane lipoprotein to result in internalization of the virion. Thereafter the virion itself may direct removal of the protein capsid. Some viral infections have lengthy latent periods during which uncoating is delayed. Once uncoated the viral nucleic acid may incorporate into the host cell genetic material. In the case of RNA viruses, a DNA copy must first be synthesized before incorporation. Whether integrated or not, viral genetic material dictates its own replication via the host cell's biosynthetic pathways. Viral components synthesized by the host cell are gathered together or form an intact virus particle. These particles are released from the host cell either by lysing and destruction of the host cell or by budding, for example, adenoviruses and influenza viruses. During budding a virion migrates toward the host cell

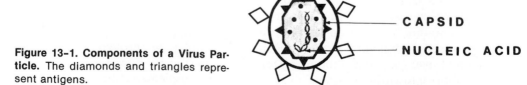

Figure 13-1. Components of a Virus Particle. The diamonds and triangles represent antigens.

ENVELOPE

CAPSID

NUCLEIC ACID

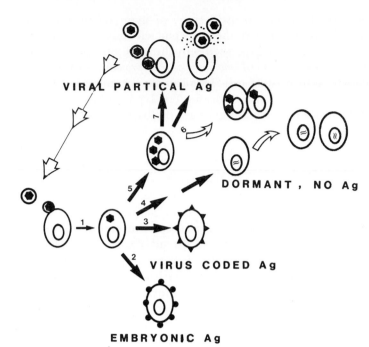

VIRAL PARTICAL Ag

DORMANT , NO Ag

VIRUS CODED Ag

EMBRYONIC Ag

Figure 13-2. Outline of Viral Infection and Resultant Antigens. *(1)* Initial attachment and entry into cell. *(2)* Induction or derepression of embryonic antigens. *(3)* Induction of virus-coded antigens. *(4)* Dormant virus with no detectable antigens. *(5)* Multiplication within infected cell. *(6)* Cell division with passage of viral genome. *(7)* Release of new viral particles by budding or lysis.

surface. When the virion reaches the membrane, an outward bulge of membrane (bud) containing the virion develops. This bulge containing the virion pinches off from the cell membrane. The period during which large masses of virions are found extracellularly in the circulation is called *viremia.* These new virions can then attach to other cells, and the process of infecting a host cell begins anew. Influenza and adenovirus are examples of viral infection spreading via budding of virions.

Several variations in the above direct infective process are well known. Once internalized some viruses undergo lengthy latent periods during which they remain coated. If the infected cell containing this latent viral particle forms an intracytoplasmic bridge with another host cell, the viral particle could be transferred to that host cell via the bridge, for example, cytomegalovirus, Epstein–Barr virus, and varicella zoster. Other viruses, once integrated into the host genetic material, will go through a dormant phase during which there is no production of new viral particles. There is no cytologic evidence that the cell is infected. If these host cells undergo meiosis or mitosis, the viral genome is passed on with host genetic material, for example, retroviruses.

Immunologically, viruses present several types of antigens that are significant. (1) Newly synthesized particles may bud out of host cell membrane and eventually be released as free particles. While associated with host cell membrane, *viral particle* antigen is available to stimulate immune responses and to react with effector elements such as antibodies and cytotoxic T cells. (2) Viruses may also dictate synthesis of *nonviral proteins* that appear on the membrane surface of the host cell. Although these host cell surface proteins are not part of the virion itself, some of them are useful in diagnosing specific viral infections. (3) Presence of the virus particle may also derepress to expression parts of the genome normally expressed only during embryonic or fetal development. This causes abnormal synthesis of *embryonic or fetal proteins*. (4) Viral particles may also induce transformation of host cell. This can be accompanied by the expression of *tumor specific antigens* on the cell membrane. The types of host cell membrane antigens discussed above and the virion antigens are the basis for immunologic assays for viral diseases.

IMMUNE RESPONSE TO VIRAL INFECTIONS AND EVASION TACTICS OF VIRUSES

Viruses induce both humoral and cellular immune responses. Although humoral immunity has proved to be protective against infection and spread of some types of virus, current data indicate that the cellular immune defense is more important. Different immune responses may be important at different stages during viral infections. Humoral immunity is important against the extracellular viral forms and prevents some infections by blocking attachment of viruses to cells. Once the virus is intracellular, cellular immunity is more important, for example, cytotoxic T cell destruction of infected cells. Generally, hypogammaglobulonemic individuals survive viral infections quite well; however, patients with deficient cellular immunity do not. There is no question that vaccinations and passive immune therapy offer protection against polio, measles, mumps, hepatitis A and B, rubella, and varicella. There is no standard method for developing vaccines or passive immune therapies for viral infections. A major difficulty in designing vaccines or passive immune therapy is that virions have many proteins that can act as antigens, and immune responses toward most of these proteins do not produce protection against infection. Exactly which proteins are important in stimulating a protective immune response is not easily determined. Viral infections have an extracellular phase and an intracellular phase. Many immune elements are not effective against intercellular parasites due to the fact that they are inaccessible when inside cells. Humoral antibodies, for example, cannot enter cells and are therefore potentially protective only during the time when the virus particles are extracellular, as during the initial exposure or during viremia and spread of the virus to other cells. Cellular immune responses, however, provide defenses toward viruses located intercellularly, which is where they are found throughout most of the infection. These cellular immune defenses recognize as foreign and attack those host cells that contain "nonself" membrane proteins that appear as a result of the presence of the intercellular virus. Effectiveness of the humoral versus the cellular immune system depends upon the particular virus involved and upon the stage of the viral infection.

Nonspecific Defenses

The body's defenses to viral infections may be divided into nonspecific and specific defenses. *Nonspecific viral defenses* include the skin and mucus, interferon, complement, inflammation, macrophages, and natural killer (NK) cells. After a new virus penetrates the skin and/or mucous membrane and enters the body, the earliest defense is interferon, which appears long before any antibody or cellular responses (Fig. 13–3). *Interferon* is a class of proteins that inhibits viral replication by mechanisms discussed below. α and β Interferons are directly antiviral and antiproliferative, whereas γ interferon, derived from T cells, is immunoregulatory and indirectly antiviral. γ Interferon inhibits B cell antibody synthesis, enhances T cell cytotoxic activities, activates macrophages, and activates NK cells. Once produced, interferons are effective over long ranges in that they can travel and act on cells some distance from the cell that produced them. Experimental data suggest that most body cells can synthesize all types of interferon and that conditions dictate which type is produced at any particular time. Interferons are target cell nonspecific but species specific. This means that any interferon is effective against viruses in general rather than against only a specific virus and that it is only effective in that species or host that originally synthesized it. For example, human interferon is not effective against viral infection of guinea pig cells. In addition to viruses, other stimulators of interferon are double-stranded polynucleotides (poly I : C), mitogens, protozoa, *rickettsiae, chlamydiae,* and bacterial endotoxins. Some of these interferon inducers have been utilized in anticancer and antiviral therapy.

Antiviral and antiproliferative activities of interferon have been found to result from several combined effects. (1) Interferon reacts with target cell–surface receptors to induce activity of 2′, 5′-oligoadenylate synthetase, which converts ATP to 2′, 5′-oligoadenylate, which activates endoribonucleases to degrade ribonucleic acid (RNA). If

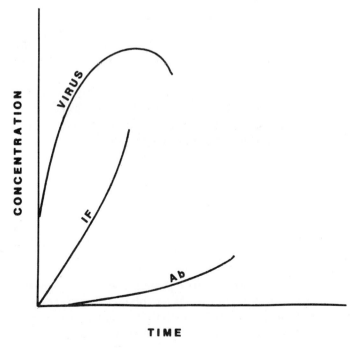

Figure 13-3. Appearance of Interferon and Antibodies in Relation to Infection by Virus.

there is reduced RNA there is reduced transcription. (2) Interferon activates a kinase that inactivates elongation factor 2 (EF-2) by phosphorylating it. Without EF-2 translation cannot proceed. (3) Interferon induces phosphodiesterase activity to cleave the 3'CCA from transfer ribonucleic acid (tRNA) to prevent attachment of amino acids. Without charged tRNA, translation halts. All three of these activities are directed toward viral replication and toward tumor cell proliferation. Therefore interferon is a nonspecific defense that inhibits viral replication and tumor cell proliferation.

Macrophages are another nonspecific defense against viral infections. These cells are activated by interferon and lymphokines to greater phagocytic activity. Macrophages will attack virus particles as well as virally infected host cells. Interferon converts resting macrophages to active macrophages that demonstrate enhanced motility, enhanced phagocytosis, increased numbers of lysosomes, and increased metabolism.

NK cells are non-B, non-T lymphocytes that will also attack and destroy foreign cells. Interferon activates these cells to increased cytolytic rates, to increased rates of recycling from target to target, and to increased synthesis of surface recognition sites.

Complement can be activated via the alternate pathway by some viruses and by-products of cell injury and inflammation. Activated complement can be an opsonin and can enhance macrophage phagocytosis of virus particles and of virus-infected cells. Activated complement can also mediate lysis of viral particles and of virus-infected cells.

Specific Defenses

All of the above defenses—interferon, macrophage, NK cell, and complement—are nonspecific defenses in that they are active toward all viruses or virus-infected cells. Their activities are not limited to a specific virus. A separate set of specific defenses may be developed as a result of infection, and these defenses are directed toward that particular virus that induced their development. The specific defenses involve both antibodies, or the humoral immune response, and sensitized cells, or the cellular immune response.

Antibodies defend the body against viral infections in several ways. Attachment of antibodies to specific complementary viral antigenic sites neutralizes or prevents that virus from infecting host cells. Antibodies covering viral antigens can prevent attachment of the virus to the host cell membrane-specific receptor for that viral antigen. Even when attachment does occur, antibody bound to a virus can prevent uncoating of the internalized viral particle. Secretory IgA is particularly important in neutralizing those viruses that infect mucosal surfaces, for example, rhinovirus, parainfluenza, and respiratory syncytial virus.

IgG and IgM antibodies activate the *complement* cascade when they bind to viruses or to virus-infected cells. This can cause steric configurational changes in the virus particles to enhance neutralization effects. Complement activation by antibody may result in lysis of viral particles and virus-infected cells.

Both complement and antibody act as opsonins to enhance *phagocytosis* of virus or virus-infected cells by macrophages and neutrophils. Macrophages have receptors for both the Fc portion of IgG and IgM and for C3b. Phagocytosis resulting from antibody opsonins is a specific defense against viral antigens that reacts with the antibody.

The macrophage can be involved in either specific or nonspecific defenses. Ingestion by macrophage is not always fatal to the viral particle nor is it always beneficial to the host. Enteroviruses are usually degraded after phagocytosis, whereas arboviruses survive and demonstrate enhanced replication.

Another specific body defense mediated via antibody attachment to virus or virus-infected host cell is antibody-dependent cell cytotoxicity (ADCC) by *K cells*. This activity, discussed in Chapter 8, does not require HLA compatibility between K cell and target cell.

Cytotoxic T cells destroy host cells infected with virus and expressing viral antigens for which the T cells have specificity. T cytotoxic cells require HLA compatibility between target and effector cells, as discussed in Chapter 8. Stimulator helper T cells secrete lymphokines that influence viral defenses in several ways. One of these lymphokines is γ interferon, which is immunoregulatory. Data suggest the following immunoregulatory activities of γ interferon (1) Interferon increases the number of DR antigens (products of the HLA-D MHC region) on accessory cells to influence the T cell immune response, which in turn enhances the B cell response. (2) Interferon increases the number of interleukin 2 (Il 2) receptor sites on lymphocytes, which in turn influences the T and B cell responses. Other lymphokines act as chemotaxins for macrophages and neutrophils. Migration inhibition factor (MIF) confines the phagocytes to a particular area. Il 2 is a lymphokine that stimulates proliferation of both T and B cells. All of the above viral defenses are specific in that they are effective only against that viral antigen that stimulated their development. Generally humoral immune defenses are more effective aganist viremia and systemic spreading of viral infections, whereas cellular immune defenses are more effective against viral infections involving dissemination via intercytoplasmic bridges and cell division.

EVASION TACTICS OF VIRUSES

In spite of all of the body's defenses, viruses infect host cells. Viruses also exhibit evasion tactics that are related to the anatomic site of the viral infection. Because viruses are obligate intracellular parasites, they are isolated from many of the body's defenses. Some viruses, for example, influenza, are notorious for their ability to *change surface antigens* by mutation or recombination. This antigenic shifting enables the virus to evade immune responses previously developed against the original antigenic structure. Along the same line, some diseases are caused by a *number of antigenically distinct types* of virus, for example, rhinoviruses. Immunity against one antigenic strain will not protect an individual from disease resulting from infection by a different antigenic strain. Some viruses have a lengthy latent period during which there are no antigens on host cell surfaces, and therefore immune mechanisms are ineffective. Some virus antigens on the host cell surface *camouflage* themselves as self by adsorbing host cell proteins, for example, herpes antigens bind the Fc portion of host antibodies. Similarly, the normal attachment of host-defense antibody to surface viral antigens can cover up antigens so that they go undetected by cytotoxic T cells and other antigenically directed cellular defense mechanisms. Viral infections may also *depress immune responses,* for example, measles decreases cellular immunity, as demonstrated by a reduction in the delayed hypersensitivity (DTH) test.

SEROLOGIC ASSAYS FOR VIRAL DISEASES

Laboratory evaluation, especially by serology and culture, is important to the diagnosis and management of viral diseases. For those laboratories that have the facilities, cell culture often provides the best means of identification for many viruses. Some laboratories cannot afford cell cultures. Some viruses are difficult or impossible to culture and proper patient specimens are not always available. Consequently serologic assay is often the clinical method for substantiating infection by a particular virus. Even when cell cultures are available, serologic methods are often used to identify the culture or to confirm its identification. Serologic assays provide data much more rapidly than cell culture and, as technology improves with the availability of more monoclonal antibodies, they are gradually replacing cell culture.

Serologic assays provide a rapid diagnosis for life-threatening viral infections, for example, *herpes encephalitis.* Because some antiviral drugs are toxic to the patient, an accurate identification of the infectious agent may prevent unnecessary discomfort and side effects of therapy. Serology can provide a rapid diagnosis of respiratory viral diseases in neonates. If a viral etiology can be determined, the patient can be isolated from other patients to prevent nosocomial spread of the virus to a particularly susceptible population. Besides the serologic assays already discussed in Chapter 4, viral serology includes additional techniques that are based on characteristics of viruses and their effects upon infected host cells.

Hemadsorption and *hemadsorption inhibition assays* are based upon the fact that some viruses will alter the host cell membranes to demonstrate receptors that adsorb erythrocytes from a particular species. The myxoviruses and paramyxoviruses—influenza, parainfluenza, rubeola, and mumps—can be identified by this technique. Antibodies to virus-induced host cell membrane receptors are capable of binding to and covering up the receptors to inhibit any subsequent hemadsorption.

Orthomyxoviruses and paramyxoviruses have receptors for specific erythrocytes and will hemagglutinate erythrocytes of that specific species when mixed with them. Antibodies to the virus may bind, add to, or cover up the specific erythrocyte receptor to prevent this agglutination. This phenomenon is the basis for *hemagglutination* and *hemagglutination inhibition* assays. These assays are somewhat analogous to the hemadsorption assays but employ viral surface receptors rather than host cell surface receptors. Hemagglutination assays for viruses should be evaluated immediately because some viruses have neuraminidase, which will cleave the erythrocytes from their receptors to give a false-negative hemagglutination. It should be emphasized that these hemadsorption and hemagglutination assays are not antigen–antibody assays but are, rather, receptor-specific assays based on properties of the virus and/or its effect on infected host cell. Patient sera may contain nonspecific inhibitors of hemagglutination that can be removed by erythrocyte adsorption prior to testing. Adequate controls are a must to detect the above interferences.

The *anticomplement immunofluorescence assay* (ACIF), which was described in Chapter 4, is more sensitive than the direct or the sandwich immunofluorescence assay. The ACIF is utilized more in relation to viral specimens than it is in relation to bacterial specimens.

Neutralization assays are based upon the binding of antibodies to specific viral antigens to inhibit that virus from infecting cultured host cells. Bound antibody prevents the virus particle from attaching to a specific host cell receptor.

There are a few general considerations and precautions pertaining to viral serologic assays. For serodiagnosis of a current infection, two samples are compared for a rise in total antibody titer. The first sample should be taken within 7 days of onset of the symptoms, and the second sample should be taken about 10 days later. A fourfold rise in titer is usually taken as indicative of current infection.

An alternative method sometimes used for diagnosing current viral infections is to assay one sample for IgM. A single sample is taken during the first week or two of onset of symptoms. Either IgM may be separated from the serum for assay, or anti-IgM indicators may be used with whole serum for assay. An important precaution is the removal of rheumatoid factor (RF), which is IgM anti-IgG. RF will combine with any IgG and may cause false-positive reactions in those assays using fluorochrome-labeled anti-IgM as an indicator of specific IgM antibody. This RF precaution should be utilized in any assay for IgM. Table 13–1 lists the possible viral etiologies for diseases or symptoms. Some of the more common viruses and methods for their serologic and immunologic diagnosis will now be presented.

TABLE 13–1. DISEASE SYMPTOMS AND RELATED VIRAL AGENTS

Symptom	Probable Viral Agents
Viral exanthema	Coxsackie, ECHO, varicella-zoster, herpes simplex, vaccinia, variola, rubella, rubeola, dengue virus
Pleurodynia	Coxsackie
CNS disease	Polio, coxsackie, ECHO, arboviruses, herpes simplex, measles, mumps, varicella-zoster, cytomegalovirus, lymphocytic choriomeningitis virus
Ophthalmic disease	Herpes simplex, varicella-zoster, adenovirus, Newcastle disease virus
Parotitis	Mumps
Upper respiratory tract illness	Influenza, parainfluenza, rhinovirus, respiratory syncytial virus, adenovirus, ECHO virus
Lower respiratory tract illness	Respiratory syncytial virus, rhinovirus, adenovirus, influenza, parainfluenza, measles, varicella-zoster, cytomegalovirus
Pericarditis, myocarditis	Coxsackie B, mumps
Enteritis	ECHO, coxsackie
Cystitis	Adenovirus
Vulvovaginitis	Herpes simplex, coxsackie B, LGV
Orchitis	Mumps, coxsackie B, lymphocytic chorio-meningitis virus
Cervicitis	Cytomegalovirus
Mononucleosis	EBV, cytomegalovirus, herpes simplex

SELECTED VIRAL DISEASES

Herpes Group

Herpes simplex virus types I and 2 (HSV-1 and HSV-2) are DNA core viruses most commonly known for their self-limited vesicular skin lesions. Herpes is known for its integration into host DNA material and subsequent passage from host cell to host cell without going through an extracellular phase. This method of spreading the virus explains the latent periods between episodes of symptoms. HSV isolated from genital sites are usually HSV-2. HSV-2 has been incriminated in the pathogenesis of cancer of the cervix. HSV-2 infection of neonates during passage through the birth canal of an infected mother can be severe and even fatal. HSV isolated from nongenital sites are usually HSV-1. HSV-1 often causes fever blisters. HSV keratoconjunctivitis can cause blindness. Once a host has been infected, HSV-1 remains in the host for life. Reactivation of latent virus as fever blisters can be initiated by sunlight, fever, trauma, or stress. Transmission of these viruses is related to their sites of infection—HSV-1 is transmitted via oral secretions and HSV-2 is transmitted venereally. Both of these herpes viruses can cause meningitis. In the case of suspected neonate infection, antibody titer, especially IgM, can be useful in diagnosis. A fourfold or greater rise in titer occurs as a result of primary infections with HSV. Thereafter, however, rises in titer of IgG or IgM are not normally seen with reinfection. Herpes varicella-zoster virus and HSV demonstrate serologic cross-reactivity and share the ability to stimulate anamnestic responses of each other. Anti-HSV antibodies in CSF may result from serum antibodies crossing a damaged blood brain barrier or from synthesis of antibodies within the CNS. Comparison of titers of paired samples of serum and of CSF is helpful in distinguishing the origin of antibodies and thus the etiologic agent during meningitis. This is called the HSV encephalitis (HSVE) antibody index, and should be less than 2 in individuals who do not have HSVE. HSV can be detected in specimens by direct IFA, RIA, and ELISA methods (see Chap. 4 for methods). HSV type can be determined with monoclonal antibodies.

Varicella-zoster is another herpes virus. It causes chickenpox (varicella) and shingles (zoster) in older adults. Primary infection results in chickenpox, followed by a latent phase. Subsequent reactivation results in episodes of shingles. Varicella is one of the four most common childhood viral diseases. This disease manifests as fever, with a papular skin rash that progresses to pustules and then to scales. Older adults suffering a primary infection may have complications such as pneumonitis and encephalitis. Zoster is a reactivation of the virus in later years. The virus travels down the sensory nerve fibers and produces a sudden onset of pain and tenderness, with mild fever, malaise, and vesicular skin lesions. Varicella zoster virus is not culturable in the laboratory but clinical symptoms usually are adequate for diagnosis. Acute and convalescent sera titers showing a fourfold increase in antibodies against this virus are indicative of primary infection. A complement fixation assay can be used to detect anti-varicella-zoster antibodies. Other laboratory assays include IFA, ELISA, and ACIF assays for specific antibody. These assays for presence or absence of specific antibodies are useful in determining the immune status of immunocompromised patients who have been exposed to the virus.

Cytomegalovirus (CMV) is another herpes virus. It was originally identified in infants with symptoms of congenital syphilis. Pregnant women can pass infections to the fetus, resulting in growth retardation, microcephaly, thrombocytopenia, hepatitis, mental retardation, and deafness. Primary infections acquired after birth are usually asymptomatic or mild. Older children and adults, when infected, sometimes develop mononucleosis-like syndromes of malaise, fever, hepatosplenomegaly, atypical lymphocytosis, and adenopathy. These individuals have a negative heterophile test. Latent CMV infections occur as they do in all other members of the herpes virus family and are usually asymptomatic. CMV infection is a complication following bone marrow and kidney transplants and blood transfusions to neonates. Severe complications have occurred following transplantation from seropositive donors to seronegative recipients. CMV has been identified as the most frequent opportunistic agent infecting AIDS patients. Passive hemagglutination with antigen-coated erythrocytes, complement fixation, ACIF, and ELISA are frequently used serologic methods for detecting CMV infection. Because CMV induces Fc receptors on infected host cells, indirect immunofluorescence microscopy using intact antibodies can give false positive results, since the antibody could attach via its Fc rather than via its specific Fab region.

Epstein–Barr virus (EBV) is also a herpes virus. It preferentially infects B cells. Primary EBV infections in young children are usually asymptomatic. In persons who remain uninfected into their teens, primary infection often is manifested as infectious mononucleosis (IM). This disease is usually self-limited. Symptoms and signs are fever, sore throat, lethargy, malaise, headache, tender lymphadenopathy, and splenomegaly. Tonsillitis, rubella infection, toxoplasmosis, influenza, hepatitis, and CMV infection may have features that resemble infectious mononucleosis, including the presence of atypical lymphocytes. EBV also causes Burkitt's lymphoma and nasopharyngeal carcinoma. EBV has been shown to depress cellular immunity. This can be detected by DTH skin tests and mitogen stimulation assays of T cells. During IM patients develop antibodies that will agglutinate sheep or horse erythrocytes and provide the basis for the *Paul–Bunnell* test (Fig. 13–4), a rapid-screening assay for IM. CMV causes IM-like symptoms but is heterophile negative. Antibodies that react with heterogeneous antigens of other species are called heterophile antibodies. In addition to IM, other conditions such as serum sickness produce heterophile antibodies that agglutinate sheep and horse erythrocytes. In the Paul–Bunnell test a *Forssman antigen* (an antigen common to several species) adsorbs out all non-IM heterophile antibodies so that any remaining agglutinins for sheep erythrocytes will be the IM-induced heterophile antibodies. In the Paul–Bunnell test, guinea pig kidney is usually used as the Forssman antigen. Bovine erythrocytes are used to specifically adsorb out the IM heterophile antibodies. The Paul–Bunnell heterophile antibody test for IM is based upon the fact that sheep erythrocyte agglutination remains after adsorption of patient serum with Forssman's antigen but disappears after adsorption with bovine erythrocyte stroma. Biological false positives may be seen in patients with rheumatoid arthritis, viral hepatitis, and leukemia. IM heterophile antibodies appear during the acute phase of the disease, reach their peak at about 2 weeks, and rapidly decrease after the fourth week, with no detection after 3 months (Fig. 13–5).

Another 10% of patients with classical IM never develop heterophile antibodies;

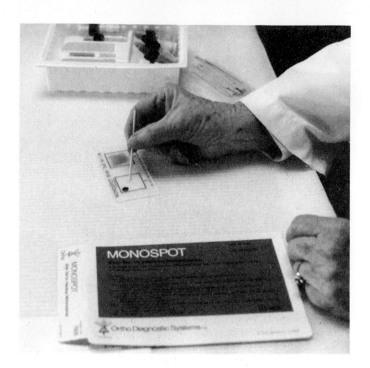

Figure 13-4. Heterophile Test for Infectious Mononucleosis.

therefore a more specific serologic test based on viral antigens has been developed. EBV has 3 major antigens that stimulate production of antibodies useful in diagnosing current or past infections (Table 13-2). There are the *viral capsid antigen (VCA)*, the *early antigen (EA)*, and the *Epstein–Barr nuclear antigen (EBNA)*.

IgM to VCA appears within a week of illness onset, peaks during the acute stage, and then disappears within 4 to 8 weeks. VCA IgM assays are especially useful if only one specimen is available. EA antibodies have a transient appearance during the acute phase and are completely gone within 3 months. IgM antibodies to EA and IgM antibodies to VCA parallel each other in occurrence and disappearance. Most IM patients who seek medical assistance already have peak titers of IgG to VCA that later decline but persist throughout life. The EBNA antibodies begin to appear later in the convalescent stage of IM, peak 2 months after the acute phase, and persist throughout life. IM antibodies associated with the EBV are measured with the indirect immunofluorescence microscopy and the ACIF assay. ACIF is used to assay for EBNA antibodies, and IFA is used to assay for EA and VCA antibodies. The antigen containing substrate for these assays is usually a lymphoid cell line that has the EBV genome and is expressing the desired EBV antigen. Interpretation of the assays is (1) past infection if EBNA and VCA antibodies are present, (2) reactivated infection if antibodies to EBNA and EA and/or IgM to VCA are present, (3) present infection if antibodies to VCA and EA but not to EBNA are present, (4) current primary infection if IgM to VCA and anti-EA are

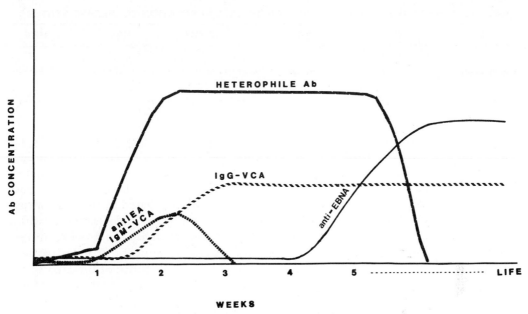

Figure 13-5. Antibodies Produced During Epstein–Barr Infection.

present, (5) recent infection if VCA antibodies in titers of 1 : 640 or greater are present, (6) current infection if VCA antibodies have risen fourfold, but not EBNA antibodies.

Hepatitis

Viral hepatitis can be classified as hepatitis A (HAV), hepatitis B (HBV), or hepatitis non-A, non-B. The infection usually begins with a low-grade fever, easy fatigability, malaise, blunted taste and smell, nausea, and vomiting. This is followed by right upper-quadrant pain with hepatosplenomegaly and jaundice. Hepatitis A, formerly known as infectious hepatitis, is the cause of most epidemic outbreaks, is passed via the fecal–oral route, and is known for its absence of sequelae after an asymptomatic infection. Hepatitis B, formerly known as serum hepatitis, is passed via parenteral routes and

TABLE 13-2. SIGNIFICANCE OF IM ANTIBODIES

Antibody	Appearance of Ab	Longevity of Ab	No Infection	Acute Infection	Past Infection	Reinfection
IgM-EA	Early	Temporary	−	+	−	+
IgM-VCA	Early	Temporary	−	+	−	+
IgG-VCA	Early	Life	−	+	+	+
Anti-EBNA	Late	Life	−	−	+	+

TABLE 13–3. HEPATITIS B ANTIGENS AND ANTIBODIES IN RELATION TO DISEASE STATES

Stage	Anti-HBe	Anti-HBc	Anti-HBs	HBe	HBs
Acute	−	+	−	+/−	+
Recovered	+/−	+	+	−	−
Chronic	−	+	−	+/−	+

also is usually asymptomatic. Hepatitis B can lead to chronic hepatitis. The HBV surface antigen (HBsAg), formerly called Australian antigen; the HBV core antigen (HBcAg); and the HVBe antigen (HBeAg) are used in laboratory serologic evaluation of patients with hepatitis (Tables 13–3 and 13–4). Other causes of viral hepatitis, such as IM, CMV, rubella, and herpes simplex, are readily differentiated by serologic assays.

In HAV infections anti-HAV IgM rises in the first 2 weeks and disappears within 3 to 4 months (Fig. 13–6). Anti-HAV IgG begins to appear about 4 to 5 weeks into the infection and persists for life. In HBV infections HBsAg appears first, with HBeAg appearing shortly thereafter. With recovery there is disappearance of the HBsAg and HBeAg as antibodies to both appear. ELISA and RIA methods are used in evaluations of antigens and antibodies. For IgM, beads coated with anti-IgM first adsorb patient antibody and then HAV is added to bind to specific IgM. Laboratory employees exposed to blood products and who screen negative for anti-HBs antibody may wish to be vaccinated to prevent infection with HBV.

Rubella

Rubella (German measles or 3-day measles) is an important and preventable cause of congenital defects including mental retardation. In children and young adults, who have the highest incidence, the disease is benign and self-limited. It usually consists of rash, lymphadenopathy, and low-grade fever. Serologic evaluation of a patient's immune status is the most important reason for rubella serology, because most people have been infected with rubella by adulthood. Pregnant women who become infected can spread the virus to the fetus. If this occurs within the first 3 months of gestation, the infection may cause congenital cataracts, deafness, heart disease, and mental retardation. Congenital infections can be confirmed by neonate IgM titers of antirubella antibodies. IgM titers rise, peak within 7 days of onset of rash, and disappear within 4 to 6 weeks. IgG rises later and remains throughout life. If women of child-bearing ages are not immune, vaccination is recommended. When a pregnant mother is ex-

TABLE 13–4. SCREEN FOR HEPATITIS A, B, OR NON-A, NON-B

Disease Stage	IgM-anti-HAV	HBsAg	Anti-HBc
Acute B	−	+	−/+
Active B	−	−/+	+
Recent A	+	−	−
Non A,B	−	−	−

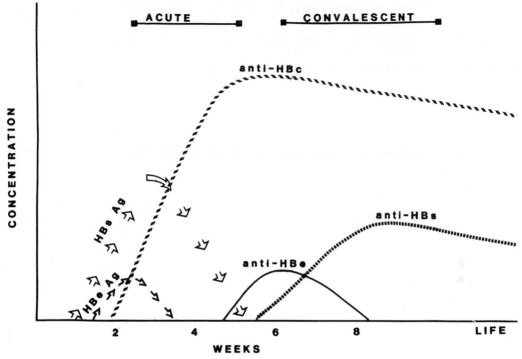

Figure 13-6. Antibodies Produced During Hepatitis A Infection.

posed to the virus and is not immune, passive immunotherapy is given. Reinfections are well documented; however, they are not accompanied by shedding of virus particles, so that pregnant women suffering reinfections present no threat of passing the virus to the fetus. Primary infections occurring within the first trimester of pregnancy are potentially dangerous to the fetus. Because cell culture takes weeks to complete, serology is the diagnostic method of choice, with HI and ELISA (see Chap. 4 for methods) being the most widely used assay methods. Rubella viral envelope contains a hemagglutinin for a wide variety of erythrocytes, including human group O erythrocytes.

Paramyxovirus Group

The paramyxovirus group of RNA viruses includes mumps, rubeola, parainfluenza, and respiratory syncytial viruses. These viruses have surface hemagglutinin receptors that provide the basis for hemagglutination and hemagglutination inhibition assays. Neuraminidase and hemolysins are also part of virus surfaces. For these reasons processing of patient sera with *receptor-destroying enzyme, kaolin adsorption,* or *erythrocyte adsorption* is necessary to remove nonspecific inhibitors before performing the hemagglutination assays.

Measles (rubeola) is a highly contagious childhood disease characterized by fever, conjunctivitis, cough, and maculopapular skin eruptions. Childhood infections are sometimes complicated by allergic encephalitis and may result in death. Adult infections are usually benign. In pregnant women it is important to distinguish between a rash caused by rubella and one caused by rubeola. Rubeola does not cause congenital defects in the fetus. Measles vaccine has greatly reduced the incidence of the disease. Diagnosis is usually easily accomplished by clinical symptoms. Serology, if ordered, is usually the HI, with antibodies inhibiting viral hemagglutination.

Mumps is another paramyxovirus and replicates in T cells. Mumps shares antigens with the parainfluenza viruses. Mumps is one of the causes of aseptic meningitis, encephalitis, and inflammation of the testes, pancreas, and ovaries. The infection is usually mild in children and is characterized by swelling of the parotid glands, some fever, and possibly headache. It is usually self-limited, with symptoms lasting for about 7 to 10 days. Infection of the central nervous system and the testes are the most important complication. Orchitis occurs in about 20% of infected adult males. Although active immunity via an attenuated live virus vaccine prevents the disease, passive immunotherapy does not. Combination vaccines of measles, mumps, and rubella (MMR) are routinely given to children at about 15 months of age. Serologic assays are useful in determining past and present infections. Antibodies to nucleocapsid antigen can be identified within 3 days after onset of clinical symptoms and disappear 3 to 4 weeks later. Antibodies to the hemagglutinin or neuraminidase develop later and persist. As with other members of the paramyxoviruses, HI is an available assay: however, since the mumps virus shares antigens with the parainfluenza viruses, the HI is not specific. Both IFA and ELISA offer specificity, and one or the other is the assay of choice. Intradermal DTH tests can be performed for cellular immunity but do not really indicate immune status, because there are cross-reactions with other paramyxoviruses. Mumps DTH is sometimes used to assess intactness of the cellular immune system because most adults have been exposed to the virus.

Parainfluenza viruses are another member of the paramyxovirus group and can cause respiratory diseases in all age groups. Four different serotypes infect humans. Types 1 to 3 can produce severe illness with primary infection. Types 1 and 2 produce upper respiratory tract inflammation, croup, or laryngotracheobronchitis. Type 3 produces pneumonia and bronchiolitis and is second only to respiratory syncytial virus as the cause for the diseases in children less than 6 months old. Type 4 does not have the potential for causing severe disease or primary infection in children. Parainfluenza viruses do not exhibit antigenic shift like the influenza viruses. Most humans have experienced all types of influenza early in their life, and subsequent infections are of lesser severity. IgA is important in the prevention of surface infections but does not give complete protection. IgE has been implicated as a possible mediator of the airway changes that cause the croup and wheezing symptoms. The only way to identify an influenza type with certainty is via culture because antibodies cross-react with each other and with mumps. If there are no culture facilities, the next best approach is to assay paired samples for increase in titer. The HI is the serologic assay most often used to type parainfluenza. Parainfluenza viruses have hemagglutinins and hemadsorption sites for specific types of erythrocytes, as do the other paramyxoviruses.

Respiratory Syncytial Virus

Respiratory syncytial virus (RSV) is, along with the parainfluenza viruses, one of the most common causes of bronchiolitis, croup, and pneumonia in infants and children. RSV is the most common cause of nosocomial infections in infants. Rapid diagnosis is made by identifying infected cells with IFA on direct nasal oropharynx swabs. Therefore serologic assays are no longer important in diagnosing RSV infection.

Rotavirus

Rotavirus is a major cause of nonbacterial gastroenteritis, especially in young children. This virus does not readily grow in cell culture; therefore immunologic diagnosis is important for diagnosis. An early diagnosis facilitates patient isolation, eliminates possible unnecessary antibiotic treatment, and allows for more objective prognosis. An ELISA assay is available for the antigen detection in stool specimens. A less sensitive rapid-detection system identifies rotavirus antigens in stool by agglutination of latex particles coated with antirotavirus antibodies.

Human T Lymphotropic Virus

Human T lymphotropic virus III (HTLV III), also called human immunodeficiency virus (HIV), causes asymptomatic infections in 65% of its victims, causes AIDS-related complex symptoms (fever, weight loss, diarrhea, fatigue, lymphadenopathy, night sweats, decrease in the T helper cells with a decreased helper/suppressor ratio, leukopenia, thrombocytopenia, lymphopenia, anemia, and an increased concentration of immunoglobulins) in 15% of its victims, and causes a lethal acquired immune deficiency (AIDS) in 20% of its victims. In the United States the majority of cases occur in homosexual males, with the next most frequent group being needle-sharing intravenous drug users. Blood products donated by HIV-carrying individuals have been determined to be a means of transmission. Incubation periods from exposure to symptoms is several years. HIV selectively eliminates T helper activity by binding to and destroying them. Patients often develop Kaposi's sarcoma, oral candidiasis, pneumocystis carinii pneumonia, and CMV infection, including retinitis. Diagnosis is made by a seropositive assay for HIV antibodies, a decrease in T helper cells, and presence of some infection predictive of a defect in cellular immunity, for example, those listed above. An ELISA is used as a screen for HIV antibodies, with confirmation by the Western blot, IFA, or RIA techniques. The Western blot consists of lysing whole virus and separating the resulting protein fragments by polyacrylamide electrophoresis. These proteins are transferred to a nitrocellulose filter to which they bind. After washing with milk proteins to make sure all nonspecific binding sites on the nitrocellulose are covered with protein, patient serum being analyzed for antibodies to viral proteins is layered over the gel. Later, radioactive protein A, which selectively binds to immunoglobulins, is layered onto the gel. Protein A attaches to any antibody that is bound to the viral protein. The gel is then layered onto a photographic film, which is later developed. Energy from the radioisotope will oxidize the silver granules and, after development of the film, will be seen as a dark area. If several bands of radioactivity develop, the serum is positive and contains the antibodies. A single-band result is questionable.

Influenza Virus

Influenza viruses are responsible for the many seasonal outbreaks of flu for which vaccines are made. As a group the influenza viruses are notorious for constantly changing their antigenic nature (the hemagglutinin antigen) and thus demanding constant updating of vaccines. Influenza is highly contagious by airborne transmission of virus-containing droplets expelled from infected persons. Most infections are asymptomatic or have trivial symptoms of mild fever with cough and muscle aches. In young children and the elderly, more severe infections can occur. Bronchiolitis or croup can resemble parainfluenza and respiratory syncytial virus infections in young children. Older patients with severe infections usually have primary viral pneumonia or secondary bacterial pneumonia. Past epidemics are the Asian and Hong Kong influenzas of 1957 and 1968. Influenza viruses are divided into 3 major groups, A, B, and C. Influenza comes from A, which has many subtypes based on variation in the hemagglutinin and neuraminidase structures. Protection is afforded by antibodies to the hemagglutinin, but antibodies to the neuraminidase have little protective effect. When using the HI to measure antibody response, neuraminidase or receptor-destroying enzyme has to be eliminated first. Interpretation of any HI result is difficult due to the fact that repeated influenza infections often cause anamnestic antibody responses to a prior influenza subtype. Thus the HI increase in paired samples may not be solely to the one causing the current infection. Complement-fixation serologic tests can be used to diagnose infections. FIA (see Chap . 4) is used to identify infected epithelial cells in nasopharyngeal swabs.

PARASITIC INFECTIONS

In the United States parasitic infections are relatively well controlled. In third world countries, however, parasitic diseases are among the most important causes of fatalities, with malaria, schistosomiasis, and leishmaniasis being the leaders. During infections parasites undergo many changes in structure and site of anatomic residence. As with viruses, the various host immunologic reactions and their importance in protection are not yet completely known. Within the past several years, however, both the knowledge of and a revived interest in parasitology have grown. During the life cycle of parasites, there are times when they are very vulnerable to elimination by the body's defenses, and there are other times when they are not. Body defenses are effective, and immune responses are stimulated only when the parasite is exposed in its extracellular or nonencysted form. When the parasite is intracellular or encysted, it is essentially isolated from the defenses. Unlike viruses, intracellularly located parasites do not signal their presence by stimulating the host cell to synthesize and exhibit an associated antigen on its surface. Therefore parasites are essentially protected from the immune defenses when they are intracellular. In addition to locating intracellularly, some parasites have developed other tactics to evade the body's defenses. The following discussion will first describe the body's defenses and immune responses to parasitic invasion, then evasion tactics used by parasites with specific examples, and finally methods for laboratory diagnosis of parasitic infections.

Body Defenses

Body defenses against parasitic infections include both immune and nonimmune mechanisms. Some of these defenses are beneficial and eliminate the parasite, while others are harmful and more detrimental to the body than the infection itself. Examples of detrimental effects are the hepatic granuloma formations and tissue damage in schistosomiasis, the immune complex deposition and resultant glomerulonephritis in malaria, and the anaphylaxis induced by hydatid cysts. There is evidence that the anemias associated with malaria, schistosomiasis, and trypanosomiasis are mediated by autoantibodies stimulated by the parasites' presence.

Nonimmune defenses include the normal physical barriers of the skin and mucosal membrane, the phagocytic cells, and the alternative pathway of complement activation. Some parasites, such as *Schistosoma mansoni,* are capable of penetrating the skin. Other parasites, such as malaria, have insect vectors that penetrate the skin and inject the parasites. Most, however, enter the body through a break in the skin or through oral ingestion with subsequent migration to the lymph, blood, and organs. Those parasites that are ingested orally may be eliminated by peristalsis and excretion. Once inside the body there are other nonimmune defenses that actively strive to eliminate the invaders. Some parasites are capable of activating complement via the alternative pathway. Complement products then act as opsonins and mediate phagocytosis or attachment by those cells (neutrophils, monocytes, and macrophages) that contain receptors for the complement on their surface. If the parasite is small enough to be ingested, postphagocytic destruction is likely; however, most parasites are in a life stage that is too large to be ingested. In this case attachment of the cell surface stimulates the phagocyte to synthesize and secrete products that injure the parasite, including the toxic products of oxygen metabolism. In addition to its opsonic activity, C3b binds to parasites and activates the membrane attack complex, leading to lysis of the organism. To date the NK cell, which is so important in body defenses against viral infections, has not been found to be important in protection against parasitic invasion.

Immune defenses toward parasites are stimulated by and directed toward those stages of its life cycle during which it is exposed to lymphocytes and their products. Antibodies that play important roles in defenses against parasites include IgM, IgG, and IgE. Attached antibody can cover the parasite's binding site, which is required for infecting host cells, and thus prevent infection. IgG or IgM attachment to parasites can activate the complement system via the classical pathway and lead to lysis of the parasite. This occurs in plasmodia and trypanosome infections. Attachment of antibody also enhances phagocytosis through its opsonic activity. Phagocytes with membrane receptors for the Fc portion of antibodies and/or for C3b actively attach to the coated (opsonized) parasites. Thereafter destruction may be either by phagocytosis or by synthesis and secretion of the toxic products that act on the unengulfed parasites.

Seemingly unique to helminth worm infections is the defensive ADCC activity of the eosinophil. Anti-parasite IgE first binds to mast cells. These cells degranulate upon subsequent exposure to parasite antigen. One of the mast cell products is eosinophil chemotactic factor (ECF). Chemotactic activity of the ECF calls many eosinophils into the area. Incoming eosinophils acquire antiparasite IgE on their membrane via Fc receptors for the Ab. This eosinophil-bound IgE will attach to parasite antigen. Eosinophils also have membrane receptors for complement and will bind complement-coated parasites. Eosinophils act as other phagocytes and injure or destroy the organisms by ingestion or by secretion of toxic products.

Cellular immune responses are important in parasite defenses. Although the cytotoxic T cell and the NK and K cells have not yet been found to play definable roles, the T cell is essential. Lymphokines are important mediators of cellular immunity against parasites. Activation of macrophages by MAF is one of the results of T cell stimulation. This mechanism has been found to play a key role in stimulating macrophage phagocytosis for the control and killing of plasmodia, leishmania, trypanosomes, and schistosomes. Activated T cells also secrete lymphokines that are chemotaxins for eosinophils and macrophages. This multiplies the activities provided via these cells in combating infection by parasites. T helper cells also mediate parasite infection defense in that their lymphokines and cellular interaction are essential for the B cell generation or antibodies. Some parasites are known for their ability to cause polyclonal stimulation of B cell clones. Malaria is a good example of a parasite that incites polyclonal production of malaria antibodies and of autoantibodies.

Evasion Tactics

Parasites have developed mechanisms to evade immune and other body defenses. The ability to *locate intracellularly* and to isolate themselves from the immune and nonimmune defenses has already been discussed. Trypanosomes, toxoplasma, and leishmania have mechanisms that allow them to survive in macrophages after phagocytosis. In fact, the macrophage is the host cell for trypanosomes and leishmania. Toxoplasma survive within the macrophage by inhibiting fusion of lysosomes and phagosomes and thus preventing postphagocytic degradation.

Trypanosomes, the cause of sleeping sickness transmitted by the tsetse fly, are notorious, as are the influenza viruses, for their ability to *change antigenic structure*. The life cycle of this extracellular parasite in man takes place in the blood and lymph. They reproduce by binary fission. Each new wave of parasites has a different antigenic structure. The new antigen is not susceptible to immune responses stimulated by the previous ones. Thus the older parasites succumb to the immune defenses, and the newer parasites predominate. Some malarial strains also show antigen variation.

Schistosomes are known for their *camouflaging of antigenic foreignness by absorbing host cell antigens.* Fresh water snails release the parasite, which penetrates the skin and invades the body of individuals who come into contact with water. Thereafter it travels through the blood to the lungs and liver, where it matures. The traveling parasites camouflage their foreignness by adsorbing host blood group or host MHC antigens and thus evade the body's immune and other defenses. Some of the adult worms around the portal vein or in the mesentery of the bladder or intestines release eggs that enter the lumens of the intestines and bladder, where they are excreted to begin a new cycle as they hatch in water. Other eggs travel through the blood to the liver, where they remain and incite T cell-mediated granulomas around themselves.

There is evidence that parasites nonspecifically *suppress the immune response.* For example, *Trichinella spiralis,* which infects man via intake of raw pork, secretes a lymphotoxic substance.

Laboratory Diagnosis

Laboratories generally have limited immunologic and serologic assays for parasites due to the low occurrence of infections and due to the more general diagnostic practice of demonstrating parasites by direct microscopic examination of specimens. The Communicable Diseases Center makes all serologic assays available through local state health department referrals. One of the parasitic serologic assays that many laboratories do use is the IFA for antibodies to *toxoplasm gondii.* This parasite, like rubella, CMV, and herpes, can cause congenital disease. Pregnant women are sometimes evaluated for TORCH (toxoplasma, rubella, CMV, and herpes) antibodies to determine potential danger to the fetus. Current or recurrent infection by toxoplasma, such as to a fetus, is evaluated by the IgM-specific IFA or ELISA. The IgM ELISA is more sensitive. Another laboratory assay used to diagnose toxoplasmosis is the Sabin–Feldman dye test. This test is based on the organism's absorption of dye in nonimmune serum but nonabsorption of the dye in immune serum.

CHLAMYDIAL AND RICKETTSIAL INFECTIONS

Chlamydia

Chlamydiae are obligate intracellular bacteria and are a major cause of sexually transmitted disease. Most infections are asymptomatic. Symptomatic infections are characterized by conjunctivitis, urethritis, or cervicitis. Chlamydial infections in pregnant women are important to detect, since they can be transmitted to the neonate and can result in conjunctivitis. This closely mimics gonococcal conjunctivitis. Chlamydia are a most important cause of blindness in underdeveloped countries and are implicated as an important cause of sterility. To eradicate *chlamydia,* it is essential to define and treat the asymptomatic carriers. Laboratory diagnosis is by monoclonal FIA on urethral or cervix swabs. This assay provides a rapid diagnosis of active infection and can be used as a general screening method. CF and ELISA assays (see Chap. 4) for antibodies and cell culture for identification are also used.

Rickettsia

Rickettsiae are also obligate intracellular parasites. They infect arthropods and mammals, which are vectors and reservoirs, respectively, for human infections. *Rickettsiae* cause several febrile diseases, the most common of which is Rocky Mountain spotted fever transmitted via ticks. Other rickettsial diseases include epidemic typhus, Brill–

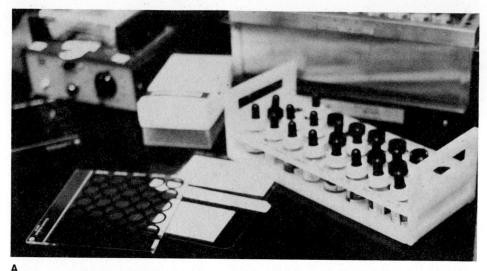

A

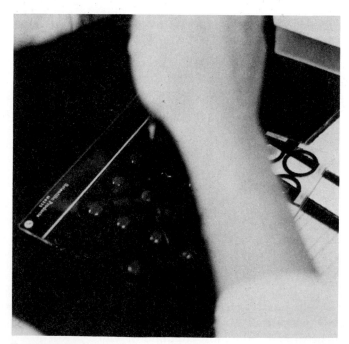

B

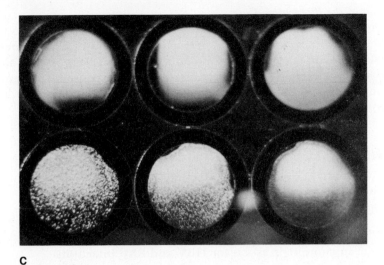

C

Figure 13-7. Weil-Felix Assay for Rickettsial Infection. (A) Reagent latex particles and ringed slide. **(B)** Application of reagents and serum. **(C)** Top row = negative agglutinations; bottom row = positive agglutinations.

Zinsser disease, endemic typhus, and scrub typhus. These infections induce production of antibodies that cross-react with various strains of *Proteus*. Rickettsiae also cause Q fever and rickettsial pox; however, these do not induce cross-reacting antibodies to *Proteus*. The *Weil–Felix* slide agglutination assay (Fig. 13–7) utilizes *Proteus vulgaris* antigens OX-19 and OX-2 and *Proteus mirabilis* antigen OX-K to test for rickettsial antibodies (Table 13–5). A rapid, sensitive method for diagnosing Rocky Mountain spotted fever is the latex slide agglutination or the skin biopsy FIA.

TABLE 13-5. CHARACTERISTIC PATTERNS OF PROTEUS CROSS-AGGLUTINATION IN RICKETTSIAL DISEASES

	OX-19	OX-2	OX-K
Rocky Mountain spotted fever	+ + + +	+	0
Epidemic typhus	+ + + +	+	0
Murine typhus	+ + + +	+	0
Scrub typhus	0	0	+ + +
Q fever	0	0	0

Discussion of the Illustrative Case

Serologic tests are used to diagnose congenital toxoplasmosis. As in the illustrative case, the mother typically does not have symptoms of toxoplasma infection. Serial serum samples are best for confirming the diagnosis. A single, high, toxoplasma-specific IgM titer is diagnostic, but this may not be present in infants with congenital toxoplasmosis if they are sampled too early or too late (several months) in relation to delivery.

QUESTIONS

1. Outline the infective process for a virus.
2. List and discuss the types of viral antigens.
3. Discuss the immune and nonimmune defenses toward viruses.
4. Describe the immunologic assays for HBV and EBV infections.
5. List some of the evasive mechanisms and the respective parasites that have developed them.
6. Give the logic of the Weil–Felix assay, and explain its significance.
7. Why are chlamydial assays important?
8. Define TORCH.

Suggested Readings

REVIEW ARTICLES

Bottazzo GF, Todd I, Mirakian R, et al: Organ-specific autoimmunity: A 1986 overview. Immunol Rev 94:137–169, 1986.

Cronenberger JH: Physiologic responses to infection. J Med Tech 4:150–153, 1987.

Dalmasso AP: Complement in the pathophysiology and diagnosis of human diseases. CRC Crit Rev Clin Lab Sci 24:123–183, 1986.

Dinarello C, Mier J: Interleukins. Annu Rev Med 37, 1986.

Foon KA, Todd RF: Immunologic classification of leukemia and lymphoma. Blood 68:1–31, 1986.

Foon KA, Gale RP, Todd RF: Recent advances in the immunologic classification of leukemia. Semin Hematol 23:257–283, 1986.

Henkart PA: Mechanisms of lymphocyte-mediated cytotoxicity. Ann Rev Immunol 3:31–58, 1985.

Herberman R: Natural killer cells. Annu Rev Med 37, 1986.

Jelinek DF, Lipsky PE: Regulation of human B lymphocyte activation, proliferation, and differentiation. Adv Immunol 40:1–59, 1987.

Kalden JR, Rollinghoff M: Clinical applications of lymphokines. Immunobiology 172, 1986.

Kishimoto T: Factors affecting B-cell growth and differentiation. Ann Rev Immunol 3:133, 1985.

Kronenberg M, Sin G, Hood LE, Shastri N: The molecular genetics of the T-cell antigen receptor and T-cell antigen recognition. Ann Rev Immunol 4:529–591, 1986.

Marrack P, Kappler J: The antigen-specific, major histocompatibility complex-restricted receptor on T-cells. Adv Immunol 39:1–30, 1986.

Masur H, Lane C: The acquired immunodeficiency syndrome. Curr Clin Top Infect Dis 6:1–39, 1985.

Melchers F, Andersson J: Factors controlling the B-cell cycle. Ann Rev Immunol 4:13–36, 1986.

Naama JK, Niven IP, Zoma A, et al: Complement, antigen-antibody complexes and immune complex disease. J Clin Lab Immunol 17:59–67, 1985.

Needleman P, Turk J, Jakschik B, et al: Arachidonic acid metabolism. Annu Rev Biochem 55: 69–102, 1986.

Paul WE, Ohara J: B-Cell stimulatory factor. Annu Rev Immunol 5:429–459, 1987.

Pestka S, Langer JA: Interferons and their actions. Annu Rev Biochem 56:727–777, 1987.

Rosen SM, Buxbaum JN, Frangione B: The structure of immunoglobulins and their genes, DNA rearrangement and B-cell differentiation, molecular anomalies of some monoclonal immunoglobulins. Semin Oncol 13:260–274, 1986.

Salvidio G, Andres G: Immune deposits and immune complex disease. Clin Exp Rheumatol 4:281–288, 1986.

Tosato G, Blaese M: Epstein-Barr virus infection and immunoregulation in man. Adv Immunol 38:99–150, 1986.

Wilson CB, Smith AL: Rapid tests for the diagnosis of bacterial meningitis. Curr Clin Top Infect Dis 7:134–156, 1986.

BOOKS

Bellanti JA: *Immunology III.* Philadelphia: Saunders, 1985.

Bernal JE: *Human Immunogenetics: Principles and Clinical Applications.* Philadelphia: Taylor & Francis, 1986.

Bryant NJ: *Laboratory Immunology and Serology.* Philadelphia: Saunders, 1986.

Clark WR: *The Experimental Foundations of Modern Immunology.* New York: Wiley, 1986.

Collins WP (ed): *Alternative Immunoassays.* New York: Wiley, 1985.

Fox CF (ed): *UCLA Symposia on Membrane-Mediated Cytotoxicity.* New York: AR Liss, 1986.

Goidl EA: *Aging and the Immune Response.* New York: Marcel Dekker, 1987.

Gordon DS (ed): *Monoclonal Antibodies in Clinical Diagnostic Medicine.* New York: Igaku-Shoin, 1985.

Grieco MH, Meriney DK: *Immunodiagnosis for Clinicians: Interpretation of Immunoassays.* Chicago: Year Book, 1983.

Hokama Y, Nakamura RM: *Immunology and Immunopathology: Basic Concepts.* Boston: Little, Brown, 1982.

Kaplan LA, Pesce AJ: *Clinical Chemistry.* St. Louis: CV Mosby, 1984.

Lennette EH: *Laboratory of Viral Infections.* New York: Marcel Dekker, 1985.

Lennette EH, Balows A, Hausler WJ, Shadomy HJ (eds): *Manual of Clinical Microbiology, 4th ed.* Washington, DC: Am Soc Microbiol, 1985.

Lewis GP: *Mediators of Inflammation.* Wright, Briston, 1986.

McCarty GA, Valencia DW, Fritzler MJ: *Antinuclear Antibodies: Contemporary Techniques and Clinical Application to Connective Tissue Diseases.* Oxford: Oxford University Press, 1984.

Oriel D, Ridgway G, Schachter J, et al: *Chlamydial Infections.* Cambridge: Cambridge University Press, 1986.

Roitt IM: *Essential Immunology, 5th ed.* Oxford: Blackwell Scientific, 1984.

Roitt IM, Brostoff J, Male DK: *Immunology.* St. Louis: CV Mosby, 1985.

Rose NR, Bigazzi PE (eds): *Methods in Immunodiagnosis, 2nd ed.* New York: Wiley, 1980.

Rose NR, Friedman H, Fahey JL: *Manual of Clinical Immunology, 3rd ed.* Washington DC: Am Soc Microbiol, 1986.

Schook LB: *Monoclonal Antibody Production.* New York: Marcel Dekker, 1987.

Sternberger LA: *Immunocytochemistry, 3rd ed.* New York: Wiley, 1986.

Stites DP, Stobo JD, Wells JV (eds): *Basic and Clinical Immunology, 6th ed.* Norwalk, CT: Appleton & Lange, 1987.

Tietz NW (ed): *Textbook of Clinical Chemistry.* Philadelphia: Saunders, 1986.

Thompson RA (ed): *Techniques in Clinical Immunology.* Oxford: Blackwell Scientific, 1981.

Thompson RA (ed): *Laboratory Investigation of Immunological Disorders.* Philadelphia: Saunders, 1985.

Virella G, Goust J, Patrick CC, Fudenberg HH: *Medical Immunology.* New York: Marcel Dekker, 1987.

Weir DM: *Handbook of Experimental Immunology.* Boston: Blackwell Scientific, 1986.

Wick G, Traill KN, Schauenstein K: *Immunofluorescence Technology: Selected Theoretical and Clinical Aspects.* New York: Elsevier Biomedical, 1982.

Index